Cardiology at its Core

Cardiology at its Core

Peysh A. Patel
Consultant Cardiologist, Queen Elizabeth Hospital
University Hospitals Birmingham NHS Trust
UK

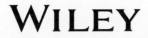

Library of Congress Cataloging-in-Publication Data is applied for
Paperback ISBN: 9781119893141

Cover Design: Wiley
Cover Image: © Yurchanka Siarhei/Shutterstock

Set in 9.5/12.5pt STIXTwoText by Straive, Pondicherry, India
Printed and bound by CPI Group (UK) Ltd, Croydon, CR0 4YY

C9781119893141_270323

To my late grandparents, Pema and Amba Kanji, who surpassed grave adversity to provide stability for the family. To my parents, Dhansukh and Daksha Pema, for supporting and nurturing every venture I embarked upon. To my wife Suhanya for her unwavering support, and to my son Sachin who is the joy of my life.

Contents

Contents

About the Author

Dr Peysh A. Patel, PhD is a consultant cardiologist and honorary associate clinical professor based in Birmingham, UK. He studied natural sciences at Cambridge University with an additional subinternship at Harvard University. His specialist interests are in heart failure, cardio-oncology and cardiac devices, with international board accreditation in the latter (CCDS). He also has a fervent interest in teaching, with over 100 publications and completion of a postgraduate certificate in clinical education (with distinction). These contributions have culminated in appointment as a Fellow of the Higher Education Academy (FHEA). He lives in West Midlands with his family and enjoys cooking, reading and racquet sports in his spare time. He is also subcommittee lead for Pace4Life (www.pace4life.org), a charitable organisation that sources, reconditions and distributes pacemakers to countries with limited healthcare access.

Foreword

Cardiology is a fascinating sub-speciality of medicine, combining many of the elements from medical school teaching, such as anatomy, physiology, pharmacology, biochemistry, embryology, histology and molecular medicine/genetics, into a rapidly evolving acute speciality. It is also one of the most evidence-based specialities and provides the satisfaction of knowing that many of the treatments offered achieve real reductions in death and/or disability. In addition, with so many sub-speciality areas of cardiology, including prevention, imaging, congenital heart disease, electrophysiology and devices, inherited cardiac conditions, and coronary and structural intervention, there is something to suit every personality and interest, making it an exciting career choice and one that is open to everyone.

This readable and authoritative guide will be an asset to both cardiology and general internal medicine trainees throughout their core medical training and specialist training years. The author has done a superb job distilling modern cardiology concepts into a readable and enjoyable text. Each chapter is disease-focused and reviewed by experienced consultant cardiologists with the input of senior trainees, giving it just the right balance of complexity needed for core medical training. As well as covering the core knowledge in the cardiology curriculum, each chapter also contains Hot Points, References, Further Reading and Self-assessment questions (multiple choice questions), useful for those considering the European Exam in Core Cardiology (EECC).

All of the major disease areas have been comprehensively covered, including ischaemic heart disease, heart failure, cardiomyopathies, valvular heart disease and arrhythmias. Some of the less common aspects of cardiovascular disease, such as adult congenital heart disease, aortopathies and cardiac tumours, may need additional further reading. Appreciating that it is exceptionally challenging to cover every topic of cardiovascular disease in a single text, the author has done an excellent job and produced a book that can be highly recommended as a core cardiology text for both general medicine and cardiology trainees alike.

Professor John Greenwood, MBChB, PhD, FRCP, FACC, FSCMR
Professor of Cardiology, University of Leeds & Leeds
Teaching Hospitals NHS Trust, UK
President, British Cardiovascular Society

Preface

Education is the kindling of a flame, not the filling of a vessel.

Socrates

Cardiovascular medicine as a speciality is enthralling and challenging in equal measure, mandating a firm grounding in anatomy, physiology and pathology so that principles can be translated into clinical practice. Although there are several excellent books in the field, they often neglect the crucial integration from bench to bedside.

The modus operandi of this book is to offer a unique merger between handbook and textbook, conceptualising core topics using a 'first principles' framework but with retention of brevity and clarity. It has deliberately been written in prose to aid digestibility of content and is interspersed with unique figures and tables to facilitate long-term recall. Relevant and landmark clinical trials are highlighted and summarised succinctly at the end of each chapter, with the addition of 'Hot Points' and 'Self-assessment' sections to consolidate learning. It is primarily targeted at postgraduate clinicians who are preparing to embark on specialist training or in their early formative years. As content is broadly aligned with the European Society of Cardiology (ESC) core curriculum, it should also provide a contemporary revision aid for those undertaking speciality assessments (EECC).

I am grateful to my colleagues for their expertise and meticulous feedback at every stage. Of course, I shall be eternally grateful to Wiley-Blackwell for supporting this endeavour and enabling a seamless transition from concept to production. It is my hope that this book is not perceived as a quixotic endeavour, but one that instills intellectual curiosity and catalyses a thirst for learning that can be applied perennially to postgraduate training and beyond.

Dr Peysh A. Patel MA(Cantab) MB BChir MRCP (2011)
PGD (Health Res) PhD PGC (Clin Ed) FHEA CCDS
Consultant Cardiologist, Queen Elizabeth Hospital, Birmingham, UK

Acknowledgements

Dr Noman Ali
Consultant Cardiologist, Leeds Teaching Hospitals NHS Trust, Leeds, UK.

MCQs: Chapter 1 (*Electrophysiological principles*), Chapter 6 (*The cardiac pump*), Chapter 7 (*Arterial and venous system*), Chapter 9 (*Coronary vasculature*), Chapter 10 (*Stable angina and non-invasive testing*), Chapter 11 (*Ischaemic heart disease*).

Dr Sudantha Bulugahapitiya
Consultant Cardiologist, Bradford Teaching Hospitals NHS Trust, Bradford, UK.

Reviewer: Chapter 10 (*Stable angina and non-invasive imaging*).

Dr Amrit Chowdhary
Clinical Research Fellow, University of Leeds & Cardiology Registrar, Leeds Teaching Hospitals NHS Trust, Leeds, UK.

MCQs: Chapter 13 (*Valvular disease*), Chapter 14 (*Cardiomyopathies*).

Figures: 10.6 (*Stable angina and non-invasive testing*), 14.2, 14.4, 14.5, 14.10 (*Cardiomyopathies*).

Dr Joseph de Bono
Consultant Cardiologist, University Hospitals Birmingham NHS Trust, Birmingham, UK.

Reviewer: Chapter 2 (*Atrial fibrillation*).

Dr Sudhakar George
Consultant Cardiologist, University Hospitals Birmingham NHS Trust, Birmingham, UK.

Reviewer: Chapter 7 (*Arterial and venous system*).

Dr Karina Gopaul
Consultant Cardiologist, Leeds Teaching Hospitals NHS Trust, Leeds, UK.

Reviewer: Chapter 8 (*Regulation of the circulatory system*).

Dr Manish Kalla
Consultant Cardiologist, University Hospitals Birmingham NHS Trust, Birmingham, UK.

Reviewer: Chapter 3 (*Narrow complex tachycardias*).

Dr Dibbendhu Khanra
Electrophysiology Clinical Fellow, University Hospitals Birmingham NHS Trust, Birmingham, UK.
MCQs: Chapter 4 (*Broad complex tachycardias*).

Prof Francisco Leyva-Leon
Consultant Cardiologist, University Hospitals Birmingham NHS Trust, Birmingham, UK.
Reviewer: Chapter 12 (*Congestive heart failure*).

Dr Ben Mercer
Consultant Cardiologist, Leeds Teaching Hospitals NHS Trust, Leeds, UK.
Reviewer: Chapter 4 (*Broad complex tachycardias*).

Dr Ramesh Nadarajah
Clinical Research Fellow, University of Leeds & Cardiology Registrar, Leeds Teaching Hospitals NHS Trust, Leeds, UK.
MCQs: Chapter 5 (*Bradycardias and conduction disease*), Chapter 8 (*Regulation of the circulatory system*), Chapter 12 (*Congestive heart failure*).
Figures: 3.6, 3.9 (*Narrow complex tachycardias*), 4.3, 4.6 (*Broad complex tachycardias*), 11.8 (*Ischaemic heart disease*), 13.4, 13.11 (*Valvular disease*), 14.6 (*Cardiomyopathies*).

Dr Vikrant Nayar
Consultant Cardiologist, Mid Yorkshire Hospitals NHS Trust, Wakefield, UK.
Reviewer: Chapter 8 (*Regulation of the circulatory system*).

Dr James O'Neill
Consultant Cardiologist, Leeds Teaching Hospitals NHS Trust, Leeds, UK.
Reviewer: Chapter 13 (*Valvular disease*).
MCQs: Chapter 2 (*Atrial fibrillation*), Chapter 3 (*Narrow complex tachycardias*), Chapter 4 (*Broad complex tachycardias*).
Figure: 13.11, 13.12 (*Valvular disease*).

Dr Ramkumar Ramachandra
Consultant Cardiologist, South Tyneside and Sunderland NHS Foundation Trust, Sunderland, UK.
Reviewer: Chapter 9 (*Coronary vasculature*).

Dr Anshuman Sengupta
Consultant Cardiologist, Leeds Teaching Hospitals NHS Trust, Leeds, UK.
Reviewer: Chapter 14 (*Cardiomyopathies*).

Dr Alexander Simms
Consultant Cardiologist, Leeds Teaching Hospitals NHS Trust, Leeds, UK.
Reviewer: Chapter 1 (*Electrophysiological principles*).

Dr Ravi Vijapurapu

Post-CCT Heart Failure & Device Fellow, Sheffield Teaching Hospitals NHS Trust, Sheffield, UK.

Figures: 13.7, 13.14 (*Valvular disease*).

Prof Stephen Wheatcroft

Consultant Cardiologist, Leeds Teaching Hospitals NHS Trust, Leeds, UK.

Reviewer: Chapter 11 (*Ischaemic heart disease*).

Prof Klaus Witte

Senior Lecturer, University of Leeds & Consultant Cardiologist, Leeds Teaching Hospitals NHS Trust, Leeds, UK.

Reviewer: Chapter 5 (*Bradycardias and conduction disease*), Chapter 6 (*The cardiac pump*).

Abbreviations

ACE	angiotensin-converting enzyme
Ach	acetylcholine
ACM	arrhythmogenic cardiomyopathy
ACS	acute coronary syndrome
AD	autosomal dominant
ADH	antidiuretic hormone
ADP	adenosine diphosphate
AF	atrial fibrillation
AHRE	atrial high-rate episode
ALS	advanced life support
ALT	alanine transaminase
AMD	arrhythmia-modifying drug
AMVL	anterior mitral valve leaflet
ANP	atrial natriuretic peptide
ANS	autonomic nervous system
AP	accessory pathway
AP	action potential
AR	aortic regurgitation
AR	autosomal recessive
ARB	angiotensin II receptor blocker
ARNI	angiotensin receptor-neprilysin inhibitor
ARVC	arrhythmogenic right ventricular cardiomyopathy
AS	aortic stenosis
ASD	atrial septal defect
AT	atrial tachycardia
ATP	adenosine triphosphate
ATP	anti-tachycardia pacing
AV	aortic valve
AV	atrioventricular
AVA	aortic valve area
AVN	atrioventricular node
AVNRT	atrioventricular nodal reentrant tachycardia
AVR	aortic valve replacement
AVRT	atrioventricular reentrant tachycardia
BAV	bicuspid aortic valve
BAV	balloon aortic valvuloplasty

BBB	bundle branch block
BCT	broad complex tachycardia
BD	twice daily
BMI	body mass index
BMS	bare metal stent
BNP	b-type natriuretic peptide
BP	blood pressure
BSA	body surface area
BTS	british thoracic society
CABG	coronary artery bypass grafting
cAMP	cyclic adenosine monophosphate
cGMP	cyclic guanosine monophosphate
CBT	cognitive behavioural therapy
CCC	cardiovascular control centre
CHB	complete heart block
CHF	congestive heart failure
CI	chronotropic incompetence
CLS	closed loop stimulation
CNS	central nervous system
CO	cardiac output
COPD	chronic obstructive pulmonary disease
COX	cyclo-oxygenase
CPAP	continuous positive airway pressure
CPEX	cardiopulmonary exercise
CPVT	catecholaminergic polymorphic ventricular tachycardia
CRP	c-reactive protein
CRT	cardiac resynchronisation therapy
CRT-P	cardiac resynchronisation therapy (pacemaker only)
CRT-D	cardiac resynchronisation therapy (with defibrillator)
CS	coronary sinus
CSA	cross-sectional area
CT	computed tomography
CT	crista terminalis
CTCA	computed tomography coronary angiography
CTI	cavo-tricuspid isthmus
CVP	central venous pressure
CW	continuous wave
Cx	circumflex
DAD	delayed after-depolarisation
DCCV	direct current cardioversion
DCM	dilated cardiomyopathy
DCT	distal convoluted tubule
DES	drug-eluting stent
DM	diabetes mellitus
DOAC	direct oral anticoagulant
DPD	deoxypyridinoline
DSE	dobutamine stress echocardiography
DT	deceleration time

EAD	early after-depolarisation
ECG	electrocardiogram
ECMO	extracorporeal membrane oxygenation
ED	emergency department
EDV	end-diastolic volume
EF	ejection fraction
EGE	early gadolinium enhancement
EP	electrophysiology
EROA	effective regurgitant orifice area
ERP	effective refractory period
ESC	european society of cardiology
ESV	end-systolic volume
ETT	exercise tolerance testing
EV	eustachian valve
FBC	full blood count
FFR	fractional flow reserve
GFR	glomerular filtration rate
GORD	gastro-oesophageal reflux disease
GTN	glyceryl trinitrate
GTP	guanosine triphosphate
HCM	hypertrophic cardiomyopathy
HCN	hyperpolarisation-activated cyclic nucleotide-gated
HDL	high-density lipoprotein
HFmrEF	heart failure with mid-range ejection fraction
HFpEF	heart failure with preserved ejection fraction
HIV	human immunodeficiency virus
HLA	human leucocyte antigen
HOCM	hypertrophic obstructive cardiomyopathy
HR	heart rate
IABP	intra-aortic balloon pump
IAS	interatrial septum
ICC	inherited cardiovascular conditions
ICD	implantable cardioverter-defibrillator
ICP	intracranial pressure
iFR	instantaneous wave-free ratio
IHD	ischaemic heart disease
INR	international normalised ratio
INTERMACS	interagency registry for mechanically assisted circulatory support
ISMN	isosorbide mononitrate
IST	inappropriate sinus tachycardia
IVC	inferior vena cava
IVRT	isovolumic relaxation time
IVS	interventricular septum
IVUS	intravascular ultrasound
JET	junctional ectopic tachycardia
JVP	jugular venous pressure
LA	left atrium
LAA	left atrial appendage

LAD	left anterior descending
LAD	left axis deviation
LAF	left anterior fascicle
LBB	left bundle branch
LBBA	left brunch branch area
LBBB	left bundle branch block
LCA	left coronary artery
LCC	left coronary cusp
LDL	low-density lipoprotein
LFT	liver function test
LGE	late gadolinium enhancement
LIMA	left internal mammary artery
LMS	left main stem
LMWH	low–molecular–weight heparin
LPF	left posterior fascicle
LV	left ventricle
LVAD	left ventricular assist device
LVEDD	left ventricle end-diastolic diameter
LVEDP	left ventricle end diastolic pressure
LVESD	left ventricule end-systolic diameter
LVF	left ventricular failure
LVH	left ventricular hypertrophy
LVOT	left ventricular outflow tract
LVOTO	left ventricular outflow tract obstruction
LVSD	left ventricular systolic dysfunction
LVSF	left ventricular systolic function
MACE	major adverse cardiac events
MAP	mean arterial pressure
MAT	multifocal atrial tachycardia
MI	myocardial infarction
MINOCA	myocardial infarction with non-obstructive coronary arteries
MMP	matrix metalloproteinase
MPG	mean pressure gradient
MPI	myocardial perfusion imaging
MR	mitral regurgitation
MRA	magnetic resonance angiography
MRI	magnetic resonance imaging
MS	mitral stenosis
MV	mitral valve
MVA	mitral valve area
MVP	mitral valve prolapse
NA	noradrenaline
NCC	non-coronary cusp
NCT	narrow complex tachycardia
NDHP CCB	non-dihydropyridine calcium-channel blocker
NO	nitric oxide
NOAC	novel oral anticoagulant
NOS	nitric oxide synthase

NPJT	nonparoxysmal junctional tachycardia
NPV	negative predictive value
NSAIDs	non-steroidal anti-inflammatory drugs
NSR	normal sinus rhythm
NSTEMI	non-st elevation myocardial infarction
NSVT	non-sustained ventricular tachycardia
NYHA	new york heart association
OCT	optical coherence tomography
OD	once daily
OM	obtuse marginal
OSA	obstructive sleep apnoea
PA	posteroanterior
PA	pulmonary artery
PAC	premature atrial complex
PaCO$_2$	partial pressure of carbon dioxide
PaO$_2$	partial pressure of oxygen
PASP	pulmonary arterial systolic pressure
PCC	prothrombin complex concentrate
PCI	percutaneous coronary intervention
PCR	polymerase chain reaction
PCT	proximal convoluted tubule
PCWP	pulmonary capillary wedge pressure
PDA	posterior descending artery
PE	pulmonary embolus
PET	positron emission tomography
PHT	pressure half-time
PISA	proximal isovelocity surface area
PJRT	permanent junctional reciprocating tachycardia
PLAX	parasternal long-axis
PMC	percutaneous mitral valve commissurotomy
PND	paroxysmal nocturnal dyspnoea
PNS	parasympathetic nervous system
PoTS	postural orthostatic tachycardia syndrome
PPV	positive predictive value
PS	pulmonary stenosis
PSAX	parasternal short axis
PTL	pre-test likelihood
PV	pulmonary valve
PV	pulmonary vein
PVC	premature ventricular complex
PVI	pulmonary vein isolation
PVR	pulmonary vascular resistance
PW	pulsed wave
RA	rheumatoid arthritis
RA	right atrium
RAA	renin–angiotensin–aldosterone
RAA	right atrial appendage
RAD	right axis deviation

RAP	right atrial pressure
RBB	right bundle branch
RBBB	right bundle branch block
RCA	right coronary artery
RCC	right coronary cusp
RCT	randomised controlled trial
ROS	reactive oxygen species
RyR	ryanodine receptor
RV	right ventricle
RVF	right ventricular failure
RVOT	right ventricular outflow tract
RVSD	right ventricular systolic dysfunction
RVSF	right ventricular systolic function
RVSP	right ventricular systolic pressure
RWMA	regional wall motion abnormality
SAM	systolic anterior motion
SAN	sinoatrial node
SCAD	spontaneous coronary artery dissection
SCD	sudden cardiac death
SCT	stem cell transplantation
SE	stress echocardiography
SGLT2	sodium-glucose cotransporter 2
SIDS	sudden infant death syndrome
SLE	systemic lupus erythematosus
SND	sinus node dysfunction
SNP	sodium nitroprusside
SNRT	sinus node reciprocating tachycardia
SNRT	sinus node recovery time
SNS	sympathetic nervous system
SPECT	single photon emission computed tomography
SR	sarcoplasmic reticulum
STEMI	st elevation myocardial infarction
SV	stroke volume
SVC	superior vena cava
SVI	stroke volume index
SVR	systemic vascular resistance
SVT	supraventricular tachycardia
TAVI	transcatheter aortic valve implantation
TB	tuberculosis
TDI	tissue doppler imaging
TdP	torsades de pointes
TFB	trifascicular block
TIA	transient ischaemic attack
TIBC	total iron-binding capacity
TOE	transoesophageal echocardiogram
ToT	tendon of todaro
tPA	tenecteplase
TPR	total peripheral resistance
TR	tricuspid regurgitation

TTR	time in therapeutic range
TV	tricuspid valve
U&E	urea and electrolyte
UK	united kingdom
VEGF	vascular endothelial growth factor
VF	ventricular fibrillation
VSD	ventricular septal defect
VSMC	vascular smooth muscle cell
VT	ventricular tachycardia
VTI	velocity time integral
vWF	von willebrand factor
WACA	wide area circumferential ablation
WPW	wolff–parkinson–white

1

Electrophysiological Principles

1.1 Learning Objectives

- Generation of action potentials in pacemaker and non-pacemaker cells.
- Anatomical overview of the electrical conduction system.
- Principles that underpin normal ECG morphology.
- Common ECG abnormalities in the context of diseased states.

Cardiology at its Core, First Edition. Peysh A. Patel.
© 2023 John Wiley & Sons Ltd. Published 2023 by John Wiley & Sons Ltd.

1.2 Cardiac Action Potential

Every single cell in the heart has the ability to generate action potentials (AP). However, in normal electrophysiology, cardiac AP originate from the sinoatrial node (SAN), which has no true resting potential but instead generates spontaneous AP during diastole. The rate of this **automaticity** determines intrinsic heart rate (HR) and is mediated by cell permeability through hyperpolarisation-activated cyclic nucleotide-gated (HCN) channels via the inward mixed sodium–potassium funny current (I_f). Automaticity is an inherent feature of pacemaker cells located in the SAN, internodal conduction tracts, atrioventricular node (AVN), bundle of His, bundle branches and Purkinje network. The SAN is the dominant pacemaker as its rate of automaticity is highest, at 60–100 beats min^{-1} (bpm). Each time these cells generate an electrical current, the distal slower-firing subsidiary cells are depolarised before they can do so automatically ('overdrive suppression of automaticity'). However, if there is SAN dysfunction or disease of the conduction system, the subsidiary cells can assume pacemaker function in a phenomenon termed **escape pacing**, albeit typically at slower rates (AVN 40–60 bpm, bundle branches 30–40 bpm, Purkinje system 30–40 bpm).

A schematic representation of AP originating in the SAN is provided in Figure 1.1. In the resting state, the high concentration of extracellular sodium and intracellular potassium ions results in an overall negative electrical potential of around −70 mV. When I_f activation reduces potential to a critical membrane threshold of −35 mV (phase 4), there is activation of 'all-or-nothing' long-lasting, dihydropyridine-sensitive calcium channels ('L type'). Opening results in a slow, sustained influx (phase 0). Once the cells have fully depolarised, repolarisation occurs via efflux of potassium ions with a return to resting state (phase 3). Cells do not need to return to resting potential before they can depolarise again, assuming that the membrane threshold is reached. Depolarisation of one cell acts as an electrical impulse on adjacent cardiac cells and enables propagation of current in the direction of depolarisation. Cells in the AVN also have intrinsic pacemaker activity and mechanism of propagation is comparable. Notably, AP are directly susceptible to neural influence. For instance, adrenaline can increase I_f current (i.e. rate of phase 4) with effects on the rate of spontaneous firing. Parasympathetic mediators have contrasting effects.

In comparison, non-pacemaker myocytes demonstrate maintenance at the resting potential without spontaneous depolarisation. Indeed, atrial and ventricular extrasystoles (ectopy) most typically occur because excitability is triggered by adjacent Purkinje cells. Additionally, there are crucial

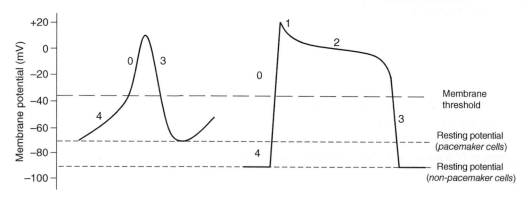

Figure 1.1 Schematic representation of action potential in pacemaker (left) and non-pacemaker (right) cardiac cells. AVN, atrioventricular node; CS, coronary sinus; CT, crista terminalis; CTI, cavo-tricuspid isthmus; EV, Eustachian valve; IAS, inter-atrial septum; IVC, inferior vena cava; RAA, right atrial appendage; SVC, superior vena cava; ToT, tendon of todaro; TV, tricuspid valve.

differences in morphology of AP which are depicted in Figure 1.1. The resting potential is more negative, in the region of -90 mV. Influx in phase 0 is determined by fast sodium channels as opposed to L type calcium channels resulting in a higher rate of depolarisation. The overshoot of AP is more pronounced. There also exists a distinct plateau (phase 2) mediated by prolonged slow repolarisation secondary to influx of calcium (and sodium) and efflux of potassium ions. Indeed, it is this inward calcium current that results in ion availability to initiate the process of excitation–contraction coupling (discussed in Chapter 6). Lastly, phase 4 in non-pacemaker cells involves the activation of sodium-potassium adenosine triphosphate (ATP)ase enzyme, which transports excess sodium out of cells and potassium back in. These pumps are not essential for inherent features of automaticity in pacemaker cells, although they may play a role in modifying depolarisation rate.

1.3   Electrical Conduction System

From a functional perspective, two categories of cardiac cells can be considered: myocardial and electrical. The myocardial cells contain numerous myofibrils consisting of contractile protein filaments, namely actin and myosin. This enables contractile properties of the myocardium, referring to its ability to shorten and return to its original length upon electrical stimulation. The underlying processes are explored in Chapter 6. By contrast, the specialised cells of the electrical conduction system do not have myofibrils and hence lack the ability to contract. Instead, they demonstrate an abundance of **gap junctions** between cells that permit rapid propagation of impulses in a fashion comparable to that seen in nerve fibres. An overview of the electrical conduction system is depicted in Figure 1.2 and discussed further in this subsection.

1.3.1   Sinoatrial Node

As highlighted, impulses originate from the SAN in normal electrophysiology. This region is a crescent-shaped structure, 2–3 mm wide, which is located laterally in the right atrium (RA) at the **sulcus terminalis**, a fat-filled groove demarcating the junction between RA appendage and

Figure 1.2   Overview of electrical conduction system in the heart.

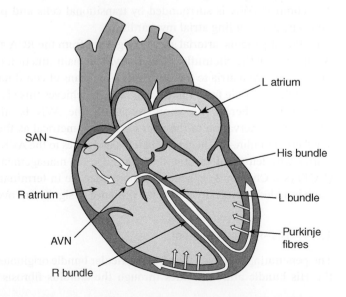

L atrium

SAN

His bundle

R atrium

L bundle

AVN

Purkinje fibres

R bundle

superior vena cava (SVC) and corresponding internally to the crista terminalis. Blood supply originates from right coronary artery (RCA) territory in approximately 60% of cases, and approaches the node in a counterclockwise direction. The SAN is also densely innervated with postganglionic adrenergic and cholinergic nerve terminals, allowing neurotransmitters to modulate electrical discharge rate via stimulation of β_1- and β_2-adrenergic and muscarinic receptors, respectively.

1.3.2 Internodal Tracts

There is anatomical evidence of three intra-atrial pathways – anterior, middle and posterior. The anterior internodal pathway curves anteriorly around the SVC to enter the **Bachmann bundle** (anterior interatrial band). This extends beyond the right upper pulmonary vein to the left atrium (LA) and provides a branch to the AVN. The middle internodal tract (**Wenckebach bundle**) travels behind the SVC to the crest of the interatrial septum and descends towards the superior margin of the AVN. Lastly, the posterior pathway (**tract of Thorel**) travels posteriorly around the SVC and along the crista terminalis to the Eustachian ridge. It proceeds into the interatrial septum above the coronary sinus where it joins the posterior portion of the AVN. Notably, these pathways do not demonstrate discrete histological features and may therefore be better referred to as internodal atrial myocardium.

1.3.3 Atrioventricular Node

The compact portion of the node is a superficial structure at the base of the atrial septum (i.e. it is an atrial structure). It is formed from merging of fibres of the right and left postero-inferior extensions, which run from the coronary sinus. The compact AVN is directly anterior to the ostium of the coronary sinus and above the insertion of the septal leaflet of the tricuspid valve (TV). It is at the apex of **Koch's triangle** (see Figure 1.3), which is bordered by the septal leaflet of the tricuspid valve anteriorly, the tendon of Todaro posteriorly and the coronary sinus inferiorly. The tendon of Todaro is absent in two-thirds of patients but, when present, originates in the AVN and passes through towards the Eustachian ridge and the rudimentary Eustachian valve. The compact AVN is surrounded by transitional cells and provides a connection between the node and surrounding atrial myocardium.

In 85% of patients, arterial supply originates from the RCA at the crux. In the remaining 15%, it is supplied by the circumflex (Cx) artery. The main function of the AVN is to modulate impulse propagation from atria to the ventricles as a means of coordinating chamber contraction and protecting the ventricle from rapid atrial rates. It achieves this via the phenomenon of **decremental conduction** whereby the more frequently the AVN is stimulated, the slower it conducts. Autonomic innervation to the nodes is not symmetrical as there is a higher abundance of right-sided efferent fibres to the SAN and left-sided fibres to the AVN. This provides some explanation to clarify why left-sided carotid sinus massage for management of narrow complex tachycardias (NCT) (see Chapter 3) is generally more effective in termination of dysrhythmias. Nonetheless, there is added complexity due to the presence of significant overlapping innervation.

1.3.4 His–Purkinje System

The penetrating region of the atrioventricular bundle originates distally from the compact AVN as the His bundle and continues through the annulus fibrosis as it penetrates the membranous

Figure 1.3 Oblique projection of RA to outline structures that define Koch's triangle.

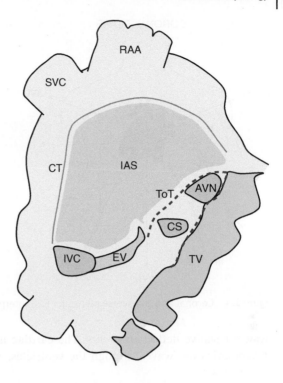

septum. The exact region that differentiates the AVN from the His bundle has not been delineated either anatomically or electrically. There is dual arterial supply from left anterior descending artery (LAD) and posterior descending artery (PDA) territories which enables greater protection from ischaemia. The bundle branches originate from the His bundle. The left bundle cascades downwards beneath the non-coronary aortic cusp and provides an anterior and posterior fascicle. The right bundle extends intramyocardially down the right side of the interventricular septum to the right ventricular apex. The terminal Purkinje fibres connect to distal bundle branches to form interweaving networks on the endocardial surface of both ventricles. This enables simultaneous and coordinated transmission of impulses to the entire left and right endocardium. The fibres terminate at synapses with myocardial cells.

1.4 ECG Morphology

1.4.1 General Principles

Electrical activity of the heart is determined routinely through a 12-lead electrocardiogram (ECG) derived from 10 electrodes. Use of specific leads with distinct anatomical distribution provides the ability to distinguish between normal and abnormal electrophysiology. Conventional lead placement occurs in two planes: transverse and coronal (see Figure 1.4). In the transverse plane there are six chest leads (V1–V6) which correspond roughly to anteroseptal (V1–V2), anteroapical (V3–V4) and anterolateral (V5–V6) territories. Leads in the coronal plane are I/aVL (left lateral surface), II/III/aVF (inferior) and aVR (right atrium). Each lead therefore provides a different perspective of electrical activity and corresponds to a differing ECG pattern. If overall activity is in the direction of the lead, a predominantly positive deflection occurs. Conversely, if it is predominantly directed

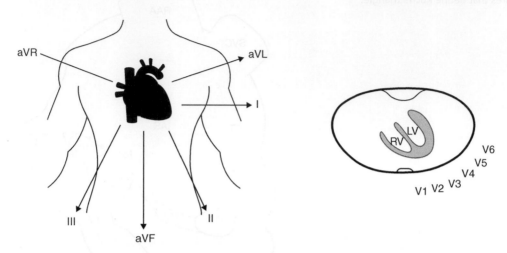

CORONAL PLANE   TRANSVERSE PLANE

Figure 1.4 Coronal and transverse planes for ECG interpretation.

away, a negative deflection occurs. The **cardiac axis** refers to the average direction of spread of depolarisation waves through the ventricles. A normal axis in the coronal plane is from $-30°$ to $+90°$.

On a 12-lead ECG, electrical activity in corresponding anatomical segments can be differentiated (see Figure 1.5). The initial positive deflection (P wave) relates to atrial depolarisation. The subsequent deflection (QRS complex) results from ventricular depolarisation and, finally, the T wave due to ventricular repolarisation when ventricles are refractory to excitability. As inferred, the PR interval constitutes duration between atrial and ventricular depolarisation and is normally in the region of 120–200 ms. It is mediated by the AVN. The QT interval refers to the duration

Figure 1.5 Morphology of normal ECG complex.

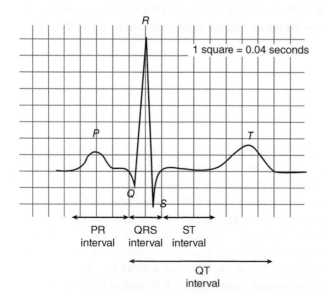

1 square = 0.04 seconds

between the onset of the QRS complex and the end of the T wave. It is adjusted for the resting HR and is presented more meaningfully as a corrected QT interval (QTc), equal to the QT interval divided by √RR interval. QTc is roughly < 440 ms for men and < 460 ms for women.

1.4.2 P Wave

Propagation of impulses from the SAN through the atria results in atrial depolarisation and a corresponding P wave. This activation begins superolaterally in the RA and proceeds simultaneously towards the LA, via the Bachmann bundle, and inferomedially towards the AVN. Hence, the P wave is usually upright in inferior leads (i.e. II/III/aVF) and inverted in aVR. If these characteristics are absent, the sinus node is unlikely to have initiated the impulse or the leads have been misplaced. Atrial activity is often best seen in leads V1 and II. Overall, RA precedes LA activation, which continues even once RA activation is complete. Normal P wave duration is < 120 ms with an amplitude < 0.25 mV. The electrical potentials generated by atrial repolarisation are rarely observed due to a combination of low amplitude and superimposition on the QRS complex.

1.4.3 QRS Complex

The earliest sites of ventricular activation are the centre of the left side of the septum and at the anterior and posterior paraseptal walls of the left ventricle (LV). This generally corresponds to the sites of insertion of the left bundle branch. Septal activation hence commences on the left and spreads to the right, and from apex to base. Subsequent wavefronts spread to activate the anterior and lateral walls of the LV, with the posterobasal segment the last to be activated. Excitation of the right ventricle (RV) begins similarly at the insertion point of the right bundle branch, in close proximity to the base of the anterior papillary muscle with spreading to the lateral wall. The final regions to be activated are posterobasal and the pulmonary infundibulum. Hence, in both ventricles, excitation begins in the septal region and is directed down to the apex before migrating to the free wall and posterobasal regions in an apex to base direction. Wavefronts are propagated from endocardium to epicardium via direct conduction between individual myocytes.

The initial negative deflection in the QRS complex is the Q wave, followed by a positive deflection as the R wave and a subsequent negative S wave. A second upright wave following the S wave is termed prime (depicted as R′). This pattern of ventricular activation can be deciphered by simplifying the process into septal and subsequent free wall activation. Initial conduction in the interventricular septum corresponds to directionality from left to right (coronal plane) and posteriorly to anteriorly (transverse plane). Hence, there is an initial positive deflection (R wave) in right-sided leads, with an initial negative deflection (Q wave) in left-sided leads. Subsequent components of the QRS complex reflect LV and RV free wall activation. However, RV mass is significantly lower than that of LV and its negligible contribution mandates consideration only of septal and LV activation. In a right-sided lead, there is subsequent downward deflection (S wave) as the bulk of the LV is depolarised. Conversely, in a left-sided lead, there is an upward deflection (R wave). Thus, QRS complexes in the chest leads demonstrate gradual progression from being predominantly negative (in V1) to positive (in V6). The normal duration of a QRS complex is < 120 ms. It is also worth mentioning that Q waves should be distinguished as physiological or pathological. In the context of the latter, they will generally be > 0.04 s and exceed 25% of the amplitude of the subsequent R wave.

1.4.4 T Wave

As highlighted, this region of the ECG complex is generated during ventricular repolarisation. It is generally positive in all leads except aVR, V1 and III. It can also be negative in V2 in younger patients and V3 in Afro-Caribbeans. Occasionally, a small U wave of 0.5 mm in amplitude may be observed following the T wave with the same overall polarity. It is best seen in leads V2–V3. Notably, prominent U waves (> 1–2 mm or >25% of T wave amplitude) may be associated with pathological states such as hypokalaemia, severe bradycardia and digoxin toxicity.

1.5   ECG Abnormalities

1.5.1   Peaked and Bifid P Waves

RA depolarisation usually precedes that of the LA. The combined wave, denoted by the P wave, is < 120 ms wide and < 2.5 mm in amplitude. If the RA is dilated, such as in the context of pulmonary hypertension or tricuspid regurgitation, RA depolarisation is longer in duration and its waveform extends to the end of LA depolarisation. This results in a P wave that is of greater amplitude but of normal duration (P-pulmonale or 'peaked' P wave – see Figure 1.6). In LA enlargement, secondary to left ventricular diastolic dysfunction or mitral regurgitation, for instance LA depolarisation lasts longer. Hence, the P wave amplitude is unaffected but is of prolonged duration and may be associated with a notch near its peak (P-mitrale or 'bifid' P wave).

1.5.2   P Wave Inversion

The presence of P wave inversion in the inferior leads (II/III/aVF) is indicative of retrograde conduction and a non-sinus origin for atrial depolarisation. If the PR interval is < 120 ms or there are P waves after the QRS complex, the source of electrical activity lies within the AVN and is often defined as a 'junctional rhythm'. If the PR interval is > 120 ms, the origin is within the atria and associated with premature activity (ectopy).

1.5.3   Left Ventricular Hypertrophy

Left ventricular hypertrophy (LVH) is associated with conditions such as systemic hypertension, aortic stenosis and some cardiomyopathies. In general, the QRS amplitude is increased and is directed more posteriorly. Hence, negative QRS complexes predominate in the right-sided leads. Various diagnostic criteria exist with good specificity and reasonable sensitivity, such as the **Cornell voltage criteria**. Broadly speaking, the most characteristic feature is the presence of tall R waves laterally (V5–V6) and deep S waves anteriorly (V1–V2).

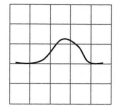 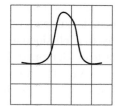 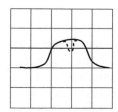

Figure 1.6   Morphology of P waves in right atrial (middle) and left atrial enlargement (right).

1.5.4 Axis Deviation

From the coronal view, as shown in Figure 1.7, the depolarisation wave normally spreads through the ventricles from 11 to 5 o'clock and is defined by a usual axis between −30° and +90°. This results in overall negative deflections in lead aVR and positive in lead II. The average direction of propagation defines the axis and normality can be defined simply by assessing for predominantly positive deflections in leads I, II, and III. If there is right axis deviation (RAD), lead I will be predominantly negative and corresponds coronally with a shift in axis ranging between +90° and +180°. Causes include right ventricular hypertrophy or strain. If there is left axis deviation (LAD), leads II and III will become negative and correlate with a coronal axis situated between −30° and −90°. Causes include LVH, right ventricular pacing and left bundle branch block (LBBB).

1.5.5 Bundle Branch Block

To appreciate the mechanisms underpinning bundle branch block (BBB), it is important to first remember that the septum is normally depolarised from left to right. Second, the left ventricle exerts more influence on the ECG than the right due to its substantial muscle mass. In BBB, there is a conduction delay resulting in QRS complex > 120 ms (see Figure 1.8).

1.5.5.1 Right Bundle Branch Block

In right bundle branch block (RBBB), the septum is depolarised from the left side as per usual, resulting in a small r wave in V1 and a small q wave in V6. Excitation subsequently spreads to the left ventricle and causes a S wave in V1 and R wave in V6. There is delayed excitation of the right ventricle resulting in a second wave (R′) in V1 and a deep s wave in V6. Some find it helpful to recall this pattern of excitation as 'M' in V1 and 'W' in V6. Of note, this pattern may exist in the context of a normal QRS duration, i.e. < 120 ms. This is defined as 'partial RBBB' and not deemed to be of pathological significance.

Figure 1.7 ECG axis interpretation.

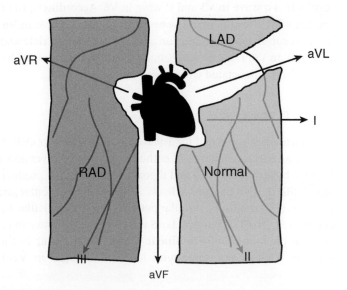

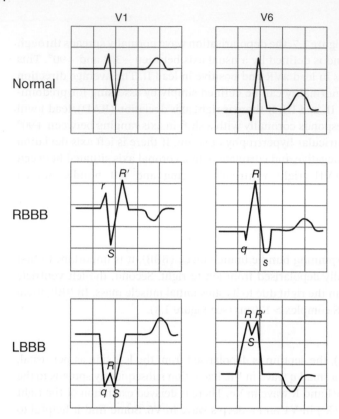

Figure 1.8 Morphology of QRS complexes in the RBBB and LBBB.

1.5.5.2 Left Bundle Branch Block

By contrast, the existence of LBBB irrespective of duration should always be considered abnormal. If there is a conduction defect in the left bundle, the septum depolarises from right to left. This results in a q wave in V1 and R wave in V6. Accordingly, the right ventricle is depolarised before the left which results in a R wave in V1 and an S wave in V6 (often appearing only as a notch). There is subsequent late depolarisation of the left ventricle and it is this that causes a S wave in V1 and an R' in V6. The classical pattern of LBBB may helpfully be recalled as 'W' in V1 and 'M' in V6. It can also be associated with lateral T wave inversion.

1.5.6 T Wave Inversion

As indicated, it is normal for T waves to be inverted in aVR, V1, III, V2 (young patients) and V3 (Afro-Caribbeans). Causes of pathological T wave inversion include ischaemia/infarction, ventricular hypertrophy, BBB and digoxin toxicity. LBBB produces T wave inversion in lateral leads and RBBB in right precordial leads. Acute right ventricular strain secondary to saddle pulmonary embolus (PE) produces a similar pattern to right ventricular hypertrophy and may manifest as the classical SI QIII TIII pattern, i.e. S wave in lead I, Q wave in lead III and T wave inversion in lead III. The phenomenon of **biphasic T waves** can occur in the context of significant ischaemia, such as Wellens syndrome with localised changes in V2–V3 that are strongly indicative of proximal, critical LAD artery stenosis. In such contexts, a positive deflection precedes the negative deflection. The opposite biphasic appearance, i.e. negative before positive, is suggestive of severe hypokalaemia. Indeed, there may be coexistence of a second positive deflection after the T wave (i.e. U wave).

1.5.7 Miscellaneous

There are a multitude of distinct ECG abnormalities that have not been explored in this section. Abnormalities include sinus node dysfunction (SND), AVN conduction disease, fascicular block and ST segment changes. These will be explored individually in other chapter subsections and discussed in the context of specific disease states.

Hot Points

- The SAN has the highest rate of inherent automaticity and enables dominant pacemaker characteristics.
- A key difference between action potentials in non-pacemaker cells and pacemaker cells is the presence of a plateau phase (phase 2), that allows excitation–contraction coupling.
- Interpretation of 12-lead ECG involves consideration of lead placements in two planes: transverse (chest leads) and coronal (limb leads).
- A normal ventricular axis exists between −30° and +90°, with deviations manifesting as LAD (−30° to −90°) or RAD (+90° to +180°).
- The concept of BBB is based upon the premise that a) the ventricular septum is depolarised from left to right, and b) the LV exerts more influence than RV.

1.6 Self-assessment Questions

1 In relation to cardiac action potentials, which is the correct statement?

    A In the resting state of the SAN, high concentration of extracellular potassium and intracellular sodium ions results in overall negative electrical potential of around −70 mV.

    B The term 'overdrive suppression of automaticity' describes the means by which the AVN acts as a dominant pacemaker within the heart.

    C Following generation of an action potential, pacemaker cells need to return to resting potential prior to further depolarisation.

    D Activation of the sympathetic nervous system enhances I_f current, allowing membrane threshold to be reached more rapidly in phase 4 of the AP, thus increasing HR.

    E In contrast to pacemaker cells, non-pacemaker myocytes have no true resting potential; instead, they generate spontaneous AP during diastole.

2 Regarding the electrical conduction system, select the correct statement.

    A The SAN is a crescent-shaped structure located laterally in RA at the Eustachian ridge, a fat-filled groove which corresponds internally to the crista terminalis.

B Anatomically, three pathways connecting SAN to AVN are recognised (anterior, middle, and posterior intermodal tracts). However, due to lack of discrete histological features, these may be better referred to as internodal atrial myocardium.

C The AVN is situated at apex of Koch's triangle and is bordered by anterior leaflet of the tricuspid valve anteriorly, tendon of Todaro posteriorly and coronary sinus inferiorly.

D In 65% of patients, arterial supply for the AVN originates from RCA, whilst in the remaining 35%, it is supplied by Cx artery.

E The His–Purkinje system receives dual arterial supply from Cx artery and PDA, enabling protection from ischaemia.

3 Regarding ECG morphology, which of the following is the correct statement?

A The cardiac axis refers to average direction of spread of depolarisation waves through the ventricles, and a normal axis in the coronal plane is between $-30°$ and $-90°$.

B QTc represents the QT interval adjusted for resting heart rate and is calculated by dividing the QT interval by the RR interval.

C An upright P wave in the inferior leads is indicative of retrograde conduction and non-sinus origin for atrial depolarisation.

D Ventricular activation spreads from epicardium to endocardium via direct conduction between individual myocytes.

E T wave inversion in V3 can be non-pathological in Afro-Caribbean patients.

4 Regarding ECG abnormalities, select the correct statement.

A P-pulmonale generally results from LA enlargement and is associated with pulmonary hypertension.

B Tall R waves in lateral leads and deep S waves in anterior leads are characteristic ECG findings in patients with LVH.

C Causes of LAD include LVH, left ventricular pacing and LBBB.

D An RSR′ pattern in the context of normal QRS duration is termed 'partial RBBB' and is thought to predict development of right ventricular dysfunction.

E Wellens syndrome is characterised by T wave inversion in leads V2–V3 and suggestive of critical left main stem stenosis.

5 Please select the correct statement.

A Phase 4 of the action potential in non-pacemaker cells involves activation of sodium–potassium guanosine triphosphate (GTP)ase enzyme, which transports excess sodium out of cells and potassium into cells.

B Right-sided carotid sinus massage is generally more effective in dysrhythmia termination due to higher abundance of right-sided efferent fibres to the AVN.

C The phenomenon of decremental conduction is a means of protecting the ventricles from rapid atrial rates.

D In the transverse plane, leads V1–V2 roughly correspond with the anterolateral segment of the left ventricle.

E The PR interval describes duration between atrial and ventricular depolarisation and is mediated by the His–Purkinje system.

Further Reading

Anderson, R.H., Yanni, J., Boyett, M.R. et al. (2009). The anatomy of the cardiac conduction system. *Clin. Anat.* 22 (1): 99–113.

Grant, A.O. (2009). Cardiac ion channels. *Circ. Arrhythm. Electrophysiol.* 2 (2): 185–194.

Padala, S.K., Cabrera, J.A., and Ellenbogen, K.A. (2021). Anatomy of the cardiac conduction system. *Pacing Clin. Electrophysiol.* 44 (1): 15–25.

Tan, N.Y., Witt, C.M., Oh, J.K., and Cha, Y.M. (2020). Left bundle branch block: current and future perspectives. *Circ. Arrhythm. Electrophysiol.* 13 (4): e008239.

van Weerd, J.H. and Christoffels, V.M. (2016). The formation and function of the cardiac conduction system. *Development* 143 (2): 197–210.

2

Atrial Fibrillation

CHAPTER MENU

2.1 Learning Objectives

- Diagnosis and classification systems for AF.
- Pathophysiological mechanisms that underpin impulse initiation and propagation.
- Associated clinical disorders.
- Clinical sequelae including thromboembolism and tachycardiomyopathy.
- Options for rate and rhythm control.
- Risk stratification.
- Pharmacotherapies to reduce thromboembolic risk with comparison of warfarin and direct oral anticoagulants.
- Role of left atrial appendage occlusion in select cohorts.

Cardiology at its Core, First Edition. Peysh A. Patel.
© 2023 John Wiley & Sons Ltd. Published 2023 by John Wiley & Sons Ltd.

2.2 Diagnosis and Classification

Atrial fibrillation (AF) is the commonest dysrhythmia and affects approximately 10% of patients aged > 80 years. Clinical AF is diagnosed when there is the presence of AF on a single-lead ECG tracing for greater than 30 s, or the full duration of a standard 12-lead ECG recording. It can be symptomatic or asymptomatic. Subclinical AF refers to the detection of atrial high-rate episodes (AHREs) on an implanted device. This is without symptoms attributable to AF but confirmed by assessment of intracardiac electrogram or ECG-recorded rhythm.

Various systems are available for categorisation of AF, with the classical approach relying upon anatomical distinction between 'valvular' and 'non-valvular' aetiologies. An approach based upon temporal characteristics can also be considered with distinction into several subgroups:

1) First diagnosed AF – initial new-onset presentation that is irrespective of duration.
2) Paroxysmal AF – self-terminating episode of less than seven days' duration.
3) Persistent AF – episode lasting between seven days and one year but terminating with rhythm control.
4) Long-standing persistent AF – duration greater than one year but potential for rhythm control.
5) Permanent AF – persistent dysrhythmia despite attempts at rhythm control with adoption of rate control.

'Lone' AF is defined by presence of AF that is not associated with underlying disease and is utilised as a diagnosis of exclusion.

2.3 Pathophysiology

Broadly speaking, initiation and propagation of AF occurs as a result of rapid firing of foci within the pulmonary veins resulting in a disorganised atrial rhythm. This results in overdrive suppression of the SAN with a compensatory pause of usually 1–1.5 s after termination prior to onset of normal sinus rhythm (NSR). Stabilisation of AF occurs through atrial remodelling secondary to pressure and volume overload. Concurrent fibrosis is also a significant contributor and is implicated in several of the clinical disorders strongly associated with AF (see Section 2.4). This correlates with progressive evolution of temporal characteristics from paroxysmal to persistent. An overview of broad pathophysiological mechanisms is provided in Figure 2.1.

Ectopy may arise from enhanced automaticity at the site of the pulmonary veins as a result of reduced resting potential. Alternatively, it can occur as a consequence of triggered activity with two broad subtypes: early after-depolarisation (EAD) and delayed after-depolarisation (DAD). EAD describes the occurrence of abnormal depolarisation during repolarisation (phase 3), typically as a consequence of action potential (AP) prolongation. This phenomenon underpins higher prevalence of AF in congenital long QT syndrome (see Chapter 4). DAD results from abnormal calcium release from the sarcoplasmic reticulum (SR) during diastole, such as in ischaemia and cardiac failure. The consequent extracellular shift of calcium results in exchange with sodium (3 : 1 stoichiometry) and a net inward depolarising current. Neural effects also play a role in modulation and perpetuation. For instance, sympathetic activation can potentiate diastolic calcium release from SR and promote generation of DADs. Indeed, suppression of autonomic signalling may provide some explanation for the benefits observed in AF ablation procedures.

Reentry describes re-excitation of non-refractory atrial myocardium, and there are various postulated mechanisms. In circus movement, the existence of slower conduction velocities and

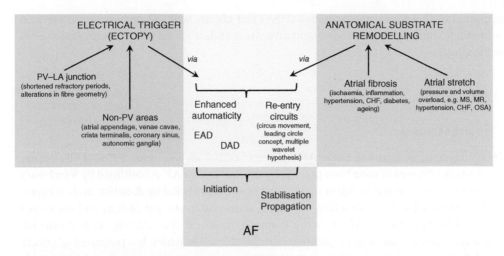

Figure 2.1 Pathophysiological mechanisms implicated in AF. LA, left atrium; MR, mitral regurgitation; MS, mitral stenosis; PV, pulmonary vein.

shortened refractory periods enable recovery of excited tissue after prior activation before it is reached by the next activation. The 'leading circle model' describes elements of reentry but with the absence of an anatomical substrate. Lastly, the 'multiple wavelet hypothesis' relates to fibrillation wavefronts continuously undergoing wavefront–wavetail interactions, resulting in breaks and generation of new fronts. Assuming a critical threshold is reached, there will be maintenance of the dysrhythmia. Factors that enhance stability include shortened velocity and increased tissue mass. This notion is supported by the Maze procedure conventionally used as an interventional strategy to treat AF, which results in anatomical subdivision of the atria into multiple compartments that are electrically distinct.

As alluded to, anatomical substrates play a critical role in impulse generation and stabilisation. The cardiac muscle sleeves at the interface of the pulmonary veins and left atrium are typical sites. Compared with normal atrial myocytes, cells have shorter refractory periods and, furthermore, there are abrupt changes in fibre orientation at these junctions that slow conduction velocity. Nonetheless, sites distinct from these regions can also be implicated and include the atrial appendage, venae cavae, crista terminalis, coronary sinus, and autonomic ganglia.

2.4 Associations

Atrial fibrillation is associated with a broad spectrum of clinical disorders implicated in atrial substrate remodelling. It is increasingly apparent that patients with AF, even those with true 'lone' features, have evidence of fibrotic deposition (termed **fibrotic atrial cardiomyopathy**). Age-related necrosis of atrial myocytes can contribute to this disease process. Infections such as pneumonia appear to increase incidence of AF. This may relate to elevated levels of pro-inflammatory cytokines, perturbations in haemodynamic homeostasis, catecholamine release and confounding effects of metabolic abnormalities and hypoxaemia. Atrial stretch may occur secondary to pressure overload from mitral regurgitation (MR), congestive heart failure (CHF), and systemic hypertension. Ischaemia from underlying coronary disease can also be implicated in addition to direct glucotoxic effects on atrial myocytes in the context of diabetes mellitus (DM).

The association of obstructive sleep apnoea (OSA) and obesity with AF may relate to elevated basal sympathetic tone, apnoea-induced oxidative stress and/or raised left atrial pressures from increased preload.

2.5 Clinical Sequelae

2.5.1 Thromboembolism

The primary adverse risk associated with AF is thromboembolism and around 20% of all cerebro-vascular events are deemed to have been potentially precipitated by AF. As outlined by **Virchow's triad**, thrombus formation is dependent upon blood stasis, endothelial dysfunction and/or hyper-coagulability. Impaired atrial contractility results in stasis within the left atrium and associated appendage (LAA), the latter of which is the dominant source if the aetiology is non-valvular. Endocardial remodelling results in progressive chamber dilatation which has potentiating effects. Endothelial dysfunction may arise from chronic inflammation secondary to reduced nitric oxide (NO) bioavailability. Elevated levels of von Willebrand factor (vWF) have also been demonstrated with sequelae due to hypercoagulability that is independent of underlying structural disease. Importantly, left atrial thrombus formation is a dynamic process in which blood flow, shear stress, turbulence and platelet count influence clot architecture and constituents. White thrombi consist of varying amounts of cellular debris, fibrin and platelets, whereas red thrombi are composed mainly of erythrocytes with some fibrin. Generally, thrombi within the atria are predominant in fibrin and therefore anticoagulants tend to be more effective than anti-platelets.

2.5.2 Tachycardiomyopathy

The atria play a crucial role in augmenting stroke volume (SV), by up to 20%. The loss of 'atrial kick' in the context of AF occurs because the chambers are fibrillating rather than contracting in a coordinated fashion. This has direct negative inotropic effects through impairment of filling. Additionally, the fast ventricular response results in a shortened diastolic phase, lower end-diastolic volumes and elevated pressures. Coronary flow reserve is also affected and can result in ischaemic insult. In addition, rate-related intraventricular and interventricular dyssynchrony has perpetuating effects. Chronic tachycardias can result in a phenomenon termed **tachycardiomyo-pathy,** even in structurally normal hearts. It describes impairment of ventricular function which is partially or completely reversible once rate control is achieved. Nonetheless, CHF can occur in the context of an irregular rhythm despite adequate rate control.

The relationship between AF and ventricular dysfunction is bidirectional. Elevated end-diastolic pressures result in atrial stretch and fibrosis due to pressure and volume overload with nidus for impulse initiation and propagation. Moreover, dysregulation of intracellular calcium handling and neurohormonal activation with elevated levels of catecholamines and angiotensin II have been strongly implicated. This provides rationale for neurohormonal blockade with angiotensin-converting enzyme (ACE) inhibitors and aldosterone antagonists in the context of cardiac failure (see Chapter 12).

It is apparent that AF and ventricular dysfunction do not simply coexist. Rather, the existence of positive feedback mechanisms result in continuous perpetuation. The augmentation of cardiac output (CO) via atrial contractility provides impetus to seek restoration of sinus rhythm in patients with symptomatic paroxysmal or persistent AF and significant ventricular impairment [1]. Nonetheless, there is delayed return of atrial contractility after cardioversion ('atrial stunning') and this necessitates a period of anticoagulation for at least four weeks post-procedure and long term if inherent risk dictates (see Section 2.6.3.2).

2.6   Management Strategies

The management of AF is complex and multi-faceted but a generalised overview is provided in Figure 2.2. Broadly, as with all narrow complex tachycardias (NCTs), it is first imperative to establish if there is evidence of associated haemodynamic compromise, although this typically occurs in the context of a precipitant such as sepsis or pulmonary embolus (PE). In these instances, acute electrical cardioversion is mandatory. It is also vital that underlying factors such as infection are scrupulously identified as targeted management often leads to full resolution of symptoms and physiological parameters. In cases without haemodynamic instability, an informed decision is required based on age, comorbidities and intrusiveness of symptoms to clarify whether a rate or rhythm control strategy is best adopted. In both instances, pharmacotherapy plays an important role although specific cases may require consideration of an interventional strategy such as ablation. An approach to stratify risk of thromboembolism is also required based on quantification using the **CHA₂DS₂-VASc** criteria. This determines whether a patient would benefit from long-term

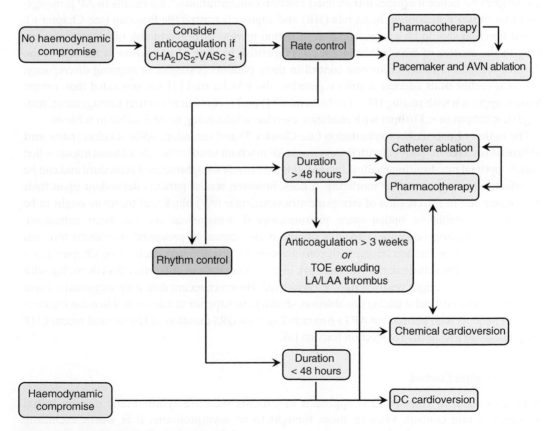

Figure 2.2   Management algorithm for AF.

anticoagulation or consideration of a LAA closure device if deemed to have clear intolerance to anticoagulation or high bleeding risk.

2.6.1 Rate Control

Control of the ventricular rate is an effective first-line management strategy in AF, particularly in elderly patients with minimal or absent symptoms. There are three broad options beta-blockers, non-dihydropyridine calcium channel blockers (NDHP CCB) and digoxin. All exert chronotropic influence by slowing conduction of the atrioventricular node (AVN) and, to a variable extent, the SAN. Bisoprolol is the most commonly used beta-blocker although alternatives with shorter half-lives such as atenolol or metoprolol may be considered if concerns exist regarding tolerability, such as in patients with emphysema. Nonetheless, they are absolutely contraindicated in patients with brittle asthma, significant hypotension and/or acute pulmonary oedema due to risks associated with negative inotropy. NDHP CCB have similar caveats but can be safely administered in patients with asthma.

Lastly, digoxin has positive inotropic effects and can be utilised irrespective of haemodynamic status. This is of particular benefit in the elderly who are ambulatory or in the context of critical illness. It may also be considered as first-line strategy instead of beta-blockers in those with permanent AF and symptoms of CHF due to potential benefits on quality of life with fewer adverse events [2]. Its primary mechanism is by inhibiting sodium–potassium adenosine triphosphatase (Na/K-ATPase). This increases intracellular sodium levels, reduces activity of the sodium/calcium exchanger and hence increases intracellular calcium concentrations. This results in AP prolongation that causes reduction in heart rate (HR) and augments contractile function (see Chapter 6). Renal function should be assessed prior to initiation in view of inherent risk of toxicity, particularly in the context of hypokalaemia due to competitive binding of potassium at the site of the digoxin receptor. The target for rate control in these patients is subject to ongoing discrepancy. Whereas earlier trials advocated strict regulation, the RACE2 trial [3] has suggested that a more lenient approach with resting $HR < 110$ beats min^{-1} [bpm] is equivalent to strict management, resting $HR < 80$ bpm or < 110 bpm with moderate exercise, whilst being more feasible to achieve.

The option of pacemaker implantation (see Chapter 5) and secondary AVN ablation (**pace and ablate**) is reserved for patients with symptomatic AF in whom ventricular rate remains uncontrolled despite optimal rate-limiting medical therapy. It is a relatively straightforward procedure and can be an effective strategy to reduce morbidity. It does, however, render patients dependent upon their pacemaker due to the creation of iatrogenic atrioventricular (AV) block and therefore ought to be considered a palliative option once pharmacological armamentarium has been exhausted. Conventionally, single-chamber pacing is advised in the context of preserved ventricular function (defined as ejection fraction ≥50%) with consideration for biventricular pacing (see Chapter 12) if there is concurrent ventricular impairment [4]. In those with narrow, intrinsic QRS His pacing with a backup lead in the right ventricle may be considered. However, recent data have suggested a lower threshold for biventricular pacing pre-ablation, shown to be superior to rate control in reducing mortality in patients with permanent AF (> 6 months), narrow QRS duration (≤110 ms) and recent CHF hospitalisation irrespective of ejection fraction [5].

2.6.2 Rhythm Control

It is reasonable to consider this approach in patients who are symptomatic despite initial attempts at rate control. Even in those thought to be asymptomatic, it is worth excluding unconscious adaptation through a rhythm control strategy, such as electrical cardioversion, to see if clinical profile is AF-related. In patients with early AF who have been diagnosed for less than 12 months, rhythm control with either anti-arrhythmics or ablation (see Section 2.6.2.2) appears to be associated with a lower risk of adverse outcomes [6]. In cases where the primary precipitant of the dysrhythmia is a reversible cause, such as infection or hyperthyroidism, a strategy for rhythm control is equally appropriate. Lastly, in patients with significant ventricular dysfunction (left ventricular ejection fraction [LVEF] ≤35%), New York Heart Association (NYHA) class II–IV symptoms and coexistent paroxysmal or persistent AF, attempts at reversion into NSR can be beneficial in reducing CHF hospitalisation and potentially improving survival [1]. Exploration of this strategy requires an individualised approach with nuanced considerations that include age, aetiology of ventricular dysfunction and temporal trend in LVEF after reversion of rhythm.

2.6.2.1 Electrical Cardioversion

In those with a first diagnosis of AF that presents clearly within 48 hours of symptom onset, acute cardioversion can be safely performed without the need for pre-procedure anticoagulation. This can be achieved via intravenous pharmacotherapy, such as amiodarone or flecainide, or through electrical cardioversion. If presentation exceeds this cut-off, a transoesophageal echocardiogram (TOE) is required to confidently exclude presence of intracardiac thrombus. Otherwise, patients can be managed conservatively with anticoagulation and rate-control therapy with scheduled electrical cardioversion electively once they have been in therapeutic range for at least three weeks. There is no evidence of benefit from early cardioversion except when patients are haemodynamically compromised. Success rates are improved by concurrent therapy with arrhythmia-modifying drugs (AMDs). Overall, cardioversion is achieved in 70–80% of cases albeit with 50% risk of recurrence within one year. Factors associated with failure include arrhythmia duration, left atrial size and presence of risk factors such as alcohol excess and raised body mass index (BMI). If there is a clear precipitant that is successfully treated, the risk of recurrence is significantly lower.

2.6.2.2 Chemical Cardioversion

Long-term therapy with AMDs is generally reserved for patients with symptomatic, paroxysmal AF. An overview of the most common agents is provided in Table 2.1. In patients with preserved left ventricular function and no history of coronary disease, flecainide is most commonly used. It can be taken as a regular medication or using a 'pill-in-the-pocket' approach where a dose is administered at the onset of AF symptoms. If flecainide is administered, there is a risk of organisation into atrial flutter (see Chapter 3). Flecainide also reduces atrial conduction velocity, resulting in relatively slow rates of 190–240 bpm as opposed to 300 bpm. As flecainide does not significantly block the AVN, patients with 'slow flutter' may conduct in a 1 : 1 fashion to the ventricles, resulting in ventricular fibrillation (VF) and cardiac arrest. Hence, patients must have concomitant AV blockade prior to administration. In those with a history of coronary disease without left ventricular dysfunction, sotalol is an acceptable option. It has dual properties of rate and rhythm control via beta-blockade and class III anti-arrhythmic effects. Notably, it can cause QTc prolongation in a dose-dependent fashion and so it is necessary to perform ECG monitoring when initiating therapy and following every dose alteration. In patients with ventricular dysfunction, amiodarone is typically used and can be highly effective in the elderly. However, it has potential side-effects, including skin photosensitivity, and requires close monitoring of thyroid, liver and pulmonary function.

Table 2.1 Overview of oral AMDs used for AF.

	Class	Mechanism of action	Side-effects	Contraindications (absolute and relative)
Amiodarone	III	Potassium channel blockade resulting in phase 3 AP prolongation (reduced efflux),	Hypotension, thrombophlebitis, thyroid dysfunction, pulmonary fibrosis, photosensitivity, interaction with warfarin, QTc prolongation	Thyroid disease, chronic liver or lung disease, pregnancy
Flecainide	Ic	Sodium channel blockade resulting in phase 0 AP prolongation (reduced influx)	Pro-arrhythmias, acute pulmonary oedema (negatively inotropic), central nervous system effects, QTc prolongation, risk of conversion into atrial flutter with 1:1 conduction	Impaired ventricular function, significant coronary artery disease, pregnancy, resting left bundle branch block
Sotalol	III	Potassium channel blockade resulting in phase 3 AP prolongation (reduced efflux), suppresses spontaneous depolarisation during phase 4, non-selective (β_1 and β_2) adrenoceptor antagonist	QTc prolongation, hypotension, fatigue	Impaired ventricular function, peripheral vascular disease, asthma, pregnancy

2.6.2.3 Catheter Ablation

In those with paroxysmal or persistent AF with refractory symptoms despite rate control and/or AMDs (typically one class I or III agent), referral to an electrophysiologist for consideration of ablation is warranted. The awareness that ectopy typically arises at the pulmonary vein–left atrium interface provides a rationale for pulmonary vein isolation (PVI) to create electrical dissociation from surrounding myocardium. This involves application of radiofrequency, cryothermal, laser or pulsed electric field energy to eradicate cells that are the nidus for impulse initiation and propagation. With expanded understanding that now also implicates ganglionic plexi in genesis, an approach of wide area circumferential ablation (WACA) is adopted as routine practice. Depending on the substrate, additional interventions such as roof line, lateral mitral line and posterior wall box isolation can be performed.

Success rates in paroxysmal AF are in the region of 70–80%, falling to between 50 and 70% in persistent AF. The procedure is generally performed on uninterrupted anticoagulation to reduce the risk of subclinical cerebrovascular events. Nonetheless, inherent procedural risks include cardiac tamponade, pulmonary vein stenosis, phrenic nerve palsy (transient or persistent), and oesophageal perforation/fistula. Of relevance, there have been no prospective studies to date with proven mortality benefit from the procedure, and accordingly, intrusive symptoms are generally a prerequisite for referral. Caution is also warranted if there is prolonged duration (typically more than two years), $BMI > 35 \, kg \, m^{-2}$, untreated OSA, persistent alcohol excess, severe left atrial dilatation ($> 55 \, mm$) or failed direct current cardioversion (DCCV) on AMDs.

2.6.3 Anticoagulation

2.6.3.1 Mechanisms

To conceptualise the mechanisms that underpin anticoagulant therapy, it is first beneficial to understand the processes implicated in normal haemostasis (see Figure 2.3). This refers to wound

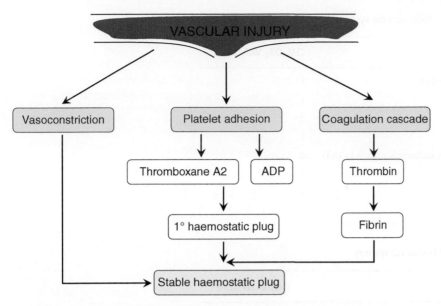

Figure 2.3   Overview of mechanisms implicated in normal haemostasis.

healing as a response to injury of the vascular endothelium. In this context, exposure of underlying collagen initiates the haemostatic process. Platelet adhesion and a release reaction produces thromboxane A2, inhibited by aspirin, and adenosine diphosphate (ADP), which is inhibited by thienopyridines such as clopidogrel and prasugrel (see Chapter 11). This results in platelet aggregation and the formation of a primary haemostatic plug. A separate pathway involves activation of the coagulation cascade that ultimately results in the formation of thrombin from prothrombin. This converts fibrinogen into fibrin, which is integrated and produces a stable haemostatic plug. Local vasoconstrictive effects at the site of endothelial injury impair blood flow and have enhancing effects. **Warfarin** operates primarily via inhibition of vitamin K-dependent clotting factors II, VII, IX, and X. By contrast, the direct oral anticoagulants (DOACs) function by direct inhibition of prothrombin/factor II (dabigatran) or factor Xa (**rivaroxaban, apixaban, edoxaban**). A comparison of warfarin and different DOACs is given in Section 2.4.

2.6.3.2   Scoring Systems

In patients who have clinical AF, a decision is required regarding suitability for long-term anticoagulation to abrogate thromboembolic risk. This should be applied irrespective of whether the patient subsequently reverts into sinus rhythm. It is not yet established what qualifies as the minimum duration of AF, and similarly, it is unclear whether anticoagulation confers benefit in patients with subclinical AF that has been detected solely on an implantable device.

Irrespective of this, a primary distinction relies on clarifying whether AF is 'valvular' in origin. Currently, this is defined as the presence of a prosthetic mitral valve or at least moderate mitral stenosis. In these instances, anticoagulation with warfarin is advocated in all cases. For those with 'non-valvular' AF, the CHA$_2$DS$_2$-VASc scoring criteria is utilised to clarify risk. Its evolution from the preceding CHADS2 scoring system is mainly to identify those individuals with true 'low risk' who do not require anticoagulation. The composite parameters are outlined in Table 2.2. CHF refers to recent decompensation irrespective of ventricular function or the presence of moderate-to-severe impairment on imaging even if asymptomatic. Vascular disease can include angiographically significant coronary disease, previous myocardial infarction (MI), peripheral vascular disease

Table 2.2 CHA$_2$DS$_2$-VASc scoring system.

Risk factor	CHA$_2$DS$_2$-VASc score
Congestive heart failure	1
Hypertension	1
Age $\geq$ 75 yr	2
Diabetes mellitus	1
Stroke (or transient ischaemic attack [TIA])	2
Vascular disease	1
Age 65–74 yr	1
Sex category (female)	1

Table 2.3 HAS-BLED scoring system.

Risk factor	HAS-BLED score
Hypertension (uncontrolled)	1
Abnormal renal or liver function	1
Stroke	1
Bleeding (history of)	1
Labile INRs	1
Elderly (age > 65 yr or extreme frailty)	1
Drugs or alcohol	1

or aortic plaque. Female patients with gender as an isolated risk factor would be considered as 'low risk' and scored as 0. A score of 1 or more suggests the need for formal anticoagulation.

A balanced approach comparing the benefits of thromboprophylaxis with the potential for major bleeding needs to be established in each patient to stratify individual risk. Bleeding risk is conventionally assessed using the HAS-BLED scoring system (see Table 2.3), which has good predictive value. Uncontrolled hypertension corresponds with systolic blood pressure consistently > 160 mmHg. Abnormal renal function includes those with creatinine > 200 μmol/l or those rendered dialysis- or transplant-dependent. Bleeding propensity may include major haemorrhage, anaemia or severe thrombocytopenia. Labile international normalised ratios (INRs) refer to time in therapeutic range (TTR) < 60% in those on warfarin therapy. Drugs considered as risk factors for bleeding include anti-platelets and non-steroidal anti-inflammatory drugs (NSAIDs), with alcohol excess defined as > 14 units per week. It is worthy of note, however, that a significant HAS-BLED score ($\geq$ 3) does not automatically exclude but instead justifies a more cautious approach with regular monitoring. An alternative strategy involves use of the ORBIT bleeding risk score, which incorporates gender, age, bleeding history, renal function, and anti-platelet therapy.

2.6.3.3 Warfarin vs DOACs
Conventional means of anticoagulation have relied upon therapy with warfarin. As stipulated, it operates via inhibition of vitamin K-dependent clotting factors II, VII, IX, and X. It also has

inhibitory effects on protein C and protein S, which ordinarily act as inhibitors of the coagulation cascade. Hence, warfarin is deemed to be initially procoagulant and patients who are loaded with warfarin require coadministration of therapeutic low-molecular-weight heparin (LMWH), such as enoxaparin or dalteparin, for the first 72–96 hours until therapeutic levels are achieved.

Patients with AF have a five-fold increased risk of thromboembolism and warfarin can mitigate this risk by approximately 66%. Nonetheless, warfarin has well-established drawbacks. It requires regular INR monitoring to ensure that the patient is within therapeutic range (conventionally 2–3), with a TTR ≥ 66% deemed most effective in stroke prevention. It is also dependent on dietary intake of vitamin K and there is a potential for interaction with a wide range of pharmacological agents and alcohol. For this reason, there have been extensive efforts to identify novel agents and DOACs are one such example (see Table 2.4). They have rapid onset of action, predictable pharmacokinetics with no requirement for monitoring and lower dependence on dietary intake. However, they have significant interactions, particularly with anti-cancer agents, antibiotics, anti-fungals, and certain anti-arrhythmics, which limit their use in particular patients. They can broadly be considered as suitable first-line option in patients with non-valvular AF. If AF is deemed secondary to valvular disease, all patients require anticoagulation and there is no substitute for warfarin.

Table 2.4 Comparison between warfarin and DOACs.

	Warfarin	Dabigatran	Rivaroxaban	Apixaban	Edoxaban
Primary mechanism	Inhibition of vitamin K-dependent clotting factors (II, VII, IX, X)	Inhibition of factor II (prothrombin)	Inhibition of factor Xa	Inhibition of factor Xa	Inhibition of factor Xa
Time to peak effect	3–5 d	3 h	3 h	3 h	1–2 h
Dose	Variable	150 mg BD (or 110 mg BD)	20 mg OD (or 15 mg OD)	5 mg BD (or 2.5 mg BD)	60 mg OD (or 30 mg OD)
Administration	OD	BD	OD	BD	OD
Renal clearance	0%	80%	35%	25%	40%
Bioavailability	100%	6%	70%	50%	62%
Monitoring	Required	Not required	Not required	Not required	Not required
Antidote	Vitamin K, prothrombin complex concentrate (PCC)	Idarucizumab	Andexanet alfa	Andexanet alfa	None currently
Special considerations		Absorption pH-dependent and reduced in patients taking proton pump inhibitor	Requirement to take with food, affects INR the most	Affects INR the least	

Abbreviations: BD, twice daily; OD, once daily.

Dabigatran was the first DOAC to demonstrate effectiveness in AF thromboprophylaxis, based upon the RELY trial [7]. A lower dose (110 mg twice daily) was non-inferior to warfarin with regard to stroke and systemic embolism and resulted in less major haemorrhage. At a higher dose (150 mg twice daily), there was lower incidence of stroke and systemic embolism but this was counteracted by higher bleeding risk and without a difference in all-cause mortality. The ROCKET-AF trial compared rivaroxaban with warfarin in AF and found it to be non-inferior with respect to stroke and systemic embolism and comparable in terms of mortality risk [8]. However, a subsequent retrospective analysis observed increased burden of gastrointestinal haemorrhage. The subsequent ARISTOTLE trial showed apixaban use to reduce systemic embolism in addition to major bleeding events [9]. Indeed, this was the first clinical trial to exhibit mortality benefit of DOAC therapy compared with warfarin. Edoxaban is the newest addition to the DOAC repertoire, with the ENGAGE-AF-TIMI trial showing non-inferiority compared with warfarin in terms of systemic embolism [10]. Incidence of major bleeding was reduced with the notable exception of gastrointestinal haemorrhage in the context of high-dose edoxaban.

2.6.3.4 Left Atrial Appendage (LAA) Occlusion

The LAA is considered the primary site of thrombogenesis in the context of AF, and indeed, complex LAA morphology may itself be an independent predictor of stroke. Consequently, occlusion of this anatomical region via closure devices is an attractive cryptogenic alternative in select patients. Specifically, it is relevant in those who fulfil the criteria for long-term anticoagulation (warfarin or DOAC) but in whom a clear intolerance or high risk of bleeding exists, although robust data for these subgroups is lacking. It should not simply be offered as alternative first-line therapy for patients who are reluctant to engage with long-term anticoagulation. The PROTECT-AF [11] and PREVAIL [12] trials, which compared the Watchman device to warfarin in patients eligible for anticoagulation, found LAA occlusion to be non-inferior to warfarin in stroke prevention whilst possibly lowering bleeding risk. There is however, no data providing direct comparison of LAA devices with DOACs. Use of LAA closure devices also introduce a procedural risk that is avoidable with pharmacotherapy, and antiplatelet therapy for at least three months is required subsequent to device deployment. Overall evidence base remains limited and further trials are necessary before clear incorporation into routine practice.

Hot Points

- AF typically arises from either ectopy formation (enhanced automaticity or triggered activity) and/or reentry circuit formation.
- The primary adverse risk associated with AF is thromboembolism. Chronic tachycardias may also result in ventricular dysfunction, termed 'tachycardiomyopathy'.
- Management options include rate and rhythm control, with determination of long-term anticoagulation using the CHA_2DS_2-VASc criteria in cases of non-valvular AF.
- Pharmacological options for anticoagulation include warfarin and DOACs with an individualised approach.
- LAA occlusion may be considered in select cases where anticoagulation is indicated but there is intolerance or high bleeding risk.

2.7 Self-assessment Questions

1 Which of the following factors are not associated with maintenance of AF?
   A Left atrial enlargement
   B Digoxin toxicity
   C Reduced atrial refractoriness
   D Myocardial fibrosis
   E Autonomic dysfunction

2 Which of these statements is correct?
   A DC cardioversion can safely be performed without anticoagulation if onset of AF is within seven days.
   B Pacemaker insertion and AV node ablation (pace and ablate) form an appropriate strategy in patients wishing to avoid long-term pharmacotherapy.
   C Flecainide is the arrhythmia-modifying drug of choice in patients with coronary disease.
   D In ambulatory patients requiring rate control, digoxin is an effective treatment.
   E Pulmonary vein isolation should be considered in patients with asymptomatic, paroxysmal AF.

3 Which of the following conditions is not associated with development of AF?
   A Obstructive sleep apnoea
   B Atrial flutter
   C Chronic lung disease
   D Diabetes mellitus
   E Hyperlipidaemia

4 Which of these statements is correct?
   A Anticoagulation should be avoided in patients with HAS-BLED score ≥ 3.
   B Patients in sinus rhythm can be considered for left atrial appendage occlusion.
   C In patients with AF and severe aortic stenosis, the recommended anticoagulant is warfarin.
   D Anticoagulation should continue indefinitely in patients with CHA_2DS_2-VASc score > 1 who undergo successful AF ablation.
   E An abnormal coagulation screen suggests that a patient is non-compliant with DOAC.

5 What is the most appropriate treatment for a patient with pre-excited AF who is haemodynamically unstable?
   A Intravenous metoprolol
   B Oral bisoprolol
   C Intravenous adenosine
   D Oral amiodarone
   E Electrical cardioversion

References

1 Marrouche, N.F., Brachmann, J., Andresen, D. et al. (2018). Catheter ablation for atrial fibrillation with heart failure. *N. Engl. J. Med.* 378 (5): 417–427.

2 Kotecha, D., Bunting, K.V., Gill, S.K. et al. (2020). Effect of digoxin vs Bisoprolol for heart rate control in atrial fibrillation on patient-reported quality of life: the RATE-AF randomized clinical trial. *JAMA* 324 (24): 2497–2508.

3 Van Gelder, I.C., Groenveld, H.F., Crijns, H.J. et al. (2010). Lenient versus strict rate control in patients with atrial fibrillation. *N. Engl. J. Med.* 362 (15): 1363–1373.

4 Curtis, A.B., Worley, S.J., Adamson, P.B. et al. (2013). Biventricular pacing for atrioventricular block and systolic dysfunction. *N. Engl. J. Med.* 368 (17): 1585–1593.

5 Brignole, M., Pentimalli, F., Palmisano, P. et al. (2021). AV junction ablation and cardiac resynchronization for patients with permanent atrial fibrillation and narrow QRS: the APAF-CRT mortality trial (published correction appears in *Eur. Heart J.* 2021) (published correction appears in *Eur. Heart J.* 2021). *Eur. Heart J.* 42 (46): 4731–4739.

6 Kirchhof, P., Camm, A.J., Goette, A. et al. (2020). Early rhythm-control therapy in patients with atrial fibrillation. *N. Engl. J. Med.* 383 (14): 1305–1316.

7 Connolly, S.J., Ezekowitz, M.D., Yusuf, S. et al. (2009). Dabigatran versus warfarin in patients with atrial fibrillation (published correction appears in *N. Engl. J. Med.* 2010;363(19):1877). *N. Engl. J. Med.* 361 (12): 1139–1151.

8 Patel, M.R., Mahaffey, K.W., Garg, J. et al. (2011). Rivaroxaban versus warfarin in nonvalvular atrial fibrillation. *N. Engl. J. Med.* 365 (10): 883–891.

9 Granger, C.B., Alexander, J.H., McMurray, J.J. et al. (2011). Apixaban versus warfarin in patients with atrial fibrillation. *N. Engl. J. Med.* 365 (11): 981–992.

10 Giugliano, R.P., Ruff, C.T., Braunwald, E. et al. (2013). Edoxaban versus warfarin in patients with atrial fibrillation. *N. Engl. J. Med.* 369 (22): 2093–2104.

11 Reddy, V.Y., Doshi, S.K., Sievert, H. et al. (2013). Percutaneous left atrial appendage closure for stroke prophylaxis in patients with atrial fibrillation: 2.3-year follow-up of the PROTECT AF (watchman left atrial appendage system for embolic protection in patients with atrial fibrillation) trial. *Circulation* 127 (6): 720–729.

12 Holmes, D.R. Jr., Kar, S., Price, M.J. et al. (2014). Prospective randomized evaluation of the Watchman Left Atrial Appendage Closure device in patients with atrial fibrillation versus long-term warfarin therapy: the PREVAIL trial (published correction appears in *J. Am. Coll. Cardiol.* 2014;64(11): 1186). *J. Am. Coll. Cardiol.* 64 (1): 1–12.

Further Reading

Brignole, M. (1998). Ablate and pace: a pragmatic approach to paroxysmal atrial fibrillation not controlled by antiarrhythmic drugs. *Heart* 79 (6): 531–533.

De Caterina, R. and Camm, A.J. (2014). What is 'valvular' atrial fibrillation? A reappraisal. *Eur. Heart J.* 35 (47): 3328–3335.

Gage, B.F., Waterman, A.D., Shannon, W. et al. (2001). Validation of clinical classification schemes for predicting stroke: results from the National Registry of Atrial Fibrillation. *JAMA* 285 (22): 2864–2870.

Hindricks, G., Potpara, T., Dagres, N. et al. (2020). ESC guidelines for the diagnosis and management of atrial fibrillation developed in collaboration with the European Association for Cardio-Thoracic Surgery (EACTS): the task force for the diagnosis and management of atrial fibrillation of the European Society of Cardiology (ESC). Developed with the special contribution of the European Heart Rhythm Association (EHRA) of the ESC (published correction appears in *Eur. Heart*

J. 2021;42(5):507) (published correction appears in Eur. Heart J. 2021;42(5):546–547) (published correction appears in *Eur. Heart J.* 2021;42(40):4194). *Eur. Heart J.* 2021 42 (5): 373–498.

Hohnloser, S.H., Kuck, K.H., and Lilienthal, J. (2000). Rhythm or rate control in atrial fibrillation – Pharmacological Intervention in Atrial Fibrillation (PIAF): a randomised trial. *Lancet* 356 (9244): 1789–1794.

Kotecha, D. and Piccini, J.P. (2015). Atrial fibrillation in heart failure: what should we do? *Eur. Heart J.* 36 (46): 3250–3257.

Lip, G.Y. (2011). The role of aspirin for stroke prevention in atrial fibrillation. *Nat. Rev. Cardiol.* 8 (10): 602–606.

Mont, L., Bisbal, F., Hernández-Madrid, A. et al. (2014). Catheter ablation vs. antiarrhythmic drug treatment of persistent atrial fibrillation: a multicentre, randomized, controlled trial (SARA study). *Eur. Heart J.* 35 (8): 501–507.

Schotten, U., Verheule, S., Kirchhof, P., and Goette, A. (2011). Pathophysiological mechanisms of atrial fibrillation: a translational appraisal (published correction appears in *Physiol. Rev.* 2011; 91(4):1533). *Physiol. Rev.* 91 (1): 265–325.

Wyse, D.G., Waldo, A.L., DiMarco, J.P. et al. (2002). A comparison of rate control and rhythm control in patients with atrial fibrillation. *N. Engl. J. Med.* 347 (23): 1825–1833.

3

Narrow Complex Tachycardias

Cardiology at its Core, First Edition. Peysh A. Patel.
© 2023 John Wiley & Sons Ltd. Published 2023 by John Wiley & Sons Ltd.

3.1 Learning Objectives

- Outline of terminology.
- Types of narrow complex tachycardias.
- Mechanisms, diagnostic strategies and management options for sinus tachycardia, atrial flutter, atrioventricular nodal reentrant tachycardia, atrioventricular reentrant tachycardia, atrial tachycardia, and junctional tachycardia.

3.2 Nomenclature

There is often confusion regarding nomenclature that pertains to narrow complex tachycardias (NCTs). This uncertainty arises because the term is used interchangeably with supraventricular tachycardias (SVTs), which is itself considered synonymous with circuits that rely on an accessory pathway (AP) such as in Wolff–Parkinson–White (WPW) syndrome. From a conceptual perspective, SVT ought to be strictly defined as any electrical impulse that is initiated at an anatomical site at or above the atrioventricular node (AVN). As propagation is via normal conduction pathways, i.e. AVN and the His–Purkinje system, this results in a QRS complex of normal duration (i.e. 'narrow complex'). However, there are notable exceptions such as in SVT with antidromic atrioventricular reentrant tachycardia (AVRT). The term SVT may therefore be better placed as an umbrella term encompassing various aetiologies. For the purposes of this section, exploration of different subtypes of regular NCT shall be provided based on those deemed most clinically relevant. Atrial fibrillation is the most common form of irregular NCT and has already been discussed in Chapter 2.

3.3 Categorisation

There are various approaches to categorise NCTs (see Figure 3.1). It is generally beneficial to distinguish between regularity and irregularity as differential diagnoses are very different. Moreover, electrophysiologists advocate assessment of the RP interval, i.e. the duration between ventricular and

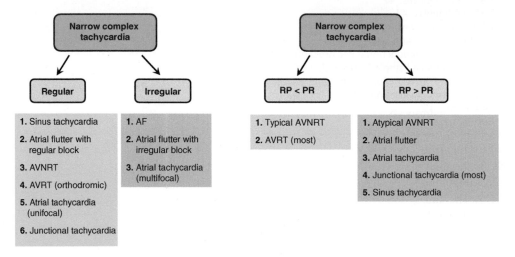

Figure 3.1 Categorisation of narrow complex tachycardias.

atrial depolarisation. This can be defined as prolonged if it is greater than the PR interval, or if the absolute interval is > 100 ms when the heart rate is > 160 beats min^{-1} (bpm). Although P wave visualisation can be challenging, determining the relative difference can provide useful indications and aid clarification.

3.4 Sinus Tachycardia

Sinus tachycardia is the most common form of regular NCT. It can be defined as a resting heart rate >100 bpm in adults, where each QRS complex is preceded by a P wave. There are a wide range of precipitants, including anxiety, pain, exercise, caffeine, infection, and hyperthyroidism. Pharmacotherapy with beta-agonists and recreational drug use such as cocaine and amphetamines may also be implicated. A separate entity, known as **inappropriate sinus tachycardia (IST)**, describes abnormal elevation of resting heart rate (HR) without a clear identifiable cause. Impulses are deemed to originate from the sinoatrial node (SAN) with genesis possibly related to autonomic dysregulation. It is not considered life-threatening *per se* but can be associated with intrusive symptoms and significant morbidity. Ivabradine, either as monotherapy or in conjunction with a beta-blocker, may be considered in those who are symptomatic. Catheter ablation can be offered in refractory cases but is associated with relatively poor outcomes [1]. This is primarily because the SAN is protected by a dense matrix of surrounding connective tissue, the thick crista terminalis and cooling effects of the nodal artery.

It can be challenging to distinguish IST from a separate condition, namely **postural orthostatic tachycardia syndrome (PoTS)**. This also results from episodic perturbations of the autonomic nervous system (ANS), but is characterised by increased HR on standing upright ($\geq$ 30 bpm from rest or absolute value $\geq$ 120 bpm) and without a concurrent drop in blood pressure (BP). It has a strong female preponderance, being five-fold more prevalent than in men, and is thought to be associated with joint hypermobility syndromes. A tilt-table test is beneficial for diagnostic purposes, and in addition, Holter monitor with histogram profiling of heart rate variability can help distinguish PoTS from IST. Treatment options are currently limited to conservative strategies such as adequate hydration, increased salt intake and elastic support stockings. Ivabradine may be considered but efficacy has not been established. Sertaline has been shown to confer positive benefit and cognitive behavioural therapy (CBT) may also be helpful in certain cohorts to reduce disease burden.

3.5 Atrial Flutter

3.5.1 Mechanisms

The most common form of atrial flutter arises because of a counter-clockwise macro reentrant circuit in the right atrium (RA) (see Figure 3.2). It is limited anteriorly by the tricuspid orifice and posteriorly by the inferior vena cava (IVC) and Eustachian valve. The activation wavefront proceeds caudocranially along the septal aspect of the RA and returns down towards the cavo-tricuspid isthmus (CTI). The same circuit occurs in clockwise flutter in a smaller proportion of cases, around 15%. 'Typical' flutter, be it clockwise or counter-clockwise, indicates that the reentry circuit is dependent on the CTI. 'Atypical' flutter arises from complex mechanisms that may include surgical scarring, prior left atrial ablation and atrial changes arising as a result of cardiomyopathies such as hypertrophic cardiomyopathy (HCM). The potential for reentry circuit formation is

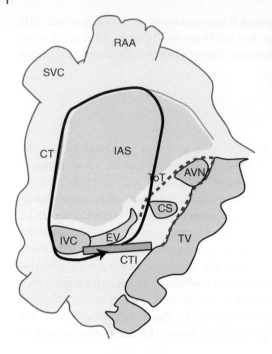

Figure 3.2 Reentry circuit in 'typical' counter-clockwise atrial flutter. CS, coronary sinus; CT, crista terminalis; CTI, cavo-tricuspid isthmus; EV, Eustachian valve; IAS, interatrial septum; IVC, inferior vena cava; SVC, superior vena cava; ToT, tendon of todaro; TV, tricuspid valve.

present in all hearts but the dysrhythmia only stabilises and propagates when the RA is able to accommodate a circulating wavefront which does not collide with the tail while in its refractory period. Hence, there is often the need for RA dilatation or regions of reduced conduction secondary to fibrosis.

3.5.2 Diagnosis

Atrial flutter is associated with increasing age, CHF, chronic obstructive pulmonary disease (COPD) and obesity. It may also occur secondary to surgery, ischaemic heart disease (IHD) and pneumonia. 'Lone' atrial flutter without underlying cardiovascular or respiratory disease is rare; however, it is not infrequent for flutter to coexist with atrial fibrillation (AF) in view of shared precipitants. Patients classically describe palpitations, which may be paroxysmal in nature, breathlessness or chest pain. These symptoms may be worsened by physical exertion. In counter-clockwise flutter, atrial waves are observed on ECG as initial negative deflections in inferior leads. These become positive as the reentry loop rotates and reverses direction, resulting in a characteristic **sawtooth** morphology (see Figure 3.3). The atrial rate is typically 300 bpm and corresponds with rate of spontaneous discharge from the SAN. As the AVN has a refractory period, not all impulses

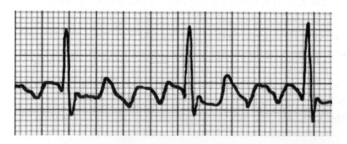

Figure 3.3 Single-lead ECG appearance of atrial flutter with sawtooth appearance.

are propagated and this results in a sequential block such as 2 : 1 (ventricular rate of 150 bpm) or 3 : 1 (ventricular rate of 100 bpm).

3.5.3 Management

3.5.3.1 Pharmacotherapy

There can often be ambiguity about the diagnosis, particularly since the classical sawtooth baseline may not be clearly distinguishable. In this instance, the ECG will be consistent with a regular NCT. As with all such dysrhythmias, initial management would depend on identification of adverse features. If there is suggestion of chest pain resulting from myocardial ischaemia due to impaired ventricular filling, pulmonary congestion, hypotension or syncope, the patient requires urgent cardioversion. If the patient is relatively stable, it is sensible to transiently enhance AVN blockade. This will result in slower ventricular rates, for instance 75 bpm if there is a 4 : 1 block, and enable assessment of underlying rhythm. Nonetheless, in the context of atrial flutter, it is unlikely to cause reversion into normal sinus rhythm (NSR) as the macro reentrant circuit can persist unabated. AVN blockade may be achieved through vagal manoeuvres such as carotid sinus massage or the Valsalva manoeuvre. If this is unsuccessful, pharmacological options include intravenous adenosine. This has a notably short half-life of 10–15 s but requires administration into a large-calibre vein with a fluid bolus to ensure that it has a targeted effect. Patients should be maintained on a rhythm strip with defibrillator pads at all times and should be clearly warned of transient symptoms including chest discomfort and dizziness. It should be avoided in any patient with a history of asthma or risk of bronchospasm.

Once a diagnosis of atrial flutter is established, a focused approach to address underlying precipitants should be implemented. AVN blockade with agents such as beta-blockers and calcium channel antagonists is beneficial provided that contraindications are explored. Digoxin works well in combination with other agents, especially in atypical flutter. If presentation has clear symptom onset within a 48-hour window, chemical cardioversion using amiodarone or electrical cardioversion can be considered. If flecainide is to be considered, patients need to be concurrently treated with AVN blockade. This is because flecainide retards atrial conduction velocity (i.e. reduced flutter rate) but does not significantly affect nodal conduction with subsequent risk of 1 : 1 propagation and ventricular fibrillation. Long-term risk of thromboembolism in patients with flutter is lower than AF as mechanical contractility of the atria is more organised. No formal risk stratification via the CHA_2DS_2-VASc criteria is recommended; however, most patients are considered for long-term anticoagulation in a similar manner. This is based on the premise that existence of flutter does result in enhanced embolic risk and, additionally, that approximately 50% of patients with flutter have alternating AF or will develop this during long-term follow-up. Likewise, similar precautions to management of AF are advocated in the context of acute and elective electrical cardioversion.

3.5.3.2 Catheter Ablation

In patients with recurrent, paroxysmal cases or with refractory symptoms, the preferential treatment of choice is radiofrequency ablation. This creates a line of electrically inert, bidirectional block at the CTI, i.e. between the tricuspid valve and the IVC or Eustachian ridge. Success rates are 95–100% with two-year recurrence < 15% [2]. If the critical component of the macro reentry pathway is distinct from this region, localisation requires use of electro-anatomical computerised mapping systems to allow targeted therapy. This may involve additional assessment of the LA via a trans-septal puncture. Success rates are comparable but recurrence rates are higher and patients may require adjunct AMDs or repeat ablation.

3.6 Atrioventricular Nodal Reentrant Tachycardia (AVNRT)

3.6.1 Mechanisms

Atrioventricular nodal reentrant tachycardia involves a congenital abnormality present in around 20% of the general population whereby the AVN is functionally dissociated into 'fast' and 'slow' pathways with differing electrophysiological properties, termed **dual AVN physiology**. The majority of cases are observed in females. The fibres of the right and left postero-inferior extensions that merge to form the compact AVN (see Chapter 1) are thought to be the substrate for the 'slow' pathway. The antero-superior 'fast' pathway is probably formed by transitional fibres connecting the interatrial septum with the compact AVN at the apex of Koch's triangle, which itself is bounded by the septal leaflet of the tricuspid valve, tendon of Todaro and coronary sinus (see Figure 3.4). The fast pathway is anatomically distinct from the slow pathway with a separation of around 15 mm.

The typical subtype of AVNRT utilises the slow pathway anterogradely and the fast pathway retrogradely (**slow-fast** – see Figure 3.5). Less commonly, the atypical **fast-slow** pathway occurs where there is a reversal. Most rarely, a **slow-slow** pathway may exist. It is unclear whether the upper segment required to complete the reentry loop and connect the two distinct pathways is atrial myocardium or true intranodal specialised tissue. The lower segment is usually the bundle of His but may occasionally be intranodal.

The typical reentry circuit is induced because the fast pathway has a higher conduction velocity but longer anterograde refractory period in comparison to the slow pathway. In NSR, impulses are conducted simultaneously down both pathways, but in view of varying propagation velocities, the impulse transmitted down the fast pathway is propagated to the ventricles but also the distal region of the slow pathway, enabling them to cancel out. A premature atrial complex (PAC) may arrive whilst the fast pathway is still refractory and, if this occurs, it will be preferentially conducted down the slow pathway. On reaching the lower segment, the impulse can return retrogradely if

Figure 3.4 Boundaries of Koch's triangle.

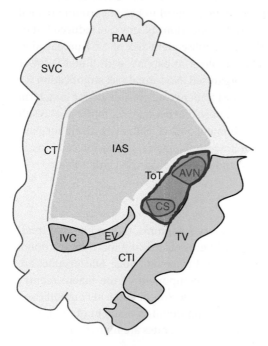

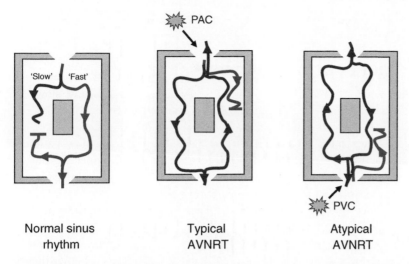

Figure 3.5   Reentry circuits implicated in typical (slow-fast) and atypical (fast-slow) AVNRT.

sufficient time has elapsed to allow recovery of the fast pathway so that it is no longer refractory. This initiates a circular reentry circuit whereby impulses continually cycle around the two pathways, activating the bundle of His anterogradely and the atria retrogradely. A similar principle exists for the atypical circuits implicated in fast-slow AVNRT, albeit precipitated by a premature ventricular complex (PVC).

3.6.2   Diagnosis

Approximately 70% of patients are females and this preponderance may be related to the presence of generally wider terminal portions of the coronary sinus. Symptoms of chest pain are possible. If present, dizziness and syncope often occur at the onset of tachycardia due to a drop in blood pressure or at termination when there is a compensatory pause. Patients have coincidental atrial and ventricular contraction and may therefore complain of neck pulsations. Assessment of the jugular venous pressure (JVP) may show the 'a+c' pattern with the presence of cannon waves. Nonetheless, ECG interpretation is often challenging (see Figure 3.6).

In the typical subtype, A : V ratio during AVNRT is usually 1 : 1. Retrograde P waves may not be visible, buried within the QRS complex or at the end ('pseudo-R' pattern). The PR interval is prolonged due to conduction along the slow pathway but with a shortened RP interval due to retrograde conduction along the fast pathway. In view of retrograde atrial activation, P waves are negative in the inferior leads. In the atypical subtype, the RP interval is prolonged and the PR interval is shortened. P waves may be visible between QRS and T waves. In slow-slow AVNRT, the P waves can appear before the QRS complex and thus mimic sinus tachycardia. Electrophysiological testing can be of benefit in formulating an accurate diagnosis. This is achieved primarily by establishing the presence of 'entrainment', which represents capture or resetting of the circuit via pacing-induced activation. Each pacing stimulus that is initiated creates an antegrade wavefront and increases the rate of the tachycardia. If there is an accessory pathway, this can conduct the wavefront retrogradely and result in collision with the orthodromic wavefront of the previous beat. These interactions create typical electrophysiological features that are indicative of a reentrant mechanism and provide the ability to localise anatomically.

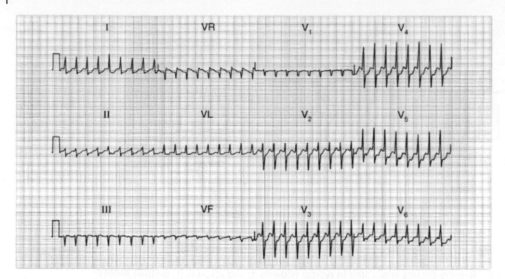

Figure 3.6   12-lead ECG indicative of AVNRT. There is evidence of a regular NCT at a rate of 220 bpm, with retrograde P waves probably buried within the QRS complex. Accompanying rate-related ischaemia is evident in the anterolateral leads.

3.6.3   Management

Paroxysmal AVNRT is nearly always terminated by transient AVN blockade using agents such as adenosine, beta-blockers, and verapamil. They function by inducing block in the anterograde slow pathway. Intravenous administration of class I anti-arrhythmics such as flecainide can also inter-rupt the reentry circuit by blocking the fast pathway. If symptoms are infrequent with clear onset, a 'pill in the pocket' approach using oral flecainide is appropriate and highly effective, although it is contraindicated in patients with significant coronary disease or left ventricular dysfunction [3]. Rate-limiting agents that interrupt the slow pathway are less effective at long-term maintenance. Rather, the definitive treatment of choice is catheter ablation of the slow pathway. The procedure has a 98% success rate with low risk of peri-procedural permanent AVN blockade in the region of < 0.5% [4]. Propensity for late pacemaker implantation is higher at around 1–2%, with similar inci-dence irrespective of ablation technique [5].

3.7   Atrioventricular Reentrant Tachycardia (AVRT)

3.7.1   Mechanisms

Atrioventricular reentrant tachycardias refer to circuit formation by the existence of a relatively fast-conducting aberrant accessory pathway (**bundle of Kent**). This connects atria and ventricles at sites where they should be electrically isolated. An accessory pathway typically arises from a con-genital defect in atrioventricular (AV) segmentation and development of the fibrous AV rings. Hence, they breach the insulation typically provided by fibrofatty deposition in the AV groove and fibrous annulus of the mitral and tricuspid valves. They are found most frequently in the left lateral regions (see Figure 3.7). Most of the pathways are constructed of functional myocardium with nor-mal gap junctions as opposed to histologically discrete cells. Impulse transmission initiated from the SAN is ordinarily via both the AVN–His axis and accessory pathway simultaneously, albeit with

Figure 3.7 Anatomical distribution of accessory pathways in AVRT. A, anterior; P, posterior; L, left; R, right.

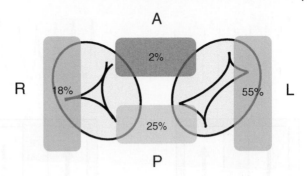

differing velocities and variable preference. This is in the context of patent pathways which conduct sequentially from atria to ventricles (A : V).

However, **concealed** pathways also exist and refer to the absence of pre-excitation on ECG in a patient with an existing accessory pathway. This may relate to weak antegrade conduction, sole retrograde conduction (i.e. V : A) or latent pathway which is anatomically distant from the SAN and AVN. A separate example of a latent pathway relates to permanent junctional reciprocating tachycardia (PJRT) (see Section 3.9.1). In addition, a rare and unique right-sided accessory pathway (Mahaim) has been identified that exhibits features of decremental conduction in close proximity to the right bundle branch and conducts only antegradely [6]. It should be emphasised, however, that most pathways have the ability to be bidirectional.

3.7.2 Categorisation

There are various ways to classify AVRT. It can be useful initially to distinguish orthodromic from antidromic AVRT, with 95% of cases being the former. In these instances, an atrial ectopic beat is propagated by the AVN–His axis in the usual anterograde fashion but there is subsequent retrograde conduction via the accessory pathway (see Figure 3.8). Alternatively, a ventricular ectopic beat is propagated retrogradely as most pathways can transmit bidirectionally. This results in a NCT. In rarer cases the accessory pathway is the anterograde limb with use of the AVN retrogradely. In view of this, there is early ventricular activation (termed **pre-excitation**) with faster conduction than via the normal AVN–His axis. However, the term describes the existence of anomalous conduction even if the velocity is no faster than usual. Because subsequent ventricular depolarisation is propagated directly via myocardial cells rather than the specialised conduction system, it will manifest as a tachycardia but with broader QRS duration. Hence, it becomes particularly challenging to distinguish this entity from ventricular tachycardia (VT) (see Chapter 4).

3.7.3 Factors Modifying Pre-excitation

The degree of ventricular pre-excitation in the context of antidromic AVRT is affected by several factors. First, the anatomical location of the accessory pathway plays an important part. The closer the accessory pathway is to the SAN or the site of atrial ectopy, the greater the degree of pre-excitation. Hence, pathways originating from the right free wall conventionally present with a shortened PR interval and wide pre-excited QRS complexes whereas left free-wall pathways mimic normal electrophysiology more closely. Invasive pacing at a region in close proximity to the pathway may enable clearer manifestation of pre-excitation. If there is existence of atrial fibrosis or enlargement, pre-excitation may not be evident in those with a left free wall pathway due to the

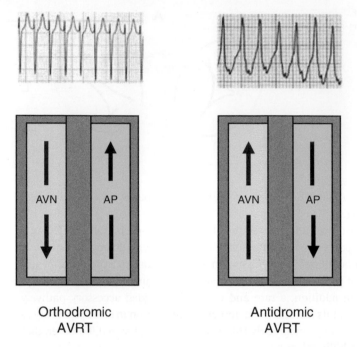

Orthodromic
AVRT

Antidromic
AVRT

Figure 3.8 Mechanisms implicated in orthodromic and antidromic AVRT.

prolonged duration of impulse propagation. Intrinsic properties of the pathway itself, namely conduction velocity and length, can affect conduction times over the pathway. For instance, there is co-association of AVRT with Ebstein anomaly where the septal and posterior leaflets of the tricuspid valve are displaced towards the right ventricular apex. In this situation multiple accessory pathways can occur and may be longer despite propagating at higher velocity. Lastly, pre-excitation is determined by relative conduction of the normal AVN–His axis so manifestation of pre-excitation would be enhanced if there is concurrent AVN blockade.

3.7.4 Diagnosis

Atrioventricular reentrant tachycardia can be described as WPW syndrome, but only if there are concurrent symptoms such as palpitations. In addition to Ebstein anomaly, there is an association with other congenital disorders such as HCM, coronary sinus diverticulum and tuberous sclerosis. However, no strong hereditary predisposition exists.

Presence of the accessory pathway may be confirmed by incidental findings on 12-lead ECG of an asymptomatic patient (see Figure 3.9). In this case, it would demonstrate a shortened PR interval, wider QRS complex and slurring of the initial segment caused by early ventricular depolarisation (**delta wave** - see Figure 3.10), which is classically associated with antidromic AVRT. Clinical presentation in the acute phase is similar to other NCTs with palpitations, breathlessness and chest pain all possible. ECG on admission will show a NCT but it can be challenging to discriminate AVRT from other differential diagnoses. Rate is usually in the region of 140–240 bpm and characteristically associated with a shortened RP interval.

Once the patient has reverted into NSR, either spontaneously or with therapy, the subsequent ECG and polarity of the delta wave, if present, can indicate anatomical location of the accessory

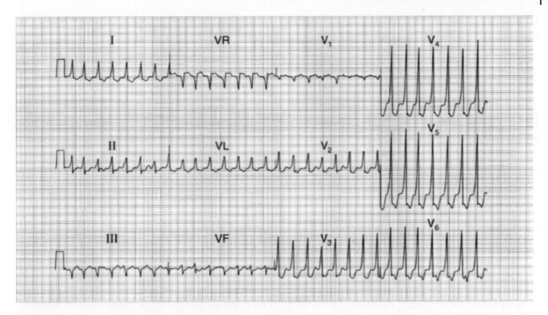

Figure 3.9 12-lead ECG indicative of antidromic AVRT. There is evidence of a regular NCT at a rate of 200 bpm, with slurred upstroke of the QRS complex and broader duration. This is indicative of antidromic AVRT with a likely septal origin (negative deflection in V1).

Figure 3.10 Sinus beat showing classic delta wave suggestive of accessory pathway.

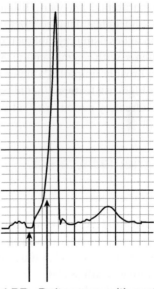

Shortened PR interval   Delta wave with prolonged QRS interval

pathway as per the Arruda localisation method [7]. If the delta wave is predominantly positive in V1, it usually originates from the left free wall. If it is negative or isoelectric in V1, the pathway is typically septal. Pathways originating from the coronary sinus or middle cardiac vein produce negative deflections in lead II. Left free-wall pathways result in predominantly negative or isoelectric complexes in lead I. As with AVNRT, triggering of entrainment via electrophysiological testing is also helpful to confirm the existence of a reentry circuit.

3.7.5 Management

For an acute episode, treatment is consistent with that of other NCTs and involves transient AVN blockade using vagal manoeuvres and/or adenosine. If there is an established history of AVRT, intravenous flecainide may be preferred. In the presence of adverse features, synchronised electrical cardioversion is warranted without the need for preceding anticoagulation. Sudden death is exceptionally rare but when it does occur, it usually relates to the coexistence of AF with 1 : 1 antegrade conduction along the accessory pathway, resulting in pre-excitation and ventricular fibrillation. In these patients, conventional AVN blockade is of direct detriment by enhancing propagation along the accessory pathway.

If symptoms are infrequent or have a clear onset, pill-in-the-pocket use of flecainide as with AVNRT is entirely appropriate on the assumption that ventricular dysfunction and significant coronary disease have been excluded. The definitive treatment option for patients with AVRT is catheter ablation. Nonetheless, flecainide, amiodarone or sotalol can be utilised as interim options if symptoms are frequent, intrusive or unlikely to respond to simple vagal manoeuvres. Success rates for ablation are > 98% with minimal morbidity and mortality [4]. Left-sided accessory pathways are usually ablated using a trans-septal approach with retrograde aortic access uncommon. By contrast, right-sided pathways require access via the venous system and are associated with slightly higher rates of recurrence due to unstable catheter position at the tricuspid annulus. Superior paraseptal and peri-Hisian accessory pathway ablation can result in iatrogenic AVN blockade and hence detailed electrode mapping pre-intervention is of paramount importance, with approaches using cryoablation or via the non-coronary cusp often preferred.

In patients with asymptomatic AVRT, risk stratification with invasive electrophysiological testing is broadly helpful. Catheter ablation is recommended when use of isoprenaline testing identifies high-risk features, including the presence of multiple pathways and/or accessory pathway effective refractory period (ERP) of ≤250 ms [8].

3.8 Atrial Tachycardia

3.8.1 Mechanisms

Atrial tachycardia (AT) is relatively rare, constituting 5–15% of all NCT. It occurs more commonly in children and adults with congenital heart disease and does not require the AVN or accessory pathways for initiation and maintenance. It is also not associated with increased risk of syncope or sudden cardiac death (SCD).

It may be predominantly focal or macro reentrant in origin (see Figure 3.11). In the former, there is clear exit of the atrial activation wavefront from which the remainder of the atrial myocardium depolarises and occurs primarily due to enhanced automaticity. There may be single or multiple sites of origin, the latter defined as **multifocal atrial tachycardia (MAT)** and strongly associated with chronic lung disease (60% of cases). Most foci originate from the RA, at sites along the crista terminalis, the tricuspid annulus or at veno-atrial junctions. Reentrant circuits may arise from regions of scar such as after corrective surgery for atrial septal defects (ASDs). **Sinus node reciprocating tachycardia (SNRT)** refers to a separate entity of lower incidence in

Figure 3.11 Subtypes of atrial tachycardia (AT).

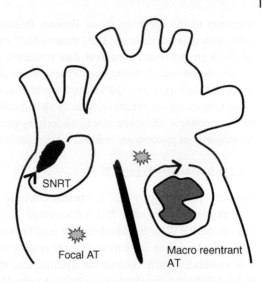

which AT arises from micro reentry and where breakthrough occurs at the crista terminalis in close anatomical proximity to normal SAN impulses.

3.8.2 Diagnosis

The main symptoms are those of paroxysmal palpitations and anxiety with sudden onset and off-set. Rarely, there may be associated dizziness, syncope or features of congestion if the tachycardia is incessant. 12-lead ECG will resemble NSR but with the exception of SNRT, P wave morphology is likely to differ due to site of origin being distinct from the SAN. Localisation of the responsible site for focal ATs can be determined by application of a revised P wave morphology algorithm [9]. In ATs that have an underlying macro reentrant mechanism, P waves similar to those observed in isthmus-dependent atrial flutter may be seen. RP interval is usually prolonged.

3.8.3 Management

In the acute phase, transient AVN blockade should be attempted. Adenosine can terminate around 10% of focal AT but not macro reentrant forms. Rate-limiting agents may be effective alone in controlling the tachycardia. However, macro reentrant AT is often refractory to traditional anti-arrhythmics such as amiodarone and flecainide. Electrical cardioversion is appropriate if it is incessant or associated with adverse features. However, definitive treatment of choice for symptomatic, intrusive AT is catheter ablation. Success rates are lower than for AVNRT/AVRT and lie in the range of 60–70%; however, use of three-dimensional electro-anatomical mapping has improved this to around 95% in experienced hands.

3.9 Junctional Tachycardia

3.9.1 Permanent Junctional Reciprocating Tachycardia (PJRT)

PJRT occurs predominantly in children. It arises from a reentry circuit using the AVN as the antero-grade limb. A slowly conducting accessory pathway that demonstrates decremental conduction is the retrograde limb, most commonly located in a right posteroseptal location with atrial insertion in proximity to the coronary sinus. Patients frequently have a long history of recurrent palpitations induced by exertion or stress. ECG shows a NCT with P waves that are negative inferiorly and RP interval that is greater than PR interval. Rate is variable as it depends upon autonomic tone, and indeed may be entirely obliterated during sleep. Frequent, spontaneous terminations may be observed that manifest on ECG monitoring as a QRS complex which is not preceded by a P wave. Vagal manoeuvres may cause temporary termination, usually by inducing retrograde block. No acute treatment is needed for these cohorts. However, due to underlying propensity for progression into tachycardiomyopathy, the majority of patients are referred for consideration of ablation regardless of symptom burden.

3.9.2 Junctional Ectopic Tachycardia (JET)

The pathophysiology of JET is unclear but burden is enhanced after cardiac surgery for disorders such as tetralogy of Fallot. If it is discovered during the first six months of life, it can be considered as a congenital disorder. Mechanisms may be related to automaticity or triggered activity, with true anatomical location from or in close proximity to the conduction system of the AVN. Nonetheless, it is associated with ventricular dysfunction, significant morbidity and carries poor prognosis. 12-lead ECG classically shows a NCT at rates of 140–300 bpm with A:V dissociation. Retrograde P waves may be observed in the terminal portions of the QRS complex (i.e. shortened RP interval). Adenosine is often effective at termination, suggesting triggered activity as the mechanism. Spontaneous resolution has been observed in young cohorts and there are reports of successful ablation in these patients whilst preserving AVN electrophysiology.

3.9.3 Non-Paroxysmal Junctional Tachycardia (NPJT)

This is a rhythm originating at the level of the AVN or bundle of His and usually observed in the context of right coronary artery ischaemia or digoxin toxicity. Indeed, short runs of this rhythm may also be observed peri-procedurally during AVNRT ablation. Enhanced automaticity of the AVN is the likely mechanism and thus 'focal junctional tachycardia' may be a more accurate description. ECG conventionally shows a NCT at rates of 70–140 bpm, unless there is pre-existent bundle branch block. The RP relationship is unpredictable. If there is retrograde block and secondary A:V dissociation, capture beats may be apparent. NPJT is usually asymptomatic and does not require specific treatment, although underlying conditions should be addressed.

Hot Points

- Narrow complex tachycardia describe rhythms that exceed 100 bpm and are of normal QRS duration.
- They may be subcategorised based upon RR regularity or RP interval (in comparison to PR interval). The most common subtype is sinus tachycardia.
- Atrial flutter usually arises from a counter-clockwise macro reentrant circuit in the right atrium.
- AVNRT results from dual AVN physiology with functional dissociation into 'slow' and 'fast' pathways.
- AVRT arises from the presence of a relatively fast-conducting accessory pathway (bundle of Kent) that is anatomically distinct from the AVN.
- Atrial tachycardias may be focal (single site or multifocal [MAT]), macro reentrant or micro reentrant (SNRT) in origin.
- Intravenous adenosine is helpful in most instances for diagnosis and/or dysrhythmia termination.

3.10   Self-assessment Questions

1   With regard to AVNRT, which of the following statements is false?
   A Up to 20% of the general population have dual AVN physiology.
   B In typical AVNRT, anterograde limb of conduction is via the slow pathway.
   C It is twice as common in females.
   D Ablation in AVNRT carries 2–3% risk of AV block requiring pacemaker implantation.
   E Symptomatic neck pulsation is highly suggestive of AVNRT.

2   With regard to typical counter-clockwise atrial flutter, which of the following statements is false?
   A It usually occurs due to a counter-clockwise macro reentrant circuit.
   B Flecainide monotherapy can be considered in patients with structurally normal hearts.
   C It causes negative P waves in the inferior ECG limb leads.
   D Catheter ablation carries success rate of > 90%.
   E Up to 50% of patients with atrial flutter will have coexistent atrial fibrillation.

3   With regard to atrial tachycardia, which of the following statements is true?
   A Focal atrial tachycardias are often sensitive to adenosine.
   B Anti-arrhythmic drugs are generally ineffective.
   C Atrial tachycardias usually cause short RP tachycardia with 1 : 1 AV conduction.
   D Catheter ablation of multifocal atrial tachycardia is considered first-line therapy.
   E Multifocal atrial tachycardias are rare in patients with chronic lung disease.

4   With regard to AVRT, which of the following statements is false?
   A Up to 10% of AVRTs are antidromic.
   B 50% of AVRTs originate from the left free wall.
   C Left-sided pathways result in greater degree of manifest pre-excitation on surface ECG.
   D Radiofrequency ablation of the accessory pathway should be considered first-line in symptomatic patients with AVRT.
   E AV nodal blocking agents should be avoided in pre-excited AF.

5   In which of the following circumstances would use of adenosine be most clinically appropriate?
   A 23-year-old male with palpitations and regular broad complex tachycardia.
   B 41-year-old female with asthma presenting with regular narrow complex tachycardia.
   C 50-year-old female with light-headedness and irregular broad complex tachycardia.
   D 82-year-old male with a history of myocardial infarction presenting with regular narrow complex tachycardia.
   E 31-year-old male presenting with breathlessness and irregular narrow complex tachycardia.

References

1 Marrouche, N.F., Beheiry, S., Tomassoni, G. et al. (2002). Three-dimensional nonfluoroscopic mapping and ablation of inappropriate sinus tachycardia. Procedural strategies and long-term outcome. *J. Am. Coll. Cardiol.* 39 (6): 1046–1054.

2 Marrouche, N.F., Schweikert, R., Saliba, W. et al. (2003). Use of different catheter ablation technologies for treatment of typical atrial flutter: acute results and long-term follow-up. *Pacing Clin. Electrophysiol.* 26 (3): 743–746.

3 Neuss, H. and Schlepper, M. (1988). Long-term efficacy and safety of flecainide for supraventricular tachycardia. *Am. J. Cardiol.* 62 (6): 56D–61D.

4 Morady, F. (2004). Catheter ablation of supraventricular arrhythmias: state of the art. *Pacing Clin. Electrophysiol.* 27 (1): 125–142.

5 Kesek, M., Lindmark, D., Rashid, A., and Jensen, S.M. (2019). Increased risk of late pacemaker implantation after ablation for atrioventricular nodal reentry tachycardia: a 10-year follow-up of a nationwide cohort. *Heart Rhythm* 16 (8): 1182–1188.

6 Ozcan, E.E., Turan, O.E., Akdemir, B. et al. (2021). Comparison of electrophysiological characteristics of right- and left-sided Mahaim-type accessory pathways. *J. Cardiovasc. Electrophysiol.* 32 (2): 360–369.

7 Arruda, M.S., McClelland, J.H., Wang, X. et al. (1998). Development and validation of an ECG algorithm for identifying accessory pathway ablation site in Wolff-Parkinson-White syndrome. *J. Cardiovasc. Electrophysiol.* 9 (1): 2–12.

8 Santinelli, V., Radinovic, A., Manguso, F. et al. (2009). The natural history of asymptomatic ventricular pre-excitation a long-term prospective follow-up study of 184 asymptomatic children. *J. Am. Coll. Cardiol.* 53 (3): 275–280.

9 Kistler, P.M., Chieng, D., Tonchev, I.R. et al. (2021). P-wave morphology in focal atrial tachycardia: an updated algorithm to predict site of origin. *JACC Clin. Electrophysiol.* 7 (12): 1547–1556.

Further Reading

Arruda, M.S., McClelland, J.H., Wang, X. et al. (1998). Development and validation of an ECG algorithm for identifying accessory pathway ablation site in Wolff-Parkinson-White syndrome. *J. Cardiovasc. Electrophysiol.* 9 (1): 2–12.

Brugada, J., Katritsis, D.G., Arbelo, E. et al. (2020). 2019 ESC guidelines for the management of patients with supraventricular tachycardia. The Task Force for the management of patients with supraventricular tachycardia of the European Society of Cardiology (ESC) (published correction appears in Eur. Heart J. 2020 Nov 21;41(44):4258). *Eur. Heart J.* 41 (5): 655–720.

Olshansky, B. and Sullivan, R.M. (2019). Inappropriate sinus tachycardia. *Europace* 21 (2): 194–207.

4

Broad Complex Tachycardias

4.1 Learning Objectives

- Key definitions and nomenclature.
- Categorisation.
- Pathophysiological mechanisms.
- Diagnostic indicators.
- Acute and chronic management options.
- Ventricular tachycardia in the context of specific clinical disorders, such as ischaemic heart disease, hypertrophic cardiomyopathy and arrhythmogenic right ventricular cardiomyopathy.

Cardiology at its Core, First Edition. Peysh A. Patel.
© 2023 John Wiley & Sons Ltd. Published 2023 by John Wiley & Sons Ltd.

4.2 Nomenclature

Broad complex tachycardias (BCTs) refer to heart rhythms that exceed 100 beats min^{-1} (bpm) and are of widened QRS duration (i.e. > 120 ms).

A **premature ventricular complex** (PVC) is characterised by early occurrence of a broad QRS complex, usually but not always exceeding 120 ms, and of a different morphology to the normal rhythm. The T wave is often similarly abnormal and usually larger than the normal wave. It is not preceded by a P wave as the impulse originates from the ventricles rather than the sinoatrial node (SAN). However, a P wave may be present as one that is either non-conducted from the atria or retrogradely conducted to the atria. If the PVC results in premature resetting of the sinus node, a subsequent pause may occur which is not fully compensatory. More frequently, there is non-propagation due to collision between the antegrade impulse from the SAN and the retrograde impulse from the PVC, resulting in a fully compensatory pause so that the timing of the basic rhythm is unperturbed. Initial investigation constitutes assessment of electrolytes, particularly potassium, calcium and magnesium, in addition to thyroid function. PVCs are not usually of prognostic relevance as they do not correlate well with progression to nonsustained ventricular tachycardia (NSVT) or ventricular tachycardia (VT). General lifestyle advice includes regulation of coffee, tea, and alcohol intake. It is also prudent to exclude a history of recreational drug use and to arrange echocardiography so that structural heart disease can be excluded. If this is confirmed and the patient is asymptomatic, PVCs are not actively treated. If troublesome symptoms occur, however, treatment with beta-blockers or calcium channel antagonists can be considered. Even in the presence of structural disease, such as that relating to infarction, treatment is often directed by occurrence of intrusive symptoms. Reassurance or rate-limiting therapy is often all that is required but adjunct therapy with arrhythmia-modifying drugs (AMD) or ablation may be considered in refractory presentations or where there is treatment intolerance.

Bigeminy refers to a repetitive pattern of sinus beat followed by a PVC. If the PVC occurs every third beat, it is termed **trigeminy**. Two PVCs in succession equals a **couplet** and three in succession is a **triplet**. If there are between four and seven PVCs in a row, this is termed a **salvo**. When there is prolonged period of ectopy with spontaneous resolution within 30 s, it is defined as **NSVT**. Conventionally, a compensatory pause occurs post-termination. If the dysrhythmia is prolonged beyond this duration, it is classically termed **ventricular tachycardia** (VT). Nomenclature extends beyond temporal characteristics and can also be based upon QRS morphology. In this case, it may broadly be subdivided as monomorphic (one focus) or polymorphic (multiple foci).

4.3 Categorisation

It is helpful to categorise BCT according to the presence or absence of rhythm regularity. An overview of the most common subtypes is provided in Figure 4.1. Regardless, any BCT should be treated as VT if there is any doubt about the underlying rhythm. A previous ECG aids in comparing morphology as mimics include narrow complex tachycardia (NCT) with aberrancy and antidromic Wolff–Parkinson–White (WPW) (see Section 4.7.4).

NCT with aberrancy is defined as abnormal intraventricular conduction of a supraventricular impulse. It occurs because of the unequal refractoriness of the bundle branches (right bundle branch [RBB] > left bundle branch [LBB]) and critical prematurity of a supraventricular impulse.

Figure 4.1 Categorisation of BCTs.

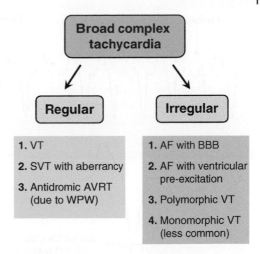

At higher rates, the impulse encounters one bundle branch that is responsive whilst the other is refractory. Thus, conduction occurs with a bundle branch block (BBB) pattern. Onset of the tachycardia with a premature P wave is indicative of a supraventricular origin. Additionally, patients may have established BBB at baseline with subsequent occurrence of SVT conducted with a pre-existent BBB. Therefore, previous ECGs are extremely beneficial to enable direct comparison.

The remainder of this chapter will explore subtypes of VT.

4.4 Mechanisms of VT

Ventricular tachycardia arises distal to the bifurcation of the His bundle, either in the specialised conduction system or in the ventricular myocardium. Broadly speaking, it may be initiated by triggered activity, i.e. early after-depolarisation (EAD) or delayed after-depolarisation (DAD) (see Chapter 2), or via reentry circuits. The latter is predominantly associated with scar tissue in the setting of structural disease such as prior myocardial infarction. A reentrant circuit is formed in relation to a region of scar where there is recurrent depolarisation and repolarisation. The **'excitable gap'** is the area of repolarised tissue that has not yet begun to depolarise, and if this region is depolarised iatrogenically such as via anti-tachycardia pacing (ATP) in the context of an implantable defibrillator VT can be terminated.

4.5 Diagnosis of VT

As accentuated, any patient with a BCT should be assumed to have VT unless an alternative diagnosis is strongly suggested. Perhaps most importantly, a history of IHD is the strongest indicator with a 95% positive predictive value (PPV). ECG interpretation can be challenging but there are certain features that favour a diagnosis of VT (see Figure 4.2).

Firstly, **A:V dissociation** may be detectable. In other words, there is evidence of atrial activity (P waves) but this is independent of ventricular activity. This is a strong indicator of VT; however, in around 25% of patients, the atria may be depolarised by the ventricles retrogradely (i.e. V:A association). VT is more likely to result in **QRS concordance** in the chest leads (V1–V6), with all being predominantly positive or negative deflections. Moreover, the presence of capture and fusion beats

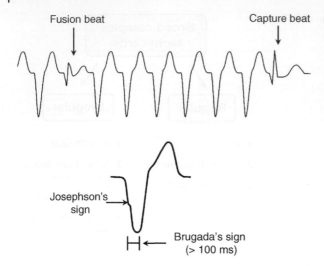

Figure 4.2 ECG characteristics indicative of VT.

are indicative of VT albeit visualised less frequently. **Capture beats** represent intermittent presence of a normal sinus beat originating from the SAN and propagating via the normal conduction system. A **fusion beat**, as the name suggests, is a result of the collision of waveforms from a sinus beat conducting via the atrioventricular node (AVN) with the waveform originating from the ventricle, resulting in a complex that is a hybrid (fusion) of sinus and VT morphology. **Josephson's sign** reflects the presence of notching near the nadir of the S wave. **Brugada's sign** refers to a distance from QRS complex onset to the nadir of the S wave that is > 100 ms. Although not routinely considered, termination of the tachycardia with vagal manoeuvres is indicative of SVT with aberrancy. A notable exception, however, is VT originating from the right ventricular outflow tract (RVOT). Lastly, VT is often associated with **extreme axis deviation** (positive QRS in aVR and negative in I/aVF), absence of typical LBBB or RBBB morphology, and presence of **RSR′ complexes** that contrast morphologically with conventional RBBB.

12-lead ECG during VT helps to identify the potential site of origin (see Figure 4.3). RBBB-like morphology suggests left-sided exit, whereas LBBB-like morphology indicates right-sided exit. If there is negative concordance in the chest leads, this is typical of VT from an apical origin. Positive concordance implies exit near the base of the ventricle, although this appearance can also occur in the context of SVT with aberrancy. A superiorly directed QRS axis (i.e. LAD) suggests inferior origin and an inferiorly directed axis (i.e. RAD) indicates superior exit as seen in VT originating from the outflow tract. VT that arises from one of the fascicles (usually posterior; see Section 4.8.2) is often of relatively narrow QRS duration.

4.6 Management of VT

4.6.1 Acute Therapy

Acute management should be in accordance with standard resuscitation guidelines for BCT using an ABCDE approach. If pulseless VT is present (i.e. electromechanical dissociation) or ventricular fibrillation (VF), urgent electrical cardioversion is indicated. In the context of pulsed VT, the presence of adverse features (chest pain due to myocardial ischaemia, pulmonary congestion, dizziness/syncope and/or hypotension) advocates a comparable approach. If there is pulsed VT without

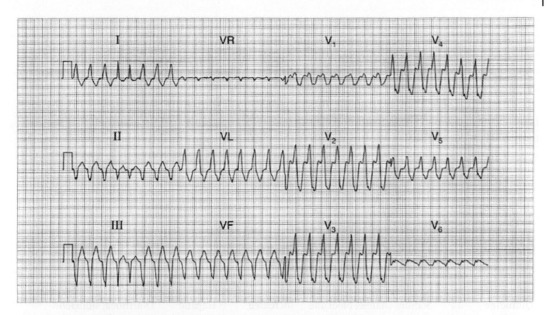

Figure 4.3 12-lead ECG indicative of VT. There is evidence of a regular BCT at a rate of 200 bpm, with capture beats (most apparent in lead I). There is positive QRS in leads I/aVL, negative QRS in II/III/aVF with early transition in V2. This is suggestive of a left inferoseptal origin.

haemodynamic compromise, it is prudent to consider potential precipitants. For this reason, urgent biochemical profiling including electrolytes and thyroid function should be performed. A careful review of the medical history is essential with specific exploration of cardiac morbidity. If available, a previous ECG is invaluable to differentiate patients with baseline aberrancy, as this aids distinction between VT and NCT with aberrancy.

Active termination of VT is commonly achieved using intravenous amiodarone. A 300 mg loading dose can be administered via a large peripheral cannula in an emergency situation, but subsequent maintenance regimen (900 mg over 23 hours) must be instituted via a central or femoral line to minimise risk of extravasation and severe tissue damage. Moreover, hypotension can be precipitated by intravenous therapy though infrequent in clinical practice and correlates more strongly with infusion rate. If there is refractory or recurrent VT, a repeat loading dose can be administered as up to 10 g may be required to achieve therapeutic levels. Adjunct options include intravenous procainamide or lidocaine with class I anti-arrhythmic properties, particularly in the context of structural heart disease. Electrical cardioversion in a more controlled manner under sedation with anaesthetist support may be warranted.

Other options include overdrive pacing, via a previously implanted cardiac device or temporary transvenous pacemaker, if the rate is below the upper threshold of device ATP. However, this is associated with inherent risk of accelerating VT into ventricular flutter or fibrillation. In the context of 'VT storm' with a monomorphic focus, referral to a specialist electrophysiology (EP) centre may be required to explore candidacy for ablation.

4.6.2 Long-term Therapy

This is directed at reducing recurrence and preventing progression to adverse sequelae, particularly sudden cardiac death (SCD). Beta-blockers are efficacious and reasonably well tolerated in the majority of cohorts. AMDs such as amiodarone or sotalol can also be considered. In refractory cases, adjunct therapy may need to be explored. However, nearly all AMDs defined by the Vaughan Williams classification require specific monitoring and can be associated with adverse events (see Table 4.1). Definitive therapy is in the form of implantable cardioverter-defibrillator (ICD), which can detect and terminate ventricular arrhythmias through anti-tachycardia pacing (ATP) or cardioversion with electrical shocks.

ATP occurs through bursts or ramps, or a combination of the two. It can be highly effective and is thought to restore rhythm in around 75% of cases [1]. If a reentry circuit is initiated in the context of VT, a depolarisation wavefront leaves the circuit and spreads through myocardium to be sensed by the implanted ICD lead. If a subsequent pacing pulse is synchronised to the sensed

Table 4.1 Overview of oral AMDs used for VT.

	Class	Mechanism of action	Effect on action potential duration	Metabolism	Side-effects
Quinidine	1a	Sodium channel blockade (moderate) resulting in phase 0 AP prolongation (reduced influx)	Increased	Hepatic and renal	Diarrhoea, stomach cramps, fever, tinnitus, rash, QTc prolongation
Mexiletine	1b	Sodium channel blockade (weak) resulting in phase 0 AP prolongation (reduced influx)	Decreased	Hepatic	Nausea, stomach cramps, blurred vision, tremor, ataxia
Propafenone	1c	Sodium channel blockade (strong) resulting in phase 0 AP prolongation (reduced influx)	No effect	Hepatic	Constipation, dizziness, headache, PR/QRS prolongation
Flecainide	1c	Sodium channel blockade (strong) resulting in phase 0 AP prolongation (reduced influx)	No effect	Hepatic and renal	Arrhythmias, acute pulmonary oedema (negatively inotropic), central nervous system effects, QRS prolongation
Bisoprolol	II	β_1 adrenoceptor antagonist resulting in deceleration of phase 4	Decreased	Hepatic and renal	Bradycardia, hypotension, bronchospasm, hypoglycaemia, fatigue
Amiodarone	III	Potassium channel blockade resulting in phase 3 AP prolongation (reduced efflux)	Increased	Hepatic	Hypotension, thrombophlebitis, thyroid dysfunction, pulmonary fibrosis, photosensitivity, interaction with warfarin
Sotalol	III	Potassium channel blockade resulting in phase 3 AP prolongation (reduced efflux), suppresses spontaneous depolarisation during phase 4, non-selective (β_1 and β_2) adrenoceptor antagonist	Increased	Renal	QTc prolongation, hypotension, fatigue

wavefront and delivered at a rate faster than the tachycardia, it stimulates the tissue in the region of the lead tip before the reentry waveform arrives. The depolarisation wavefront initiated by the lead spreads towards the approaching wavefront from the reentry circuit. These collide and the rate of depolarisation and repolarisation of the tissue between the lead and colliding wavefronts is reset. As further ATP is administered, wavefronts collide closer to the site of the reentry circuit. With correct timing and number, the tissue in the excitable gap is depolarised and blocks the reentry circuit, resulting in termination of the dysrhythmia.

In the context of secondary prevention where patients have survived VT with haemodynamic compromise or subsequent cardiac arrest, ICD is the definitive treatment of choice. It demonstrates a mortality reduction compared to conventional AMDs, and one that is maintained across all conventional subgroups [2]. In those that have an absolute contraindication or refuse device therapy, empirical amiodarone should be considered although evidence for mortality benefit is lacking [3]. A small cohort of patients with ICD in situ have incessant episodes of VT and recurrent shocks despite conventional pharmacotherapy with beta-blockers and/or AMDs, usually amiodarone. AMD treatment can result in significant side effects and, if either not tolerated or desired, catheter ablation is superior to escalated therapy in those already on amiodarone to reduce ICD therapies and associated morbidity [4]. In specific resistant cases, referral to a cardiothoracic unit for consideration of endocardial resection of substrate, such as scarred tissue from previous infarction or left ventricular aneurysm, may be considered.

ICD therapy has an additional role in primary prevention when considered in the context of congestive heart failure (Chapter 12). Historical trial data demonstrated that in patients with previous myocardial infarction (MI), severe left ventricular dysfunction (LVSD) and NSVT or inducible VT on EP testing, ICD therapy leads to improved survival compared with conventional medications [5]. In modern practice, the presence of NSVT and use of EP testing to screen for VT inducibility is rarely used for risk stratification. However, in patients with severe LVSD due to IHD without inducible VT, primary prevention ICD appears to confer mortality benefit that is entirely attributable to reductions in SCD [6]. They also have a present role in those with non-ischaemic cardiomyopathy and use is supported by current guidelines. This is subject to ongoing debate, however, and it is possible that tools will emerge to better identify cohorts most likely to derive benefit (see Section 12.7.12.1).

4.7 Structural Diseases

4.7.1 Ischaemia vs Infarction

If VT occurs in the context of IHD, it is imperative to distinguish ischaemia from infarction. These two entities differ with regard to underlying pathophysiology and management strategies are therefore discordant. In the setting of an acute event such as ST-elevation myocardial infarction (STEMI), VT can occur secondary to ischaemia in a region of myocardium supplied by the implicated coronary vessel. This typically presents within the first 48 hours of commencement of chest pain and, if present, is usually **polymorphic**, transient and self-limiting. If it is not associated with haemodynamic compromise, no further treatment is warranted and reperfusion of the occluded vessel remains the priority. Conventional beta-blocker therapy, incorporated as part of secondary prevention post-event, will further reduce propensity.

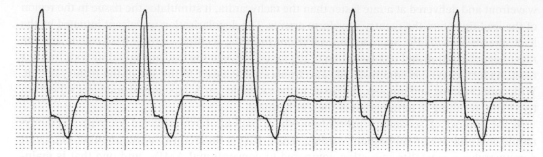

Figure 4.4 ECG strip showing accelerated idioventricular rhythm.

Indeed, the incidence of VT in the context of acute ischaemia has reduced significantly in the past decade, probably attributable to prompt revascularisation strategies and early utilisation of beta-blocker therapy.

Accelerated idioventricular rhythm is a specific type of disturbance that occurs due to enhanced automaticity in the context of acute MI, commonly during reperfusion, or in the presence of digoxin toxicity. It is characterised by a broad QRS rhythm with ventricular rates commonly between 60 and 110 bpm (see Figure 4.4). It can be regular or irregular and episodes are usually of intermittent duration, lasting a few seconds to a minute. As the rate of the ventricular rhythm closely resembles that of NSR, there is fluctuating control between these two sites for impulse initiation. As a result, fusion beats often occur at onset and termination. The rhythm is gradual in commencement and ensues when rate is greater than the sinus rate, often precipitated by autonomic modulation of the SAN or AVN. It tends to terminate spontaneously and no active intervention is usually needed as it rarely progresses. It is therefore of no prognostic value. If treatment is indicated because of symptoms or adverse sequelae, increasing heart rate via atropine or atrial pacing, for example, is often sufficient.

In patients with established infarction, the mechanism of VT relates to reentry circuit formation around and/or through a region of scar tissue. Because of this, VT related to reentrant circuit formation is **monomorphic**. Rarely, the morphology of individual complexes may exhibit subtle variability because of slightly different exit sites from the same circuit but this is the exception. In these contexts, ICD insertion is often indicated in the presence of severe LV dysfunction (as outlined earlier). In those with preserved function without haemodynamically significant VT, however, ICD implantation is often unhelpful.

4.7.2 Hypertrophic Cardiomyopathy (HCM)

Hypertrophic cardiomyopathy is a myocardial disorder of autosomal dominant inheritance. It is associated with mutations in genes encoding for cardiac sarcomeres although variations in phenotypic manifestations are substantial. Patients with HCM frequently develop problems with ventricular arrhythmias, and indeed, it is an important mode of SCD. Beyond monitoring and lifestyle measures, symptomatic individuals or those with severe disease are considered for beta-blocker or non-dihydropyridine calcium-channel blocker therapy. Although of benefit in suppressing disease progression, they do not appear to reduce pro-arrhythmic potential. By contrast, amiodarone has demonstrable efficacy although data is limited. Alcohol ablation of the septum and/or surgical myomectomy is a treatment option for patients with HCM and concurrent outflow tract obstruction, but may potentially enhance tendency for dysrhythmia. Due to the association between ventricular arrhythmias and SCD in those with HCM, ICD therapy can be considered. Risk stratification is performed with use of a validated risk model and prophylactic ICD implantation ought to be considered in the context of a five-year risk of SCD $\geq 4\%$. A more detailed exploration of this condition is provided in Chapter 14.

4.7.3 Arrhythmogenic Right Ventricular Cardiomyopathy (ARVC)

Arrhythmogenic right ventricular cardiomyopathy (ARVC) is a disorder that has a familial component, with genetic abnormalities in desmosomal proteins (involved in cell–cell junctions) and cardiac ryanodine receptors (RyR2) implicated. Pathophysiology relates to fatty or fibrofatty infiltration mediated by patchy myocarditis that preferentially occurs in the inflow/outflow tract and apex. It is a cause of SCD in athletes. Diagnosis is challenging as patients are predominantly asymptomatic and right-sided heart failure rarely manifests. Moreover, transient episodes of dysrhythmia may be well tolerated due to usual preservation of LV function.

In patients with ARVC, 'epsilon waves' may be apparent in precordial leads V1 and V2, and are visualised as terminal notches at the end of the QRS complex as a result of delayed activation through scarring in the right ventricle (see Figure 14.7). There may be evidence of incomplete or complete RBBB. If VT occurs, this tachycardia will typically arise from the right ventricle where the arrhythmogenic substrate is located. As a result, ECGs of ARVC-related VT often show a LBBB pattern. The first indication of potential underlying disease may relate to incidental echocardiographic findings of isolated RV aneurysms or enlargement without concurrent rise in pulmonary artery pressures. LV involvement can also occur. Detailed imaging using cardiac magnetic resonance imaging (MRI) aids in providing clarity on anatomy and function.

Management relies on ICD implantation either in those who have survived a cardiac arrest due to ventricular arrhythmia or as primary prevention in those deemed high-risk. There is no formal criteria for risk stratification although unexplained syncope, NSVT and ventricular dysfunction are considered predictors of poor outcome. Catheter ablation can be extremely useful in refractory cases but often requires percutaneous epicardial access to target the source of scar. A more detailed exploration of this condition is provided in Chapter 14.

4.7.4 Accessory Pathways

The classic form of AVRT relating to WPW (~95% of cases) is the orthodromic type where a reentry circuit is formed with impulses propagating down the AVN and retrogradely to the atria via the accessory pathway. However, as outlined in Chapter 3, antidromic AVRT can also occur. In this situation, antegrade impulse propagation is via the accessory pathway directly into the ventricular myocardium rather than through the specialised conduction system. Ventricular myocardium conducts electrical impulses relatively slowly in comparison to the AVN and this leads to a broad QRS complex. If there is concurrent atrial fibrillation (AF) and WPW, there can be an irregular BCT as the electrical impulses are bypassing the specialised conduction tissue. Pre-excited tachycardias can also occur if, for instance, there is coexistence of an atrial tachycardia with an accessory pathway. This will also manifest as a BCT on resting 12-lead ECG.

4.8 Idiopathic VT

This conventionally refers to the presence of **monomorphic** VT in the absence of structural disease. It constitutes around 10% of all patients with VT. The prognosis for all forms is reassuring as they tend to respond well to AMDs and are generally amenable to ablation. There are various subtypes and a succinct overview of each is provided below.

4.8.1 Outflow Tract VT

Ventricular tachycardia from the RVOT has the characteristic appearance of LBBB in lead V1 and an inferior axis in the frontal plane (see Figure 4.5). Vagal manoeuvres such as adenosine can terminate whereas sympathetic overdrive in the context of exercise or stress can initiate and perpetuate. Structural abnormalities are very unusual and conditions such as ARVC and cardiac sarcoidosis should be excluded (see Chapter 14). Treatment is only warranted if there are concurrent symptoms. Patients can present with frequent ventricular ectopics, NSVT and/or sustained VT. Beta-blockade can be useful given that adrenergic surge is an important mechanistic trigger. VT originating from the RVOT is generally amenable to catheter ablation with low complication rates. This can therefore be considered first-line if long-term medical therapy is not desirable. VT originating from the LVOT often manifest with an R wave in lead V1 and precordial transition to dominant R wave in lead V2. Ablation can be curative but success is influenced to a degree by the site of origin. ICDs are generally not indicated for idiopathic outflow tract VT given their non-compromising nature.

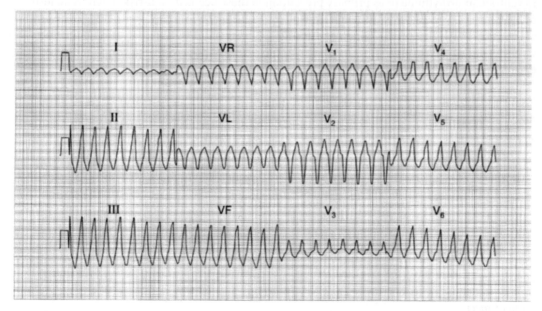

Figure 4.5 12-lead ECG indicative of RVOT VT. There is evidence of a regular BCT at a rate of 180 bpm, with LBBB-like appearance, inferior axis and transition in V3. This is typical for VT originating from the RVOT.

4.8.2 Non-outflow Tract VT

Annular VT arises from the mitral or tricuspid annulus and accounts for 4–7% of idiopathic cases. In mitral annular VT, the ECG pattern is typically RBBB with an S wave in V6. For tricuspid annular VT, foci generally originate in the septal region and this results in a LBBB pattern but of narrower QRS duration.

  Fascicular VT typically arises from the left posterior fascicle. ECG may show a relatively narrow RBBB morphology and can be of superior or inferior axis. Intravenous administration of verapamil often suppresses this type of VT whereas adenosine is rarely effective. From a mechanistic perspective, this implicates slow inward current via DAD or reentry formation. Catheter ablation is often curative and should be considered as an early interventional strategy.

  Papillary muscle VT also has RBBB morphology but is more distinct and of broader QRS duration than fascicular VT. It can be of superior or inferior axis depending on the origin and, as with fascicular VT, can arise in the context of a structurally normal heart and tends to be focal in origin. Catheter ablation can be curative but is technically challenging, usually due to relative catheter instability. Techniques such as intracardiac echocardiography can be used to aid with stable positioning.

4.9 Catecholaminergic Polymorphic VT (CPVT)

Catecholaminergic polymorphic VT (CPVT) is a rare condition that usually presents in childhood and adolescence. There is genetic predisposition with mutations in ryanodine receptor gene *RyR2* (autosomal dominant [AD]) and calsequestrin gene *CASQ2* (autosomal recessive [AR]). Patients typically present with syncope or aborted SCD with a dysrhythmia that is highly responsive to adrenaline and reproduced by exercise or stress. QTc interval is normal. Typically, exercise results in physiological sinus tachycardia. This can be accompanied by ventricular extrasystoles followed by salvos and progression into persistent, polymorphic VT. Classically, it is of a **bidirectional appearance** with beat-to-beat alternation of the frontal axis (see Figure 4.6). It is pertinent to note, however, that bidirectional VT is not commonly observed and other causes are limited but include Andersen–Tawil syndrome and

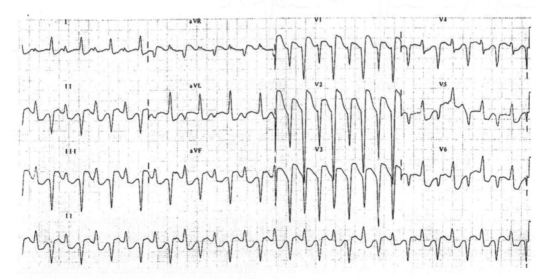

Figure 4.6 Bidirectional QRS pattern implicated in CPVT.

severe digoxin toxicity. Beta-blockers can be effective with preference for non-cardioselective agents such as propranolol to suppress exogenous adrenergic surge. Flecainide can be considered as add-on therapy if no contraindications exist. ICD implantation can be considered but a measured approach is required due to potential for electrical storm requiring recurrent discharges. Left cardiac sympathetic denervation does appear to be effective in some cases [7]. Patients should also be provided with strict lifestyle advice to avoid strenuous exercise. Empirical beta-blockers are recommended for gene-positive family members, even after negative exercise testing.

4.10   Brugada Syndrome

This is a distinct clinical entity arising from heterozygous mutations in the sodium channel α-subunit (*SCN5A*) gene encoding sodium and calcium channels. It is more common in South Asian subpopulations, with symptoms occurring predominantly at night and often induced by pyrexia. Patients may have evidence of RBBB, J-point elevation ≥ 2 mm with coved segments and T wave inversion in leads V1 or V2, although three distinct types of repolarisation patterns are described (see Figure 4.7). Use of right-sided precordial leads targeted at the RVOT can enhance diagnostic sensitivity. Sodium channel blockers such as flecainide, ajmaline, or procainamide can be used as provocative agents under strict monitoring to assist with diagnosis. Imaging typically excludes structural heart disease. In those presenting with electrical storm, quinidine or isoprenaline infusions should be considered as they can transiently activate sodium channels. Lifestyle advice includes avoidance of excess alcohol, large meals and prompt management of pyrexia in addition to withdrawal of offending agents. ICDs are the only established treatment option in these patients to prevent SCD and are indicated in the context of syncope associated with a type I ECG pattern. However, contemporary research has indicated that evidence of a fragmented QRS complex (multiple spikes) can also be useful for risk stratification [8]. Genetic testing is also applicable, particularly in guiding diagnostic work-up of family members where it contributes towards prognostic risk stratification.

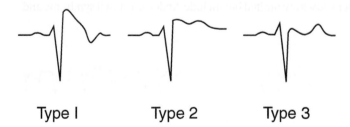

Type I   Type 2   Type 3

Figure 4.7   Distinct subtypes of Brugada syndrome.

4.11   Torsades de Pointes

4.11.1   Aetiology

Torsades de Pointes (TdP) results from prolongation and dispersion (typically epicardium to endocardium) of myocardial repolarisation with subsequent prolongation of QT interval. It is most commonly acquired and may arise secondary to chronic therapy with pharmacological agents such as tricyclics, amiodarone, sotalol, and lithium. Ischaemia and electrolyte abnormalities such as hypokalaemia and hypocalcaemia can also be implicated. This disorder can also be congenital with gene variants

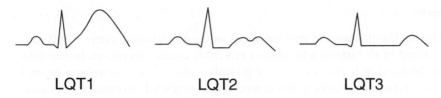

LQT1   **LQT2**   **LQT3**

Figure 4.8   Distinct subtypes of long QT syndrome.

resulting in potassium and sodium channelopathies such as Romano–Ward syndrome (AD) and Jervell and Lange–Nielsen syndrome (AR). The three most common subtypes are LQT1-3, with categorisation informed by triggers (see Figure 4.8). LQT1 appears to be precipitated by exercise, particularly swimming. LQT2 typically occurs in the context of emotional stress such as pregnancy or as a result of a sudden loud noise and is pause-dependent, unlike LQT1. LQT3 is associated with rest or sleep. LQT1 and 2 are associated with loss of function mutations in potassium channels that regulate the inward rectifier current, whereas LQT3 is associated with gain of function mutations in sodium channels that lead to a sustained late inward current and therefore prolongation of the action potential.

4.11.2   Diagnosis

Patients may present with seizures or syncopal episodes. The primary risk is of SCD, probably from degeneration of VT into VF. Diagnosis relies on assessment of the QT interval as EP studies are generally not helpful. As outlined in Chapter 1, the QT interval is inherently affected by resting heart rate (HR) and it is therefore the corrected interval (QTc) that is most informative. This can be calculated using Fridericia or Bazett methods, though the latter tends to overcorrect at faster rates. Roughly, a duration > 460 ms (males) or > 470 ms (females) is deemed abnormal with any value within 20 ms of this designated upper limit considered 'borderline'. It is best practice to manually measure QTc in multiple leads and use the one calculated to be broadest. Positive genotyping is established in around 75% of individuals with a clear phenotype but is complicated by variable disease penetrance. An individual with a confirmed pathogenic variant but without ECG changes or symptoms is still deemed to have the diagnosis. The Schwartz score can provide a useful diagnostic criterion to establish likelihood, and incorporates resting QTc duration, QTc interval at the fourth minute of recovery from exercise testing, T wave morphology, resting HR, presence of TdP, clinical history including congenital deafness and family history.

A significant prolongation in interval, usually > 500 ms, can result in the **R-on-T phenomenon**, whereby ventricular depolarisation (usually originating from a PVC) occurs during repolarisation. If it is pause-dependent, a short–long–short RR interval pattern can be observed. This can precipitate successive bursts of polymorphic VT in which QRS complexes are irregular, of varying amplitude and undulate around the isoelectric baseline, giving a typical sinusoidal appearance (see Figure 4.9).

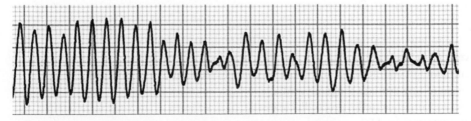

Figure 4.9   Sinusoidal ECG appearance typical of Torsades de Pointes.

4.11.3 Management

This relies on convincing identification of prolonged QTc as the precipitating event. A full electrolyte screen is required in all instances to address reversible causes. Moreover, intravenous magnesium is recommended as it provides overall protective effects on myocardium beyond reduction of dysrhythmic potential. Underpinning mechanism may relate to coronary vasodilation, reduced catecholaminergic drive and cellular magnesium–calcium interactions that restrict calcium deposition in mitochondria. In view of this, there is evidence of benefit even in patients with normal serum levels.

In congenital cases that are not pause-dependent, non-selective beta-blockade with nadolol or propranolol should be instituted with advice to avoid strenuous exercise. Sodium channel blockers such as mexiletine can be added in the context of LQT3. If the mechanism is pause-dependent, temporary pacing may be beneficial in shortening action potential (AP) duration and QT interval prior to initiation of beta-blockade. If symptomatic or asymptomatic with high-risk profile, ICD therapy may be indicated after review by a specialist. Algorithms can be set to prevent typical pauses post-PVC. In the context of acquired cases, any likely precipitants should be discontinued with close monitoring to see if QTc interval normalises. The evidence for primary prevention ICD in patients with acquired TdP and a family history of SCD but no syncope is not established. In conjunction with cardiac evaluation, genetic analysis may be useful in risk stratification of long QT syndrome patients; however, up to 25% of cases may remain genotype-elusive and hampers appropriate detection of high-risk family members.

Hot Points

- Broad complex tachycardias describe rhythms that exceed 100 bpm and are of widened QRS duration.
- The most common regular BCT is VT, which often arises from the formation of reentry circuits involving scar tissue in the context of IHD.
- Features that support diagnosis of VT include history of IHD, A:V dissociation, chest lead QRS concordance, extreme axis, capture and fusion beats.
- Structural cardiac disorders associated with VT include HCM and ARVC.
- Idiopathic VT refers to presence of a monomorphic BCT in the absence of structural disease. It is associated with a favourable prognosis and examples include outflow tract, annular and fascicular VT.
- As with NCT, management of BCT depends on the presence of adverse symptoms and signs. If these exist, electrical cardioversion is warranted.

4.12 Self-assessment Questions

1 Which of the following features is least likely to differentiate VT from SVT?
   A Positive QRS in lead aVR.
   B Shortening of QRS duration as heart rhythm changes from sinus to tachycardia.
   C P waves marching through the tachycardia.
   D Negative concordance in the precordial leads.
   E An rSR′ pattern in lead V1.

2   With regard to long QT syndrome, which of the following statements is false?
   A A QTc interval > 460 ms is a risk factor for sudden cardiac death.
   B It is inherited in an autosomal dominant pattern with incomplete penetrance.
   C It involves multiple mutations in the potassium and sodium channels.
   D The QT interval is best measured in leads II and V5.
   E Beta-blockers are considered first-line therapy in patients with inherited long QT syndrome.

3   In acute management of polymorphic VT, which of the following statements is false?
   A Urgent coronary angiography and intervention may be required.
   B Amiodarone is an effective first-line option in haemodynamically stable patients.
   C Intravenous magnesium can be considered before plasma levels are known.
   D Temporary transvenous pacing can be considered if VT is incessant.
   E Beta-blockers may help to reduce risk of recurrence.

4   With regard to VT originating from the RVOT, which of the following is true?
   A 12-lead ECG typically demonstrates RBBB-like morphology in the precordial leads with positive QRS complex in the inferior leads.
   B ICDs are not typically required.
   C Beta-blockers are commonly ineffective.
   D VT ablation should be considered as first-line therapy in symptomatic patients.
   E Abnormalities in the right ventricle are commonly observed on cardiac MRI.

5   Which of the following favours papillary muscle VT rather than fascicular VT?
   A RBBB morphology.
   B Superior axis.
   C Focal or reentry mechanism.
   D Structurally normal heart.
   E No response to verapamil.

References

1 Wathen, M.S., DeGroot, P.J., Sweeney, M.O. et al. (2004). Prospective randomized multicenter trial of empirical antitachycardia pacing versus shocks for spontaneous rapid ventricular tachycardia in patients with implantable cardioverter-defibrillators: pacing fast ventricular tachycardia reduces shock therapies (PainFREE Rx II) trial results. *Circulation* 110 (17): 2591–2596.

2 Antiarrhythmics versus Implantable Defibrillators (AVID) Investigators (1997). A comparison of antiarrhythmic-drug therapy with implantable defibrillators in patients resuscitated from near-fatal ventricular arrhythmias. *N. Engl. J. Med.* 337 (22): 1576–1583.

3 Bardy, G.H., Lee, K.L., Mark, D.B. et al. (2005). Amiodarone or an implantable cardioverter-defibrillator for congestive heart failure(published correction appears in *N. Engl. J. Med.* 2005 May 19;352(20):2146). *N. Engl. J. Med.* 352 (3): 225–237.

4 Sapp, J.L., Wells, G.A., Parkash, R. et al. (2016). Ventricular tachycardia ablation versus escalation of antiarrhythmic drugs. *N. Engl. J. Med.* 375 (2): 111–121.

5 Moss, A.J., Hall, W.J., Cannom, D.S. et al. (1996). Improved survival with an implanted defibrillator in patients with coronary disease at high risk for ventricular arrhythmia. Multicenter Automatic Defibrillator Implantation Trial Investigators. *N. Engl. J. Med.* 335 (26): 1933–1940.

6 Moss, A.J., Zareba, W., Hall, W.J. et al. (2002). Prophylactic implantation of a defibrillator in patients with myocardial infarction and reduced ejection fraction. *N. Engl. J. Med.* 346 (12): 877–883.

7 Wilde, A.A., Bhuiyan, Z.A., Crotti, L. et al. (2008). Left cardiac sympathetic denervation for catecholaminergic polymorphic ventricular tachycardia. *N. Engl. J. Med.* 358 (19): 2024–2029.

8 Morita, H., Kusano, K.F., Miura, D. et al. (2008). Fragmented QRS as a marker of conduction abnormality and a predictor of prognosis of Brugada syndrome. *Circulation* 118 (17): 1697–1704.

Further Reading

Priori, S.G., Blomström-Lundqvist, C., Mazzanti, A. et al. (2015). 2015 ESC guidelines for the management of patients with ventricular arrhythmias and the prevention of sudden cardiac death: the Task Force for the Management of Patients with Ventricular Arrhythmias and the Prevention of Sudden Cardiac Death of the European Society of Cardiology (ESC). Endorsed by: Association for European Paediatric and Congenital Cardiology (AEPC). *Eur. Heart J.* 36 (41): 2793–2867.

Schwartz, P.J. and Ackerman, M.J. (2013). The long QT syndrome: a transatlantic clinical approach to diagnosis and therapy. *Eur. Heart J.* 34 (40): 3109–3116.

5

Bradycardias and Conduction Disease

5.1 Learning Objectives

- Sinus node dysfunction.
- Atrioventricular block.
- Distal conduction disease.
- Specific indications for pacing, including neurocardiogenic syncope, acute myocardial infarction and torsades de pointes.
- Acute management strategy for bradycardias.

5.2 Overview

Bradycardia is defined as heart rate less than 60 beats min^{-1} (bpm). This may occur in normal physiology such as in those with excess vagal tone at baseline. However, it is also implicated in pathological states and may arise from defects in any region of the electrical conducting system. Broadly, it can be subcategorised based on primary abnormality of the sinoatrial node (SAN), atrioventricular node (AVN), or distal fascicles. Specific conditions in which bradycardia play a consequent role, such as neurocardiogenic syncope, shall be discussed separately. A **Stokes–Adams attack** describes transient loss of consciousness due to cerebral hypoperfusion secondary to a dysrhythmia, in which bradycardias and conduction disease are most strongly implicated. Patients with bradycardias may be entirely asymptomatic or present with adverse features such as dizziness and syncope. The remainder of this section explores potential aetiologies and acute management.

5.3 Sinus Node Dysfunction (SND)

SND is interchangeably referred to as **sick sinus syndrome** and is characterised by depressed function of the SAN with inability to generate a heart rate (HR) sufficient for physiological needs. Its prevalence increases with age. It is a class I pacing indication in symptomatic individuals and class III in those without. Although it is pertinent to assess for reversible precipitants such as rate-limiting agents, anti-arrhythmics and psychotropics, including lithium and tricyclics, it is not always possible to discontinue. There is also an association with obstructive sleep apnoea (OSA) due to hypoxaemia-induced increase in vagal tone during apnoeic episodes. In such situations, weight reduction and/or continuous positive airway pressure (CPAP) may alleviate symptoms and help to avoid invasive intervention. A summary of the broad subtypes of SND is provided below.

5.3.1 Sinus Bradycardia

This is defined as a heart rate originating from the SAN that is < 60 bpm. As alluded to, the SAN has extensive autonomic innervation such that heightened parasympathetic tone can cause marked bradycardia and prolonged sinus node recovery times (SNRTs) that may correlate with symptoms.

5.3.2 Sinus Pause/Arrest

This results from abnormal automaticity with a failure of sinus impulse generation. It is conventionally defined as a sinus pause if it is < 3 s in duration and sinus arrest if more prolonged. It is apparent on 12-lead ECG as the absence of P waves without a discernible pattern (see Figure 5.1). Degeneration and fibrosis of the node are often implicated and therefore disease of the distal conduction system may be coexistent.

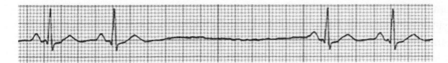

Figure 5.1   Rhythm strip showing sinus pause (< 3 s).

5.3.3   Sinoatrial Block

Sinoatrial block refers to failure of sinus impulse conduction. In such instances, impulse generation is preserved but is abnormally conducted to the perinodal region, which forms the transition
with atrial myocardium. This may arise due to infarction and/or fibrosis, for example. In **type I**
block, there is gradual prolongation of exit block which is a manifestation of calcium-sensitive
tissues, such as the SAN, that show decremental conduction. Eventually, the atrial impulse cannot
propagate and a pause results (see Figure 5.2). In **type II** block, there is again a pause with absent
P wave but in this context, the pause is an exact multiple of the R-R interval.

5.3.4   Tachy-Brady Syndrome

This syndrome refers to episodes of alternating sinus bradycardia with a tachycardia, most commonly atrial flutter or fibrillation (AF) (see Figure 5.3). Sinus node automaticity is depressed by
'overdrive suppression' resulting from the period of tachycardia, such that sinus bradycardia or
pause/arrest often follows reversion of the tachycardia. Arrhythmia-modifying agents can often
exacerbate SND, and for this reason, pacemaker insertion is usually favoured.

5.3.5   Junctional Bradycardia

Cells in or around the AVN do not exhibit automaticity (i.e. potential for spontaneous depolarisation) in normal conditions due to overdrive suppression from the SAN. However, they can act as
latent pacemakers in certain situations. This includes patients with SND as a safety mechanism
when atrial impulses do not reach the AVN. It can also occur in the context of inferior myocardial
infarction (MI) secondary to ischaemia, or in healthy athletes with heightened vagal tone that suppresses SAN automaticity. Typically, 12-lead ECG will demonstrate a regular ventricular rate in the

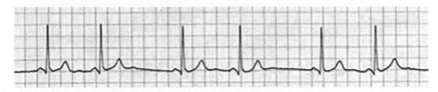

Figure 5.2   ECG appearance of type I sinoatrial block.

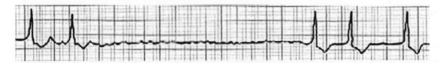

Figure 5.3   Rhythm strip showing tachy-brady syndrome.

region of 40–60 bpm. Retrograde depolarisation of the atria results in inverted P waves in the inferior leads (i.e. negative deflection) before or after the QRS wave, or it may not be visible if buried within the QRS complex due to simultaneous atrial and ventricular depolarisation. QRS interval is usually narrow unless there is coexistent intraventricular conduction delay. On a separate note, junctional tachycardia can also occur but this is a separate phenomenon unrelated to SND and is discussed separately in Section 3.9.

5.3.6 Chronotropic Incompetence

This disorder refers to inadequate rise of HR in response to physiological stress (< 85% of maximal age-predicted HR). It may occur in SND or in the context of beta-blockade, but also has distinct prevalence in patients with congestive heart failure (CHF). Correct identification is usually through use of ambulatory ECG monitoring or during exercise tolerance testing (ETT). Symptomatic chronotropic incompetence (CI) in the absence of rate-limiting agents is an indication for pacemaker implant. However, CHF results in chronic neurohumoral activation (see Chapter 12) resulting in beta-receptor downregulation and reduced sensitivity to conventional agonists. Moreover, CI in CHF is paralleled by reduced HR variability and, prior to beta-blockade, is thought to relate to disease severity. There is a significant confounder, however, as severe CHF is associated with poorer exercise tolerance and hence smaller increases in HR during exercise. Some data have suggested that for a given workload, HR in some patients with CHF may indeed be higher. Hence, the precise effects of CI on exercise capacity are not clearly established and its treatment is even more unclear. In patients with CHF suitable for device therapy, there is currently no objective evidence aside from an intuitive perspective that rate-adaptive pacing improves functional capacity [1].

5.3.7 Familial SND

Clinical presentations of familial SND are similar to non-inherited types. Cascade screening has indicated cohorts with increased susceptibility to atrial arrhythmias and channelopathies are most strongly implicated. Mutations in *SCN5A* gene results in multiple arrhythmia syndromes, including SND, long QT3, Brugada syndrome and sudden infant death syndrome (SIDS). *HCN4* channels are predominantly expressed in pacemaker cells and mutations in this gene have also been implicated.

5.4 Atrioventricular Block

5.4.1 Causes

Atrioventricular (AV) block is defined as any delay to or lack of conduction through the AVN. It may arise in multiple clinical contexts although commonly due to age-related fibrosis of conduction tissue. Acute AV block typically arises as a result of ischaemia in the context of a MI, usually due to right coronary artery (RCA) territory occlusion. This blockade is often transient and may fully resolve after a period of up to seven days. Left coronary artery (LCA) territory infarcts may also result in AVN blockade but prognosis is much poorer due to extensive myocardial involvement. Iatrogenic blockade may arise from use of conventional pharmacotherapies that increase refractory period and slow conduction velocity, such as digoxin, beta-blockers and non-dihydropyridine calcium-channel blockers (NDHP CCB). Other scenarios include biochemical perturbations such as hyperkalaemia and digoxin toxicity which can be readily excluded via blood profiling.

It can be observed in the context of dilated cardiomyopathy (DCM), particularly when gene defects such as *LMNA* or *SCN5A* mutations are present. Infiltrative cardiomyopathies such as sarcoidosis and amyloidosis are also implicated. There is an association with neuromuscular disorders such as myotonic dystrophy, Friedreich's ataxia and Kearns–Sayre syndrome. Similarly, AVN blockade can arise in connective tissue disorders such as rheumatoid arthritis, systemic lupus erythematosus (SLE) and limited cutaneous systemic sclerosis (formerly referred to as CREST syndrome).

Uncommonly, it may arise as a post-procedural complication secondary to coronary artery bypass grafting (CABG), septal myomectomy, atrioventricular nodal re-entrant tachycardia (AVNRT) ablation or surgical/transcatheter aortic valve replacement (AVR). A broad range of infections can be causative, including aortic root abscess, Lyme disease, syphilis, and myocarditis secondary to Chagas disease. Rarely, there may also be idiopathic degeneration of the conduction system such as in Lenegre's disease.

5.4.2 Types

5.4.2.1 Vagotonic
This is a specific entity that is important to exclude in all patients presenting with AVN blockade. It is common in younger patients and results from elevated parasympathetic tone with simultaneous occurrence of AV block and slowing of the sinus rate. It may manifest transiently during Holter monitoring of otherwise healthy individuals during sleep or in situations where vagal tone is heightened (e.g. athletic training, medical procedure, prolonged vomiting). Although appearances can be marked with unpredictable variability, it is generally considered benign and does not necessitate pacemaker insertion unless symptoms are resistant.

5.4.2.2 First-degree Heart Block
It is defined by a consistently prolonged PR interval ($> 200\,\text{ms}$) due to AVN delay (see Figure 5.4). Nonetheless, every atrial impulse is propagated to the ventricles resulting in no missed beats. It is most often benign and asymptomatic individuals do not require specific intervention. If symptoms occur due to atrioventricular dyssynchrony because of very prolonged PR intervals, typically $> 300\,\text{ms}$, it can mimic 'pacemaker syndrome' and pacemaker implantation can be considered to improve quality of life.

5.4.2.3 Second-degree Heart Block
This has two broad subtypes, **Mobitz type I (Wenckebach)** and **Mobitz type II**. The first is characterised by gradual prolongation in PR interval followed by a dropped beat, i.e. the P wave is not succeeded by the QRS complex (see Figure 5.5). This arises because the RP interval becomes

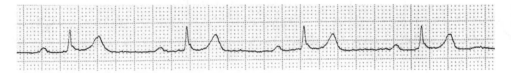

Figure 5.4 ECG appearance of first-degree heart block.

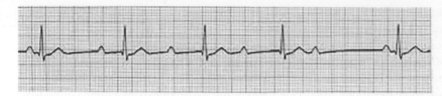

Figure 5.5 ECG appearance of Mobitz type I block.

progressively shorter until the P wave falls into the ventricular refractory period and is therefore blocked. Junctional escape beats may occur along with non-conducted P waves. A shortened PR interval occurs after the blocked sinus beat and is the cornerstone for diagnosis. Patients with symptomatic Mobitz type I should be considered for a pacemaker, or if electrophysiological testing finds the block to be located at intra- or infra-Hisian levels.

Mobitz type II block results in a stable PR interval, which may be <200 ms but with periodic blockade of the sinus P wave (see Figure 5.6). The QRS complex is often wider than in type I and may appear intermittently or with regularity. The PR interval in the first beat after the block is similar to the previous PR interval. The pause encompassing the blocked P wave is equal to twice the sinus cycle length. Any form of Mobitz type II block is a class I pacing indication irrespective of symptoms.

When 2 : 1 block is present (i.e. every other P wave is non-conducted), it is challenging to determine whether the level of block is at the node or infranodal. Although wide QRS complexes generally indicate the latter, this criterion is not reliable. If the PR interval of the conducted beats remains short and fixed, the level of block may be considered infranodal (i.e. Mobitz type II). On the other hand, if the PR interval is longer and not fixed, it is likely to be AV nodal (i.e. Mobitz type I). In addition to this observation, stress testing to assess impact of exercise on AV conduction and/or electrophysiological testing can be considered to help with decision-making regarding device implantation.

5.4.2.4 Third-degree Heart Block

Third-degree or complete heart block (CHB) refers to total absence of conduction via the AVN, i.e. complete dissociation between P and QRS complexes (see Figure 5.7). It is important to note, however, that not all patients with A:V dissociation have CHB. This is the case in patients with ventricular tachycardia (VT), for example, where dissociation arises because the ventricular rate is faster than intrinsic sinus rate (see Chapter 4).

In CHB, impulses originate from the SAN as per normal electrophysiology but are unable to propagate beyond the AVN. This results in a ventricular escape (junctional) rhythm that is regular but totally independent of atrial activity. Depending on anatomical origin, ventricular

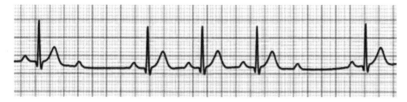

Figure 5.6 ECG appearance of Mobitz type II block.

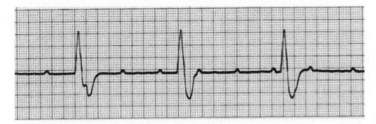

Figure 5.7   ECG appearance of third-degree heart block.

depolarisation may be of narrow or wide QRS duration. If the block is at the level of the AVN, junctional rhythm is usually in the region of 45–60 bpm. Patients usually exhibit haemodynamic stability with a HR that is responsive to exercise or atropine. When the block is infranodal, the junctional rhythm originates more distally from the His or bundle branches. Rates are usually <45 bpm and confer a higher risk of progression to asystole. They also tend to be unresponsive to exercise and atropine. In CHB, visualisation of the jugular venous pressure may show **cannon waves**. These represent prominent A waves that arise from the right atrium, contracting against a closed tricuspid valve that results in regurgitant flow into the venous system. It is a class I indication for pacing in most instances.

5.5   Fascicular Block

A reminder of the anatomy of the infranodal conduction system is provided in Figure 5.8. Definitions for the various types of fascicular block are often confusing, misplaced and result in considerable ambiguity.

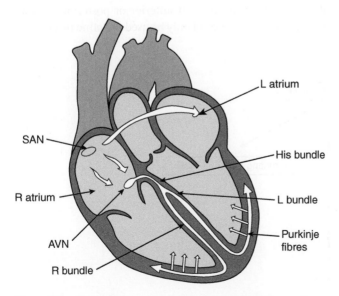

Figure 5.8   Simplistic overview of electrical conduction system.

5.5.1 Bifascicular Block

Broadly speaking, bifascicular block refers to any one of the following combinations:

1) Right bundle branch block (RBBB) and left anterior fascicular block (left axis deviation, LAD)
2) RBBB and left posterior fascicular block (right axis deviation, RAD)
3) Complete left bundle branch block (LBBB).

The presence of associated symptoms such as dizziness or syncope is a prerequisite for pacemaker implantation in the context of isolated bifascicular block. If syncope is present but unexplained, decision-making is initially guided by baseline ventricular function. If there is severe impairment defined by ejection fraction (EF) ≤35%, the patient should be considered for implantable cardioverter–defibrillator (ICD) with or without cardiac resynchronisation therapy (CRT) – see Section 12.7.12.2. If this is not the case, a pragmatic approach to pacemaker implant can be considered if the person is elderly, frail or at high risk of traumatic recurrence. Otherwise, electrophysiological testing can be considered with positivity if measured HV interval (conduction time from the proximal His bundle to the ventricular myocardium) is ≥ 70 ms.

5.5.2 Trifascicular Block

Trifascicular block (TFB) can be typically considered as **incomplete** or **complete** (see Figure 5.9). This differentiation is of clinical relevance as the overall risk of incomplete TFB progressing to CHB is relatively low. Incomplete TFB may appear as a fixed block of two of the fascicles (i.e. bifascicular block) with delayed conduction in the remaining one that manifests as first- or second-degree block (see Figure 5.10). In these situations, it is not possible to determine from the 12-lead ECG whether this disordered conduction is truly at the level of the remaining fascicle or instead at the AVN (hence technically not a true TFB). Incomplete TFB can alternatively be represented as a fixed block of one fascicle (i.e. RBBB) with intermittent failure of each of the other two (i.e. alternating LAD and RAD). If so, associated dizziness or syncope warrants pacemaker implantation.

When complete TFB occurs, the appearance is of CHB with features of bifascicular block. This arises because the escape rhythm usually originates from the left anterior or posterior fascicle distal to site of block. An alternative viewpoint is that TFB should only be used to define those with

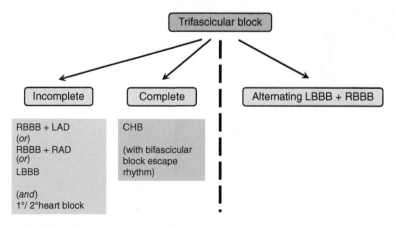

Figure 5.9 Categorisations for trifascicular block.

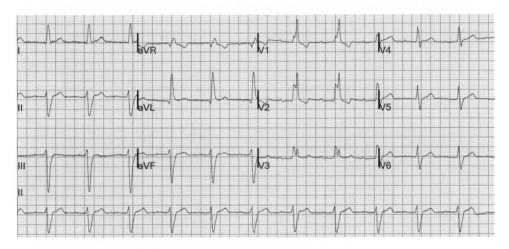

Figure 5.10 12-lead ECG depicting trifascicular block. There is evidence of significant first-degree heart block (PR 280 ms) with broad RBBB (QRS 160 ms) and LAD.

alternating LBBB and RBBB (a class I indication) or the presence of either with a prolonged HV interval. In both instances, device therapy is required even if patients are truly asymptomatic due to high inherent risk of progression to asystole.

5.6 Neurally Mediated Syncope

Neurally mediated syncope appears to result from autonomic dysregulation. This is often an exaggerated response to stimuli, such as pain, coughing or micturition. Patients often present with unexplained syncope, in which routine investigations such as ambulatory ECG monitoring, echocardiography, lying and standing blood pressure (BP) and computed tomography (CT) head are unremarkable. Diagnosis is often made by performing a **tilt test**, whereby symptoms are assessed whilst the patient is gradually elevated from a horizontal position with interval assessment of haemodynamic parameters including HR and BP. Ordinarily, elevation results in progressive pooling of blood in the lower extremities and splanchnic circulation. This triggers compensatory sympathetic activity that increases total peripheral resistance (TPR), venous return and cardiac output (CO). HR will conventionally be ≥ 10–25 bpm (unless there is evidence of CI), diastolic BP will be ≤ 5–10 mmHg and systolic BP will be ≤ 5–10 mmHg. Various abnormalities in this neural response can be observed on testing (see Figure 5.11).

5.6.1 Cardioinhibitory

This arises from enhanced parasympathetic tone and may manifest as a reduction in BP secondary to a drop in HR. In type A, HR will reduce to ≤ 40 bpm for a duration greater than 10 seconds but without asystole. In type B, there is associated asystole for ≥ 3 s. Both types are class IIa indications for pacing, particularly in patients aged > 40 years. Indeed, a recent randomised controlled trial (RCT) has shown particular benefit from dual chamber pacemaker implant with rate-responsive closed loop stimulation (CLS) [2]. This system analyses right ventricular intracardiac impedance continuously and can therefore acutely adjust pacing rate at the onset of tilt-induced bradyarrhythmia. It appeared to be highly effective in reducing symptom recurrence over a 12-month follow-up period.

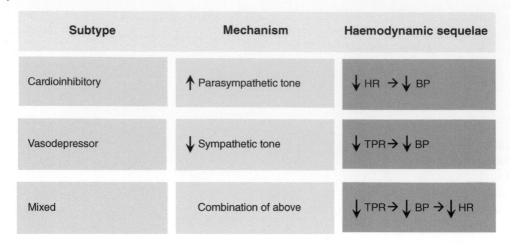

Subtype	Mechanism	Haemodynamic sequelae
Cardioinhibitory	↑ Parasympathetic tone	↓ HR → ↓ BP
Vasodepressor	↓ Sympathetic tone	↓ TPR → ↓ BP
Mixed	Combination of above	↓ TPR → ↓ BP → ↓ HR

Figure 5.11 Subtypes of neurocardiogenic syncope.

5.6.2 Vasodepressor

This is caused by suppressed sympathetic tone. It results in a drop in BP consequent to a reduction in TPR, with no dramatic changes in HR elicited. Typical examples are vasovagal syncope and postural hypotension (the latter defined by reduction in systolic BP ≥ 20 mmHg or diastolic ≥ 10 mmHg). Even if syncope ensues, HR does not fall by more than 10% of peak value. If a vasodepressor defect is diagnosed, conservative management includes adequate hydration and abstinence from alcohol to augment intravascular volume. Pacing is not indicated for these cohorts.

5.6.3 Mixed

These cases typically demonstrate both cardioinhibitory and vasodepressor components on testing. BP drops first and is followed by a reduction in HR at the time of syncope. However, rates do not tend to fall beyond 40 bpm and asystole is uncommon.

5.6.4 Postural Orthostatic Tachycardia Syndrome (PoTS)

This syndrome is most commonly observed in young women and is associated with connective tissue disorders. Its pathophysiology is not fully understood. On tilt testing, BP is maintained. However, HR increases by ≥ 30 bpm within 10 minutes of standing or there is evidence of persistent tachycardia ≥ 120 bpm. Treatment incorporates general lifestyle advice and includes adequate exercise, hydration, and salt intake. Peripheral α-adrenergic agonists such as midodrine may help by improving TPR. Beta-blockers and ivabradine have also been trialled but benefits remain inconclusive.

5.6.5 Carotid Sinus Syndrome

One variant of neurally mediated syncope is carotid sinus syndrome. A classic history involves dizziness or syncope that is precipitated by neck movements or shaving. It is predominantly cardioinhibitory in nature (i.e. mediated by excess parasympathetic tone), and can be reproduced by carotid sinus massage. If this results in systolic BP drop ≥ 50 mmHg or ventricular pause lasting ≥ 3 s (symptomatic) or ≥ 6 s (asymptomatic), there is a class I indication for pacing.

5.7 Other Indications for Pacing

5.7.1 Acute Myocardial Infarction

Indications for temporary pacing in the context of CHB secondary to acute MI depend on clinical and haemodynamic parameters. These do not necessarily correlate with indications for permanent pacing. The prognosis depends heavily on locality of conduction defect and whether it is driven by ischaemia or infarction. Generally, a transient dysrhythmia lasting < 48 hours is likely to be ischaemia-driven. SND is often reversible and permanent devices are rarely required. AV conduction disease in the context of inferior MI is also usually transient and patients are conventionally monitored for at least 5 days to allow spontaneous resolution. By contrast, second-degree block or CHB after anterior MI indicates extensive infarction and permanent pacing is usually warranted even if asymptomatic.

5.7.2 Torsades de Pointes

This is a polymorphic VT defined by sinusoidal appearance on ECG with the QRS complex undulating around its baseline. It results from prolongation and dispersion of myocardial repolarisation that prolongs the QT interval. VT is initiated by ventricular depolarisation occurring in the repolarisation phase, i.e. R-on-T phenomenon. Aside from discontinuation of pharmacological precipitants, intravenous magnesium and/or isoprenaline infusion may be indicated in acquired forms with the latter increasing resting HR, shortening action potential duration and reducing QT interval. Through similar means, overdrive pacing is occasionally warranted to enable iatrogenic increase of resting HR. A more detailed exploration of this disorder is provided in Section 4.11.

5.8 Acute Management

Standard resuscitation algorithms outline acute management of bradycardias. This commences with an ABCDE approach and advocates close monitoring of physiological parameters. Any potential reversible precipitants such as electrolyte disturbance should be identified. It is crucial to establish whether the bradycardia is associated with any adverse features, namely cardiac failure, myocardial ischaemia, shock and/or syncope. If none of these are present, risk of asystole should be stratified based on whether there is a history of recent asystole, evidence of high-grade block (i.e. Mobitz type II, CHB with broad QRS escape, ventricular pause > 3 s). If absent, a monitoring strategy is appropriate. However, if any of these features or adverse signs are present, intravenous administration of 500 μg atropine is advocated. This is a non-selective antagonist of muscarinic acetylcholine receptors (M2) implicated in parasympathetic innervation. It functions by transiently increasing SAN automaticity and conduction velocity through the AVN. Half-life of this agent is relatively short at two hours and therefore recurrent administration up to a limit of 3 mg may be indicated. Glycopyrrolate can be considered as an alternative to atropine. If symptoms are refractory, other options include isoprenaline infusion (non-selective β-adrenergic agonist), transcutaneous pacing or transvenous pacing. These are typically considered as bridge measures until definitive management in the form of permanent pacemaker implantation.

5.9 Self-assessment Questions

1 Which of the following is not a likely indication for pacing?
    A Sinus pause with symptoms.
    B Mobitz type II second-degree AV block with wide QRS rhythm without symptoms.
    C Complete heart block with symptoms.
    D Carotid sinus passage with blood pressure drop < 50 mmHg.
    E Chronotropic incompetence with symptoms.

2 Which of the following statements about fascicular block is correct?
    A Incomplete trifascicular block can consist of RBBB plus RAD and prolonged PR interval.
    B LAD between −45° and −90° is a sign of left posterior fascicular block.
    C HV interval does not predict risk of progression to complete heart block.
    D Complete trifascicular block can consist of LBBB plus second-degree AV block.
    E A patient with bifascicular block and syncope should proceed with pacemaker implantation without electrophysiological testing.

3 Which of the following conditions is not associated with AV block?
    A Kearns–Sayre syndrome.
    B Digoxin toxicity.
    C Chagas disease.
    D Amyloidosis.
    E Citalopram overdose.

4 Which of these statements is correct?
    A Patients with postural hypotension have a cardioinhibitory response on tilt testing.
    B A vasodepressor response is characterised by reduction in systolic BP ≥ 20 mmHg in the absence of significant fall in HR.
    C Postural orthostatic tachycardia syndrome is a condition that predominantly affects older males with resting heart rate > 120 bpm.
    D Patients with neurally mediated syncope will commonly show abnormalities in ambulatory ECG monitoring and echocardiography.
    E Second-degree AV block immediately after inferior MI should be treated aggressively with temporary pacing to maintain haemodynamic parameters.

5 Which of the following would not be an indication for intravenous atropine in the management of a bradyarrhythmia?
    A Shock.
    B Ventricular pause > 3 s.
    C First-degree heart block.
    D Congestive heart failure.
    E Syncope.

References

1 Lamas, G.A., Knight, J.D., Sweeney, M.O. et al. (2007). Impact of rate-modulated pacing on quality of life and exercise capacity-evidence from the advanced elements of pacing randomized controlled trial (ADEPT). *Heart Rhythm* 4 (9): 1125–1132.

2 Brignole, M., Russo, V., Arabia, F. et al. (2021). Cardiac pacing in severe recurrent reflex syncope and tilt-induced asystole. *Eur. Heart J.* 42 (5): 508–516.

Further Reading

Brignole, M., Moya, A., de Lange, F.J. et al. (2018). 2018 ESC guidelines for the diagnosis and management of syncope. *Eur. Heart J.* 39 (21): 1883–1948.

Brubaker, P.H. and Kitzman, D.W. (2011). Chronotropic incompetence: causes, consequences, and management. *Circulation* 123 (9): 1010–1020.

Bryarly, M., Phillips, L.T., Fu, Q. et al. (2019). Postural orthostatic tachycardia syndrome: JACC focus seminar. *J. Am. Coll. Cardiol.* 73 (10): 1207–1228.

Chen-Scarabelli, C. and Scarabelli, T.M. (2004). Neurocardiogenic syncope. *Br. Med. J.* 329 (7461): 336–341.

Çinier, G., Haseeb, S., Bazoukis, G. et al. (2021). Evaluation and management of asymptomatic bradyarrhythmias. *Curr. Cardiol. Rev.* 17 (1): 60–67.

Glikson, M., Nielsen, J.C., Kronborg, M.B. et al. (2021). 2021 ESC guidelines on cardiac pacing and cardiac resynchronization therapy. *Eur. Heart J.* 42 (35): 3427–3520.

Sathnur, N., Ebin, E., and Benditt, D.G. (2021). Sinus node dysfunction. *Card Electrophysiol. Clin.* 13 (4): 641–659.

6

The Cardiac Pump

6.1   Learning Objectives

- Excitation–contraction coupling.
- Overview of cardiac anatomy.
- Phases of systole and diastole.
- Factors that regulate cardiac output.
- Pressure–volume dynamics and modulating factors.
- Haemodynamics of right and left ventricle.

Cardiology at its Core, First Edition. Peysh A. Patel.
© 2023 John Wiley & Sons Ltd. Published 2023 by John Wiley & Sons Ltd.

6.2 Excitation–Contraction Coupling

Excitation–contraction coupling describes coordination between electrical excitation of the myocardium and mechanical contraction in systole. Each muscle fibre within the myocardium consists of tubular **myofibrils**. These are themselves composed of repeated regions known as **sarcomeres** that define the basic structural unit. Sarcomeres demonstrate longitudinal strands of thick **myosin** and thin **actin** filaments. Myosin has a fibrous tail and a globular head which binds to actin and also adenosine triphosphate (ATP). Contraction occurs via calcium ion-mediated exposure of actin binding sites, enabling formation of cross-bridges between the two filament types and ATP hydrolysis. This causes 'pulling' of the actin strands towards the centre of the sarcomere with the two filaments sliding upon each other (**sliding filament hypothesis**) and causing contraction of the cell and syncytium as a whole.

The sequence of events is initiated by a rise in intracellular calcium concentration (see Figure 6.1). During the plateau phase of the action potential (phase 2), calcium permeability of the cell membrane (sarcolemma) is enhanced by activation of voltage-dependent L-type calcium channels. The presence of T-tubules, intracellular protrusions of the sarcolemma that invaginate the fibres, permits rapid propagation of membrane depolarisation into the cytosol. These calcium channels are referred to as dihydropyridine receptors because of their high affinity for this group of antagonists (e.g. amlodipine, nifedipine). The primary source of extracellular calcium is the interstitium but some may also be bound to the sarcolemma or glycocalyx, a mucopolysaccharide that envelops the sarcolemma. Calcium influx *per se* is insufficient for contraction but it augments calcium release from intracellular stores in the sarcoplasmic reticulum (SR) via ryanodine receptors (RyR). Cytosolic free calcium binds to troponin C and this complex interacts with tropomyosin to unblock binding sites on actin filaments and allow the formation of cross-bridges. At the termination of systole, calcium influx ceases and the SR is no longer stimulated. Additionally, phosphorylation of troponin I inhibits the binding of calcium to troponin C, allowing tropomyosin to block interaction sites and causing muscle relaxation. Calcium is recruited back into stores within the SR through ATP-dependent SERCA enzyme activity. There is also active efflux of calcium into the interstitium in diastole by the sodium–calcium exchanger (3 : 1 stoichiometry).

There are two predominant means by which the force of contraction can be regulated: (i) altering the amplitude or duration of calcium influx, and (ii) altering myofilament sensitivity to

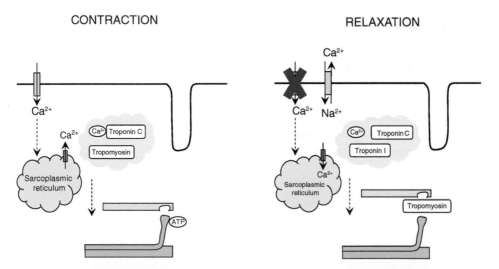

Figure 6.1 Excitation–contraction coupling in myofilament contraction and relaxation.

calcium. A higher intracellular calcium concentration results in greater abundance of cross-bridges, which determines force of contraction. This forms the basis for length-independent changes in contractility such as in the context of inotropic agents. Enhanced sensitivity correlates with increased rate of cross-bridge attachment and detachment. Myofilament sensitivity can be altered dynamically by physical stretch such as with increased preload and ventricular filling. This forms the basis for the classic **Frank–Starling mechanism** (see later).

Certain pharmacological agents have direct effects on the sequences implicated in excitation–contraction coupling. Digoxin operates as a positive inotrope to increase contractility by inhibition of the sodium–potassium pump in the sarcolemma. Net increase in intracellular sodium ions results in less efflux of calcium from the cell. By contrast, stimulation of β_1-adrenoceptors by catecholamines such as adrenaline and noradrenaline enhance contractility through cyclic adenosine monophosphate (cAMP)-dependent mechanisms that cause activatory phosphorylation of L-type calcium channels and greater release from the SR. Notably, they play a dual role in accelerating both contraction and relaxation. The latter occurs by phosphorylation of phospholamban, which in turn phosphorylates troponin I and potentiates calcium uptake into intracellular stores.

6.3 Cardiac Anatomy

The cardiac pump relies on sequenced contractility of the right ventricle (RV) and left ventricle (LV) which receive blood from the right atrium (RA) and left atrium (LA), respectively. These atria serve both as blood reservoirs and as pumps. In the pulmonary circuit, the RV receives venous blood at close to zero pressure and transmits blood to the pulmonary artery (PA) at a peak pressure of around 25 mmHg. Blood is oxygenated in the lungs and returns to the left heart via the LA. This drains into the LV which collects oxygenated blood, again at near zero pressure, and pumps at peak pressure of around 120 mmHg into the aorta and systemic circulation. During invasive assessment of intracardiac pressures, the pulmonary capillary wedge pressure (PCWP) is used as an indirect surrogate of left atrial pressure and is measured by inserting the catheter into a branch of the PA. A summary of typical cardiac pressures in each chamber and major vasculature is provided in Figure 6.2.

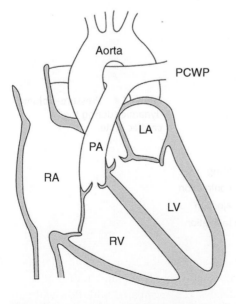

	Systole (mmHg)	Diastole (mmHg)
RA	2–8	2–8
RV	15–30	2–8
PA	15–30	4–12
PCWP	2–10	2–10
LA	2–10	2–10
LV	100–140	3–12
Aorta	100–140	60–90

Figure 6.2 Typical cardiovascular pressures.

In healthy individuals, pump efficiency is mediated by the presence of unidirectional valves. The pulmonary valves (PVs) and aortic valves (AVs), which are collectively termed semilunar, are located at the RV and LV outflow tracts. The aortic valve is usually tricuspid (right coronary cusp [RCC], left coronary cusp [LCC], and non-coronary cusp [NCC]). Its opening does not result in total adherence to the wall of the aorta and this permits unrestricted perfusion to the right and left coronary arteries that originate from the sinuses of Valsalva immediately above the valve. The two valves between the atria and ventricles are labelled as mitral (MV) and tricuspid (TV), with the former being bicuspid. Both are supported during systole by attachment to the papillary muscles in the ventricles via chordae tendinae. A detailed exploration of valve anatomy is provided in Chapter 13.

6.4 Cardiac Cycle

The cardiac pump is reliant upon orchestration of transmitted electrical activity with mechanical contraction. This results in predictable pressure and volume changes within each chamber and correlates with valve dynamics and findings on auscultation. A broad overview is provided in Figures 6.3 and 6.4, and reflects the typical cardiac cycle. For simplification, the LV is used for descriptive purposes although broadly equivalent principles apply to both ventricles.

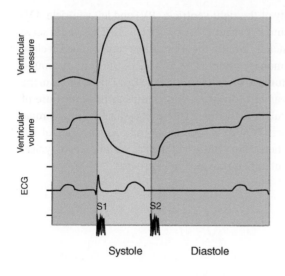

Figure 6.3 Overview of the cardiac cycle. S1 = 1st heart sound; S2 = 2nd heart sounds.

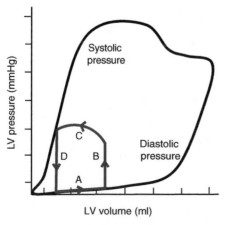

Figure 6.4 Pressure–volume dynamics during the cardiac cycle.

A   Ventricular filling
B   Isovolumic contraction
C   Ventricular ejection
D   Isovolumic relaxation

The cycle has two main components: **systole** (ventricular contraction) and **diastole** (ventricular filling during relaxation). Systole is defined as the segment between MV closure and AV closure. At rest, it represents three-eighths of total cycle duration. The remaining five-eighths is defined by diastole and strictly reflects duration from AV closure ('end-systole', end of T wave) to MV closure ('end-diastole', start of Q wave). It is typically subdivided into four distinct phases: **isovolumic relaxation**, **rapid filling**, **slow filling (diastasis)**, and **atrial systole**.

6.4.1 Systole

As alluded to, systole refers to the segment of the cardiac cycle that defines ventricular contraction. This occurs as a consequence of ventricular depolarisation as represented by the QRS complex, which terminates after repolarisation (i.e. end of the T wave). Onset occurs when LV pressure exceeds LA pressure and corresponds to the first heart sound (S1) (see Chapter 13). This is preceded by a phase of isovolumic contraction during which the LV contracts but AV remains closed. Hence, there is an increase in chamber pressure and alterations in ventricular geometry but without concomitant alterations in volume. When LV pressure exceeds aortic pressure, the AV opens and ejection occurs. This period of ejection lasts between AV opening and closure. This is most marked in the first half of systole (acceleration), but pressure crossover occurs so that in the second half, aortic pressure exceeds LV pressure and there is deceleration of forward velocities. Overall, two-thirds of the stroke volume (SV) is ejected from the LV in the first third of systole. Ventricular volumes are the smallest at end-systole.

6.4.2 Diastole

6.4.2.1 Isovolumic Relaxation
This interval occurs from AV closure, corresponding to the second heart sound (S2), to MV opening. Hence, ventricular pressure falls without an increase in volume. It is an active process that consumes ATP. Factors that affect this period of relaxation include internal and external loading conditions in addition to metabolic, neurohumoral, and pharmacological factors. An abnormal prolongation in relaxation time is a marker of early diastolic dysfunction (see Chapter 12).

6.4.2.2 Rapid Filling
This corresponds with LV pressure falling below LA pressure and mediates opening of the MV. Rapid ventricular filling results in increased chamber volumes, around two-thirds of the total within the first third of diastole. The rate and time course of filling are reliant upon ventricular compliance, a passive process which itself is dependent on shape, geometry and extrinsic influences mediated by the pericardium or pleura. Ventricular hypertrophy and infarction with secondary remodelling represent the most common cause of chamber stiffness and reduced compliance. Ventricular myocardium also exhibits a capacity for elastic recoil. This describes the storage of potential energy during systole in the form of a longitudinal gradient of circumferential rotation (twist). This is released during early diastole and augments filling.

6.4.2.3 Slow Filling (Diastasis)
During the phase of diastasis, there is equalisation of pressures between LA and LV resulting in minimal flow. However, pooled blood returning from the periphery flows into the RV and from the lungs into the LV. This contribution corresponds to a small, gradual increase in atrial and subsequent ventricular volumes in mid-diastole but without pronounced effect on cavity pressures. Duration of

diastasis is affected by heart rate (HR) and is shorter at faster rates. Indeed, in those with significant tachycardia, atrial contribution can become more marked. Diastolic reserve also becomes exhausted and this can compromise cardiac output (CO). Conversely, patients with significant bradycardia have prolongation of filling duration but as this is primarily in early diastole, the relative increase in SV is not sufficient to compensate for the lower HR and overall CO is impaired. A more detailed exploration of the primary determinants of CO is provided in Section 6.5.

6.4.2.4 Atrial Systole

Atrial contraction results in LA pressure exceeding LV pressure once more, which initiates a second phase of ventricular filling. In healthy individuals, this contribution is typically only 20% of total filling. Because there are no obstructive valves at the junctions of the venae cavae and RA, atrial systole can propel blood in both antegrade and retrograde directions. In the absence of valvular stenosis or ventricular disease limiting relaxation, inertia caused by inflow of blood prevents significant backflow of blood into the venous system.

6.5 Cardiac Output and its Regulation

6.5.1 Definitions

Cardiac output can be defined as the volume of blood ejected from the LV each minute. It is a composite of HR and SV, the latter being defined as the volume of blood ejected from the LV during each cardiac cycle. By inference, it can be calculated as the difference between end-diastole volume (EDV) and end-systole volume (ESV). This differs from calculation of ejection fraction (EF), which is detailed separately in Section 12.5. Normal SV in an adult is approximately 70 ml so assuming a resting HR of 70 bpm, this equates to CO of roughly $5 \, l \, min^{-1}$:

$$CO = (EDV - ESV) \times HR$$

Regulation of CO is dependent on the following components: preload, afterload, inotropic state (contractility), and HR. A discussion of each is provided.

6.5.2 Preload

The concept of preload can be understood by considering an unstressed muscle strip with its resting length as a starting point. Attaching a weight to one end of the strip will stretch its resting length. This length will be proportional to the weight attached and to the elastic properties of the muscle itself (which reflects the relationship between volume and pressure). This weight, or force, is defined as the preload of the ventricle. In clinical terms, the resting fibre length of the contractile unit of a myofibril, i.e. sarcomere, can be enhanced by augmenting preload and ventricular filling and is maximal at EDV. During contraction, force is generated in the ventricular wall and transferred to the blood within the cavity causing a rise in intraventricular pressure and SV. It is prudent to note that fibre length may change during this period as the ventricle assumes a more spherical shape.

This process represents an expression of heterometric autoregulation otherwise known as the **Frank–Starling mechanism**:

"The energy of contraction is a function of the length of the muscle fibre".

In other words, both the length and velocity of muscle shortening during contraction will increase in proportion to stretch in resting length (i.e. preload). It can be conceived as an intrinsic property of the ventricles that is derived from the muscle fibre itself. It is not reliant upon neural or humoral influence although these can modify intrinsic response. The mechanism plays a critical role in balancing output between RV and LV, in distribution of blood between pulmonary and systemic circulations and in adaptive states such as exercise.

Increased preload also results in direct increase in HR (**Bainbridge reflex**), exerted by the presence of stretch receptors located at the veno-atrial junctions.

6.5.3 Afterload

If a second weight is attached to the muscle strip whilst it is contracting, this results in constant tension during shortening. This represents the afterload of the ventricle. It also modulated contraction and is inversely related to the length and velocity of muscle shortening. Systemic vascular resistance (SVR) is the major contributor to afterload. At physiological arterial pressures, however, CO is relatively independent of afterload. Even with temporary reduction of SV that results from increased afterload, forces generated from RV contraction permit maintenance of LV filling (preload reserve) and restoration of left ventricular end-diastolic pressure (LVEDP). This physiological response is known as the **Anrep phenomenon**.

6.5.4 Inotropy

If preload and afterload are maintained, contractility (i.e. length and velocity of contraction) can be enhanced by increasing inotropy. This may be achieved, for instance, through sympathetic activation or use of inotropic drugs such as digoxin and adrenaline. It provides the distinct advantage of greater vigour in myocardial contractility at an equivalent EDV. Diastolic compliance is not directly affected in the absence of myocardial ischaemia or scar. If the precipitant is an increase in sympathetic tone, there will be concomitant increase in HR. In this context, SV may be limited by the shortened period of ventricular filling but the net result is usually an increase in CO.

6.5.5 Heart Rate

As stated earlier, the fourth major determinant of CO is HR. At a constant filling pressure, increased HR will reduce diastolic filling, LVEDP and SV. However, as filling predominates in the early phase of diastole, a modest increase in HR may encroach on the diastasis phase and minimise impact. If HR is increased through iatrogenic means using a pacemaker, CO will first rise but then plateau and subsequently decline at rates in the region of 120–130 bpm. This is due to proportional decrease in SV at higher HR with CO more meaningfully regulated by changes in peripheral vasodilation. If the tachycardia is occurring in physiological contexts such as exercise, the equivalent decline in CO tends to manifest at much higher rates of around 180 bpm [1]. This disparity is a combination of increased preload secondary to skeletal muscle flow and venous return in addition to direct inotropy. The promotion of inotropy (**Bowditch effect**) is deemed to be due to saturation of sodium–potassium ATPases at higher rates, resulting in accumulation of intracellular calcium via the sodium–calcium exchanger.

6.6 Pressure–Volume Relationships

The relationship between preload and SV can be depicted by the Frank–Starling function curve (see Figure 6.5). In healthy subjects who have preserved LVEDP (around 10–12 mmHg), the LV operates close to its maximum function. Any attempts to increase filling volume beyond this point lead to an increase in filling pressure but only modest improvements in SV. However, in the presence of abnormally low filling pressures, the ventricle operates on the ascending limb of the curve. Hence, increasing preload via fluid resuscitation for instance can improve pump function considerably by shifting the point on the curve to the right.

Importantly, there is no single fixed curve on which the ventricle operates. Rather, there is a spectrum of curves which are influenced by afterload and inotropy. Increased afterload or decreased inotropy will shift the curve down and to the right. At any given LVEDP, there will be a corresponding reduction in SV. If the afterload is reduced or inotropy is increased, the curve will be deflected up and to the left. Incremental pacing and physiological exercise both also shift the curve positively but relative magnitude is more significant with exercise due to adjunct effects of direct inotropy and enhanced preload as described. The capacity to increase SV in response to preload is an inherent function of normal ventricles with preserved function.

Importantly, congestive heart failure (CHF) results in a downward shift of the performance curve and therefore, at any given preload, SV will be reduced. This results in insufficient chamber emptying, higher accumulation of blood during diastole and amplified residual volume, which increases myocardial fibre stretch and induces a larger SV with the next contraction. This mechanism enables preservation of CO but its benefit as a compensatory mechanism is limited. In severe CHF, the performance curve may be nearly flat at higher diastolic volumes and elevations in LVEDP can result in pulmonary congestion.

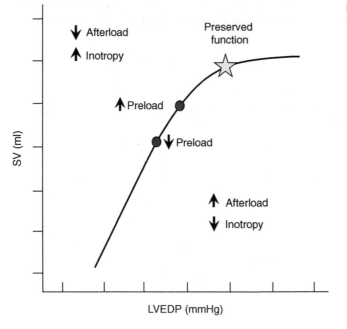

Figure 6.5 Principles of the Frank–Starling function curve.

6.7 Right Ventricle

The discussion of principles that govern the cardiac cycle and pump have been primarily centred on the LV. However, it is worth briefly providing a comparison of the RV and LV (see Table 6.1). There is a synergistic relationship between both ventricles which is pivotal for synchronicity. The ventricles share a blood supply and muscular interventricular septum that separates cavities, with myocardial bundles distributed over both. Additionally, both are encased within the same pericardium and exposed to similar perturbations of intrathoracic pressures.

However, the RV is crescent-shaped in contrast to the conical LV. The LV outflow tract exhibits a specific dyssynchrony of around 25–50 ms with the body of the ventricle, which facilitates outflow tract relaxation during inflow tract contraction and preservation of SV. Wall thickness and myocardial mass are much lower in the RV than in the LV and this reduced metabolic requirements into a lower pressure and resistance system of the pulmonary vascular bed. The corresponding reduction in intramural and intraventricular pressure results in continuous coronary arterial flow to the RV throughout the cardiac cycle. This is in stark contrast to coronaries supplying the LV where perfusion predominates in the diastolic phase. The total duration of diastole in the RV is slightly shorter due to its longer systolic period.

General principles of the Frank–Starling function curve apply to both ventricles. However, the RV is less adaptable to both acute and chronic increases in afterload. In cases of pulmonary hypertension, the RV utilises its preload reserve more readily and this causes chamber dilatation. High compliance of the thin-walled RV during diastole allows maintenance of pulmonary blood flow and LV filling without significant shift in central venous pressure. A prerequisite for this, however, is adequate preload reserve. Hence, in cases of cardiogenic shock secondary to RV infarction, adequate filling is imperative to maintain preload and CO.

It is unsurprising that there is ventricular interdependence in terms of function both in diastole and systole. Increased filling in one ventricle causes decrease in chamber compliance and filling of the other. To describe it differently, the point on the Frank–Starling function curve is shifted to the left. This interdependence is most apparent when the pericardium is intact and is typically confirmed on echocardiography as septal flattening during diastole in cases of volume overload. An example of systolic interdependence is the contribution of the LV to RV ejection. This is accomplished by pulling the RV free wall towards the septum during contraction of intertwining muscle bundles. Indeed, if the pulmonary vascular resistance was negligible, one may perceive the RV as a dispensable entity in

Table 6.1 Physiological comparison of the right and left ventricle.

Similarities	Differences
Coronary arterial blood supply	RV – crescent shape, LV – oval shape
Intertwining myocardial bundles	RV – pumps to pulmonary circulation, LV – pumps to systemic circulation
Encased within pericardium	RV – less myocardial mass
Similarly influenced by intrathoracic pressures	RV – lower metabolic requirements
Both influenced by principles of Frank–Starling function curve	RV – continuous coronary flow, LV – coronary flow predominates in diastole
Ventricular interdependence	RV – more sensitive to alterations in afterload
Cavity volumes	RV – trabeculations more coarse

cardiac pump physiology. A clinical example is in the context of a total cavo-pulmonary circulation, (e.g. post-Fontan procedure), where the RV is completely bypassed and venous blood is redirected to the pulmonary circulation to form a univentricular system.

Hot Points

- Excitation–contraction coupling describes coordination of electrical and mechanical activity during systole and relies on the 'sliding filament hypothesis'.
- Systole is defined as the segment between MV and AV closure and constitutes three-eighths of total cycle duration. The remainder is the diastolic phase.
- Diastole has four distinct phases: isovolumic relaxation, rapid filling, diastasis and atrial systole.
- CO is a composite of HR and SV.
- The Frank–Starling mechanism describes modulation of ventricular contraction in response to ventricular filling (preload).
- Both LV and RV have intertwining myocardial bundles, are encased within the pericardium and are influenced by Frank–Starling principles. There is also ventricular interdependence.

6.8 Self-assessment Questions

1   In relation to excitation–contraction coupling, select the correct statement.
   A   Muscle fibres within the myocardium consist of sarcomeres, which are themselves composed of repeated regions known as tubular myofibrils.
   B   During the process of myocardial contraction, ADP is phosphorylated to generate ATP.
   C   The two predominant means by which force of contraction can be regulated are via alterations in frequency of calcium influx and myofilament sensitivity to calcium.
   D   Digoxin operates as a positive inotrope to increase contractility by inhibition of sodium–potassium pump in the sarcolemma. The net increase in intracellular sodium ions results in less efflux of calcium from the cell.
   E   At the termination of systole, phosphorylation of troponin I activates binding of calcium to troponin C, allowing tropomyosin to block interaction sites and causing muscle relaxation.

2   In relation to cardiac anatomy, which of these statements is correct?
   A   The RV and LV pump blood to the pulmonary and systemic circulations, respectively, at a peak pressure of 120 mmHg.
   B   AV opening results in leaflet adherence to the wall of the aorta, thereby occluding origins of the coronary arteries and limiting coronary blood flow in diastole.
   C   AV and PV are collectively termed semilunar, with the MV and TV termed atrioventricular.
   D   In healthy individuals, only the PV is bicuspid whereas AV, MV, and TV are tricuspid.
   E   In healthy individuals, LA pressure of 20 mmHg in systole is within normal limits.

3   In relation to the cardiac cycle, select the correct statement.
   A Systole represents just under 40% of total cycle duration whilst the remaining proportion comprises diastole.
   B Onset of systole occurs when pressure in the LV exceeds aortic pressure.
   C Isovolumic relaxation occurs from AV closure to MV opening and is a passive process.
   D Rapid ventricular filling results in increased chamber volumes, and around one-third of total filling occurs within the first two-thirds of diastole.
   E Patients with significant bradycardia have prolonged filling time and this allows a relative increase in SV and overall CO.

4   In relation to cardiac output and its regulation, which is correct?
   A CO is a product of SV and HR, whereby SV is the sum of EDV and ESV.
   B The Frank–Starling mechanism explains why pump function can be improved by fluid resuscitation in the context of hypovolaemia.
   C Use of inotropic agents, such as digoxin and adrenaline, increase myocardial contractility and improve diastolic compliance.
   D If HR is increased through iatrogenic means such as a pacemaker, CO will first rise but then plateau and subsequently decline.
   E According to the Frank–Starling principle, energy of contraction is independent of length of muscle fibre.

5   When comparing the left and right ventricles, which of the following statements is false?
   A Both are influenced by principles of the Frank–Starling function curve.
   B The RV is composed of less myocardial mass.
   C Coronary flow to each ventricle predominates in diastole.
   D The RV is more sensitive to alterations in afterload.
   E Both are similarly influenced by intrathoracic pressures.

Reference

1 Bada, A.A., Svendsen, J.H., Secher, N.H. et al. (2012). Peripheral vasodilatation determines cardiac output in exercising humans: insight from atrial pacing. *J. Physiol.* 590 (8): 2051–2060. https://doi.org/10.1113/jphysiol.2011.225334.

Further Reading

Bers, D.M. (2002). Cardiac excitation-contraction coupling. *Nature* 415 (6868): 198–205.

Burkhoff, D., Mirsky, I., and Suga, H. (2005). Assessment of systolic and diastolic ventricular properties via pressure-volume analysis: a guide for clinical, translational, and basic researchers. *Am. J. Physiol. Heart Circ. Physiol.* 289 (2): H501–H512.

Fukuta, H. and Little, W.C. (2008). The cardiac cycle and the physiologic basis of left ventricular contraction, ejection, relaxation, and filling. *Heart Fail. Clin.* 4 (1): 1–11.

Mori, S., Spicer, D.E., and Anderson, R.H. (2016). Revisiting the anatomy of the living heart. *Circ. J.* 80 (1): 24–33.

Vincent, J.L. (2008). Understanding cardiac output. *Crit. Care* 12 (4): 174.

7

Arterial and Venous System

CHAPTER MENU

7.1   Learning Objectives

- Role of the circulatory system in pressure and volume dynamics.
- Components and determinants of systemic blood pressure.
- Central and auxiliary factors that affect the venous system.

7.2   Pressure and Volume Dynamics

Around two-thirds of total blood volume is normally in the venous system, with only one-sixth on the arterial side. However, pressure distribution differs distinctly in being almost inversely related to volume distribution. Arteries have large amounts of elastin that enable considerable expansion and storage of potential energy which can be released during elastic recoil. These arteries can therefore be considered as **'pressure storers'** of the circulation. The collecting system extends from the small venules to the venae cavae and drain blood back to the right atrium. Veins are large-capacity, thin-walled vessels with low internal pressure but intrinsic distensibility that is six- to eight-fold higher than that of arteries in normal physiology. This mediates their role as **'volume**

storers' of the circulation. Overall capacity of the venous system for blood storage is 25- to 30-fold higher than the arterial system and can reflect around 80% of total circulatory volume. Infusion of blood or fluids, therefore, is redistributed predominantly in the venous system.

7.3 Arterial System

7.3.1 Pressure Waves

Blood pressure (BP) is a measure of the force that is exerted on the walls of arteries during the cardiac cycle (i.e. systole and diastole). As highlighted in Chapter 6, approximately two-thirds of stroke volume (SV) is ejected from the left ventricle (LV) into the aorta during the first third of systole. This is followed by a sharp fall in ejection rate. At the end of systole, there is a small reversal of flow from the aorta due to perfusion of the coronary vasculature and slight regurgitation across the aortic valve (AV).

Aortic pressure is simpler to measure than flow (see Figure 7.1). Moreover, as it is anatomically situated between the heart and peripheral circulation, it provides a useful indicator of both. The ascending limb of the aortic pressure wave is due to LV ejection with secondary aortic wall distension. After a peak is reached (i.e. systolic BP), aortic pressure exceeds ventricular pressure. At this point, the AV closes with a small rebound wave (**dicrotic notch**) that marks the incisura and end of systole. Arterial distension results in storage of potential energy (Windkessel effect) which is released during elastic recoil with propulsion of blood distally and a diastolic run-off. This results in a long, declining pressure wave. The alternation of systolic and diastolic propulsion transmits flow to the peripheries and is more continuous rather than pulsatile in nature. The lowest point of the pressure wave is the diastolic BP. The difference between systolic and diastolic BP is the **pulse pressure**. It can also be used to provide a rough estimation of mean arterial BP (**MAP**), which is the single best measure of effective driving force as it reflects relative durations of each phase in the cardiac cycle. It can be quantified using the following equation:

$$MAP = \text{diastolic BP} + 1/3\left(\text{systolic BP} - \text{diastolic BP}\right)$$

The pressure values and corresponding wave configurations are altered during transmission through the arterial tree. As flow progresses distally, the corresponding dicrotic notch becomes less

Figure 7.1 Aortic pressure trace.

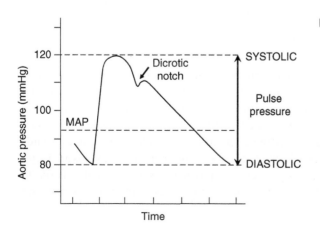

pronounced. In the descending aorta, systolic pressure is higher and the diastolic pressure lower. This is attributed primarily to resonant oscillations of
ejected blood acting on the elastic arteries and also due to reflection of pulse
waves from the distal vascular bed. However, the mean pressure is lower in
the more distal arteries. The pulsatile characteristics of the pressure wave are
usually obliterated at the level of the capillaries.

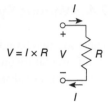

Figure 7.2 Ohm's law.

7.3.2   Determinants of Systemic BP

This can be conceived by applying **Ohm's law** (see Figure 7.2), which states that the current (I)
through a conductor between two points is directly proportional to the voltage (V) across it. If
resistance (R) is introduced as the constant of proportionality, the following equation is derived:

$$V = I \times R$$

Based upon application of these principles, MAP can be considered as a composite of cardiac
output (CO), total peripheral resistance (TPR) and central venous pressure (CVP). As defined,
CO is determined by SV and heart rate (HR). TPR is otherwise known as systemic vascular
resistance and refers to the total resistance that must be overcome to force blood through
the circulatory system and generate flow. CVP defines the pressure in the vena caval systems
and is normally a good approximate of right atrial pressure (RAP). Its absolute values are
small and can broadly be ignored for the purpose of calculating MAP. Hence, it can be defined
as follows:

$$MAP = (HR \times SV) \times TPR$$

The primary determinants of systolic and diastolic BP are outlined in Table 7.1. Reduced aortic
distensibility can arise secondary to vascular calcification such as that seen with increased age.
This will increase systolic BP and the lack of recoil will reduce diastolic BP. Hence, pulse pressure will increase. Increased SV will increase systolic BP, pulse pressure and MAP. A higher
ejection velocity will increase pulse pressure because of inadequate time for the aortic wall to
distend. An increase in TPR will augment diastolic BP and, eventually, systolic BP. Lastly, a faster
HR interrupts the diastolic decline at a higher point on the curve and diastolic BP will therefore
increase. This overview provides a conceptual perspective but in clinical terms, the presence of
coexistent disease and compensatory mechanisms makes interpretation significantly more
complex.

Table 7.1 Determinants of systolic and diastolic BP.

Systolic BP	Diastolic BP
Aortic distensibility	Systolic BP
SV	Aortic distensibility
Ejection velocity	TPR
	HR

7.4 Venous System

There are two broad factors that influence return of blood from the circulation back to the heart: mean circulatory pressure and auxiliary factors. The latter includes effects mediated by the skeletal pump, venous valves, venomotor tone, respiration, and the suction effect.

7.4.1 Mean Circulatory Pressure

The mean circulatory pressure is a static, driving pressure that represents the haemodynamic gradient for the entire systemic circulation. This can be considered as the difference between MAP and CVP.

7.4.2 Auxiliary Factors

7.4.2.1 Skeletal Pump

Upon standing, gravitational pull can result in sequestration of blood in the lower limbs and potentially reduce venous return by up to 20–25%. Skeletal muscles in the lower extremities, particularly in the calves, begin cyclical reflex contraction and relaxation that augments filling during relaxation and flow during contraction. This mechanism is also critical in physical exertion as excess blood in the extremities not only creates a deficit in circulating volume but can also hinder capillary exchange.

7.4.2.2 Venous Valves

Present in the extremities, these valves prevent retrograde flow when functioning normally. They occur at 2–4 cm intervals in the deep and superficial veins of the legs and are indispensable in optimising function of calf muscles. The walls of the veins surrounding valves are expanded into a sinus which allow cusps to separate fully without contraction of the walls and facilitates rapid valve closure.

7.4.2.3 Venomotor Function

These effects are primarily determined by the intravascular pressure. At low pressure, veins have an elliptical shape in cross-section and contraction has little effect on flow. However, at higher pressures exceeding 5–10 mmHg, veins assume a more spherical appearance and venomotor activity becomes more effective. Neural control of venous smooth muscle is exclusively sympathetic. In certain situations, such as in haemorrhagic shock, constriction of splanchnic veins shifts the pooled reservoir to increase venous return.

7.4.2.4 Respiration

This refers to the assistance given to venous return by movements during respiration. Pressures in the venae cavae and right atrium are highly dependent upon intrapleural pressure (P_{pl}), which defines pressure within the thoracic space between the organs (lung, heart, etc.) and the chest wall (see Figure 7.3). During inspiration, chest wall expansion and diaphragmatic descent result in a lower, more negative P_{pl} and expansion of lungs, cardiac chambers and veins. Right atrial expansion results in reduced RAP and enhanced pressure gradient for venous filling (i.e. preload). During expiration, the converse is true. The left side of the heart responds differently to respiratory variation. This is because lung expansion during inspiration increases the capacity of pulmonary vasculature, resulting in pooling, reduced left atrial filling and impaired SV. This effect is exaggerated in cases of constrictive pericarditis or cardiac tamponade and can be assessed on echocardiography to aid with diagnosis (see Section 14.5.5.2).

Figure 7.3 Pressure–volume dynamics of right heart during respiration.

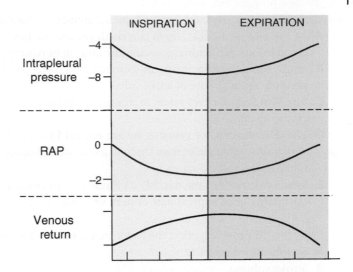

Due to the large pulmonary reservoir, left ventricular filling is less sensitive to respiratory dynamics than right ventricular filling. Additionally, haemodynamics are such that the net effect of increased rate and depth of ventilation is augmentation of SV on both right and left sides of the heart. When atypical respiratory movements are considered, such as continuous positive airway pressure (CPAP) ventilation or the Valsalva manoeuvre, these impede venous return and SV.

7.4.2.5 Suction

The ventricles also contribute directly to venous return. During systole, the atrioventricular ring is drawn downwards by the ventricles, enlarging the atria and lowering chamber pressure. This enhances flow from the venae cavae and pulmonary veins into the right and left atria, respectively. During diastole, the ventricles exert a negative pressure due to elastic recoil properties.

Hot Points

- Arteries have the ability to store potential energy (pressure storers) and veins are large-capacity vessels with distensibility (volume storers).
- Blood pressure (BP) refers to the force exerted on walls of arteries during the cardiac cycle.
- Pulse pressure is defined by the difference between systolic and diastolic BP.
- BP is determined by CO and TPR. This formula is analogous to Ohm's law.
- Venous return is modulated by lower-extremity skeletal muscles, valves, venomotor tone, respiration and the suction effect.

7.5 Self-assessment Questions

1 In relation to calculation of MAP, select the correct equation.
   A MAP = diastolic BP + 1/3 (systolic BP − diastolic BP)
   B MAP = systolic BP + 1/3 (systolic BP − diastolic BP)
   C MAP = diastolic BP + 2/3 (systolic BP − diastolic BP)
   D MAP = systolic BP + 2/3 (systolic BP − diastolic BP)
   E MAP = diastolic BP + 1/3 (systolic BP + diastolic BP)

2 With regard to the arterial system, which statement is correct?

A At the end of diastole, there is a small reversal of flow from the aorta, resulting from blood influx into coronary vasculature and slight regurgitation across the aortic valve.

B In the aortic pressure wave, the dicrotic notch corresponds to transient increase in aortic pressure upon closure of aortic valve.

C The Windkessel effect refers to storage of volume that is subsequently released during elastic recoil.

D The determinants of systemic BP are related in a way that is analogous to Watt's law, which states that the current through a conductor between two points is directly proportional to the voltage across it.

E When calculating systemic BP, CVP refers to pressure in the vena caval system and is normally a good approximate of right ventricular pressure.

3 From the list provided, select the factor that is not a determinant of diastolic blood pressure.

A Systolic blood pressure.

B Stroke volume.

C Aortic distensibility.

D Total peripheral resistance.

E Heart rate.

4 In relation to the venous system, select the correct statement.

A Mean circulatory pressure can be considered as the difference between systolic blood pressure and CVP.

B Upon standing, gravitational pull can result in sequestration of blood in the lower limbs and reduce venous return by up to 5–10%.

C Venous valves occur at 2–4 cm intervals in the deep and superficial veins and prevent retrograde flow.

D At low pressure, veins have an elliptical shape in cross-section and contraction has a significant effect on flow. However, at higher pressures exceeding 5–10 mmHg, veins assume a more spherical appearance and venomotor activity becomes less effective.

E During inspiration, lung expansion decreases capacity of pulmonary vasculature, resulting in increased left atrial filling and augmented SV.

5 With regard to the venous system, which statement is incorrect?

A The auxiliary factors that influence return of circulatory blood back to the heart are skeletal pump, venous valves, venomotor function, respiration and suction.

B The skeletal pump mechanism is critical in physical exertion as excess blood in the extremities creates a deficit in circulating volume and hinders capillary exchange.

C Walls of the veins surrounding valves are expanded into a sinus which allows cusps to separate fully without contraction of the walls and facilitates rapid valve closure.

D The effect of inspiration on SV is reduced in cases of constrictive pericarditis or cardiac tamponade.

E During systole, the atrioventricular ring is drawn downwards by the ventricles and this enlarges atria and lowers chamber pressures.

Further Reading

Bazigou, E. and Makinen, T. (2013). Flow control in our vessels: vascular valves make sure there is no way back. *Cell. Mol. Life Sci.* 70 (6): 1055–1066.

Magder, S. (2016). Volume and its relationship to cardiac output and venous return (published correction appears in *Crit. Care.* 2017 Jan 26;21(1):16). *Crit. Care* 20 (1): 271. Published 2016 Sep 10.

Monnet, X. and Teboul, J.L. (2006). Invasive measures of left ventricular preload. *Curr. Opin. Crit. Care* 12 (3): 235–240.

Strandberg, T.E. and Pitkala, K. (2003). What is the most important component of blood pressure: systolic, diastolic or pulse pressure? *Curr. Opin. Nephrol. Hypertens.* 12 (3): 293–297.

Tansey, E.A., Montgomery, L.E.A., Quinn, J.G. et al. (2019). Understanding basic vein physiology and venous blood pressure through simple physical assessments. *Adv. Physiol. Educ.* 43 (3): 423–429.

8

Regulation of the Circulatory System

8.1   Learning Objectives

- Neural mechanisms that regulate the circulatory system, including cardiovascular control centres, vasomotor tone and autonomic nervous system.
- Intrinsic and extrinsic reflexes in the context of physiology and pathology.
- Humoral influences, such as catecholamines, renin–angiotensin–aldosterone system, nitric oxide, and atrial natriuretic peptide.
- Local autoregulation of blood flow.
- Phenomenon of functional hyperaemia.

8.2 Overview

Regulation of the circulatory system to maintain a constant arterial pressure is crucial in providing adequate perfusion to meet metabolic demands of tissues. As outlined in Chapter 7, blood pressure (BP) can be considered in the context of Ohm's law, whereby BP (analogous to voltage) is directly proportional to the product of cardiac output (CO; analogous to current) and total peripheral resistance (TPR) (vascular resistance). Acute regulatory mechanisms are coordinated in the cardiovascular control centres (CCCs) in the brainstem. These coordinate efferents of the autonomic nervous system (ANS) but are also themselves influenced by impulses from other neural centres in addition to sensors both intrinsic and extrinsic to the circulation. Certain organs such as the heart, kidneys and brain have the ability to coordinate blood flow locally, i.e. to autoregulate. This allows alterations in regional perfusion without perturbations in BP.

8.3 Neural Control

8.3.1 Cardiovascular Control Centres

The CCCs of the central nervous system (CNS) are located in the lower pons and medulla oblongata (i.e. brainstem), in close proximity to the centres regulating respiration. The CCCs have two major subdivisions that innervate the heart (**cardiac control centre**) and peripheral vasculature (**vasomotor centre**), with significant anatomical and functional overlap.

The cardiac control centre can be further subdivided. The **cardioinhibitory** centre has parasympathetic vagal efferents (parasympathetic nervous system, PNS) to reduce heart rate (HR) and, to a lesser extent, atrial contractility. Activation of the **cardiostimulatory** centre increases HR (chronotropy) and myocardial contractility (inotropy) via activation of the sympathetic nervous system (SNS). The vasomotor centre also has discrete functional regions. Its **vasoconstrictor** area (C-1) contains a high concentration of neurons secreting noradrenaline (NA). This area has been proposed as one of the sites of clonidine, which binds to presynaptic α2 receptors, inhibits release of NA and reduces TPR. Neurons send vasoconstrictor fibres to the periphery via the SNS. A **vasodilator** region (A-1) inhibits activity of C-1. Finally, a sensory area A-2 receives input from cranial nerves IX and X, and efferent neurons project to vasoconstrictor and vasodilatory areas to regulate output.

The CCC also receives modulatory neural input from other discrete regions within the brain, including the motor cortex, frontal cortex and limbic system (hypothalamus, hippocampus, and amygdala), the latter being associated with emotional response. The cardiostimulatory, cardioinhibitory and vasoconstrictor areas are tonically active.

8.3.2 Vasomotor Tone

Vasomotor tone can be defined as 'the sum of muscular forces intrinsic to the blood vessel opposing an increase in vessel diameter'. This is mediated by vascular smooth muscle cells (VSMCs) in the media layer of vessel walls. Regions of endothelial cells project into this layer (myoendothelial junction) at various points along arterioles, suggesting a functional interaction between the two. VSMCs have an abundance of thin actin filaments but relatively low number of thick myosin filaments. Compared with skeletal muscle, they contract more slowly but generate higher forces with sustainable activity. Cell-to-cell conduction is via gap junctions as occurs in the myocardium.

The interaction between actin and myosin that leads to contraction is regulated by intracellular calcium concentration as with other muscle types, but molecular mechanism differs. VSMCs lack troponin and fast sodium channels. The increase in intracellular calcium arises from voltage-gated channels and receptor-mediated channels in the sarcolemma with additional release from the sarcoplasmic reticulum. Free calcium binds to calmodulin which in turn binds to myosin light chain kinase. This activated complex phosphorylates myosin cross-bridges and initiates contraction. Dephosphorylation of cross-bridges in conjunction with reduction in intracellular calcium results in relaxation.

As alluded to, vasomotor tone has various determinants including the ANS and humoral agents such as catecholamines (e.g. adrenaline), angiotensin II and nitric oxide (NO). Basal vasomotor tone is mediated by low-level, continuous impulses from the SNS (around one per second) in addition to partial arteriolar and venular constriction via VSMC contraction. Circulating adrenaline from the adrenal medulla may complement this. Basal tone is maintained at around 50% of maximum constriction. Hence, vasodilation can arise from a reduction in tonic SNS activity without directly eliciting PNS activity. The existence of basal tone results in minimal resistance to flow in the venules compared with arterioles as they are highly distensible. Nonetheless, autonomic effects influence capacitance which has direct consequence on venous return and preload.

The importance of vascular tone in regulation and maintenance of BP is reflected in clinical contexts associated with severe insults to the CNS, such as brain injury and high-level damage of the spinal cord. Trauma results in a sudden interruption of sympathetic preganglionic vasoconstrictor fibres. This causes a drastic fall in BP and a state of neurogenic shock in which only parasympathetic tone remains. Clinically, patients may appear flushed, priapic and with the inability to generate a compensatory tachycardia. If injury is above C3, a loss of neural control of the diaphragm can result in fatal respiratory arrest.

There is variability in baseline between different organs. For instance, the cerebral circulation has lower vascular tone and vasodilatory capacity compared with myocardial vasculature. Other circulations including skeletal muscle, skin and splanchnic circulations have higher resting tone.

8.3.3 Autonomic Nervous System

As indicated, the CCC modulates the ANS which itself provides direct innervation to myocardium and VSMCs. There are two complementary systems, sympathetic (SNS) and parasympathetic (PNS), with each having two interconnected neurons. Preganglionic neurons originate within the CNS but relay to the autonomic ganglion, with postganglionic neurons innervating the effector organs. In the ANS, all preganglionic neurons release the neurotransmitter acetylcholine (Ach). The neurotransmitter between postganglionic neurons and effector organs is primarily NA for the SNS and Ach for the PNS (see Figure 8.1).

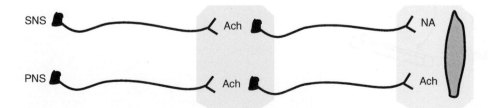

Figure 8.1 Pre- and postganglionic components of the ANS.

8.3.3.1 Heart

The ANS regulates chronotropy, inotropy, and coronary perfusion (see Figure 8.2). Stimulation of the SNS results in increased HR via β_1-**adrenergic receptors** and increased stroke volume via the stellate ganglion. Normal basal sympathetic activity maintains contractility at around 20% greater than that of a denervated heart. PNS fibres are distributed to the sinoatrial node (SAN), atrioventricular node (AVN) and atria but only minimally to the ventricular myocardium. Stimulation results in decreased rate of discharge and inhibits SAN/AVN excitability (via **M2 receptors**) and reduces HR. The right vagus nerve innervates the SAN predominantly, and the left vagus nerve the AVN, which explains why left carotid sinus massage is more likely to be effective in terminating SVTs. Because of the lack of efferent distribution to ventricles, the PNS has little effect on inotropicity.

Unlike with vasomotor tone, the heart is tonically stimulated by both SNS and PNS. The latter predominates and is most apparent in young, healthy cohorts who demonstrate resting vagal tone. For this reason, total pharmacological ANS blockade or cardiac denervation in the context of heart transplantation typically results in higher resting HR. There is a more gradual response in HR to sympathetic as opposed to parasympathetic activity and this is determined by two main factors. First, the SNS is reliant on adenylyl cyclase producing cyclic adenosine monophosphate (cAMP) as a secondary messenger in pacemaker cells as opposed to direct coupling. Second, release of the neurotransmitter NA at postganglionic nerve endings is slower than release of Ach.

In addition, cardiac afferent neurons also play a role in modulation. They can be mechanosensory, chemosensory or multimodal and can transduce release of vasodilatory neuropeptides such as substance P and calcitonin gene-related peptide. Detailed exploration is beyond the scope of this chapter.

8.3.3.2 Peripheral Circulation

The SNS dominates in regulation of vascular tone via vasoconstriction by stimulation of α_1-**adrenergic receptors**. Vasculature of the skin, kidney, spleen, and mesentery has extensive sympathetic innervation although vascular beds in the heart, brain, and skeletal muscle have less.

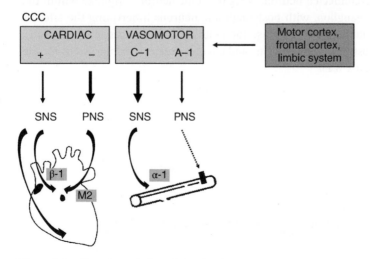

Figure 8.2   Neural regulation of the circulatory system.

By contrast, distribution of parasympathetic nerves is relatively limited with dilatation primarily achieved via receptor-mediated signalling in the endothelium (e.g. insulin).

8.3.4 Reflexes

8.3.4.1 Intrinsic

Arterial **baroreceptors** are specialised pressure-responsive nerve endings situated in the walls of the aortic arch and internal carotid artery just above the sinus (bifurcation). Afferent fibres relay with the CCC. There is basal discharge from baroreceptor afferents at physiological arterial pressure. When receptor endings are stretched, action potentials are generated and transmitted at a frequency that is roughly proportional to pressure change. Afferent input results in negative chronotropic and inotropic effects in addition to reduction in vasoconstrictor tone of arterioles and venules. Hence, increased BP provides a reflex negative feedback loop to maintain homeostasis with the greatest response when changes are in the physiological range (80–150 mmHg). Clinically, this reflex is evident acutely when standing up from a sitting position, with the kidneys playing a more prominent role in mediation of long-term pressure regulation. Reduced responsiveness can occur with age, hypertension and coronary disease. Baroreceptors are also present to a lesser extent in the atria, venae cavae, and ventricles.

The aortic and carotid bodies also contain **chemoreceptors** which respond to reduction in arterial partial pressure of oxygen (PaO_2) and increase in arterial partial pressure of carbon dioxide ($PaCO_2$). Afferent pathways are located in the same nerves as adjacent baroreceptors. Their primary function is to increase respiratory minute volume but sympathetic vasoconstriction occurs as a secondary effect.

8.3.4.2 Extrinsic

Extrinsic influences play a smaller and less consistent role in circulatory regulation. Nonetheless, they become more relevant in stress responses such as pain, CNS ischaemia, and the Cushing reflex.

Pain can produce variable effects. Mild-to-moderate severity may generate a tachycardia and increase in arterial BP mediated by the somatosympathetic reflex. Severe pain, however, may elicit bradycardia, hypotension and symptoms of shock. The CNS ischaemic response occurs when severe hypotension (mean BP < 50 mmHg) activates chemoreceptors in the vasomotor region of the CCC. A subsequent increase in SNS activity leads to profound, generalised vasoconstriction. It is a reflex for restoring cerebral blood flow in emergency states. Cushing reflex is a consequence of raised intracranial pressure (ICP) that triggers direct compression of cerebral vasculature. Resulting impairment in blood flow initiates the CNS ischaemic response and increased SNS activity as described. This reflex response to augment arterial BP is a mechanistic response to preserve adequate cerebral perfusion. However, simultaneous reduction in HR can occur and is mediated by the baroreceptor reflex.

8.4 Humoral Control

8.4.1 Catecholamines

The adrenal medulla is unique in that the gland is innervated by preganglionic SNS fibres that originate directly from the spinal cord. It secretes adrenaline and NA in response to stimulation (see Figure 8.3), which function as hormones by entering the bloodstream and exerting distant

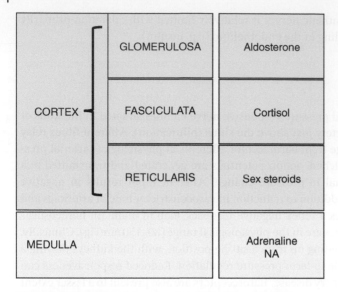

Figure 8.3 Functional components of the adrenal gland.

effects on target organs. In view of this, activity is prolonged in comparison to neurotransmitter release of NA.

8.4.2 Renin–Angiotensin–Aldosterone (RAA) System

This system does not play a significant role in health but is important in BP maintenance during periods of hypovolaemia or impaired CO when renal perfusion is compromised (see Figure 8.4).

The enzyme **renin** initiates the cascade and is secreted by juxtaglomerular cells, modified VSMCs located in the media of the afferent arteriole immediately proximal to the glomerulus. Renin secretion arises primarily due to renal hypoperfusion but can also be initiated by SNS activation of β_1-adrenergic receptors. Renin cleaves angiotensinogen, synthesised in the liver, to **angiotensin I**. This is physiologically inactive but rapidly hydrolysed by angiotensin-converting enzyme (ACE), found in high concentrations in pulmonary vascular endothelium, to form **angiotensin II**. This directly

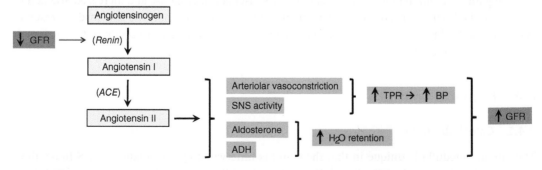

Figure 8.4 Renin–angiotensin–aldosterone system in circulatory homeostasis.

mediates arteriolar vasoconstriction in most vascular beds and stimulates SNS transmission that increase TPR and BP. It additionally results in synthesis and secretion of **aldosterone** from the zona glomerulosa of the adrenal cortex. This targets the sodium–potassium exchanger in the distal convoluted tubule (DCT) and collecting duct of nephrons to cause sodium and water retention with increase in intravascular volume. Beyond these established roles, aldosterone is thought to have direct impact on the myocardium and vasculature including hypertrophy and fibrosis. Angiotensin II is metabolised by aminopeptidases to angiotensin III. This is a less potent vasoconstrictor but has comparable influence on aldosterone secretion.

Angiotensin II also activates secretion of **antidiuretic hormone (ADH)**, otherwise known as vasopressin. This peptide is synthesised in the brainstem and transported for storage in the posterior lobe of the pituitary gland. In addition to angiotensin II, secretion is also triggered by increased plasma osmolality (detected by receptors in the hypothalamus) and decreased plasma volume (detected by receptors in the atria). ADH induces translocation of aquaporin-2 channels in collecting ducts to enhance free water permeability and resorption (anti-diuresis). ADH has additional vasoconstrictory effects which are generalised and affect most regional circulations.

8.4.3 Nitric Oxide (NO)

Nitric oxide (NO) is deemed to be one of the most important mediators of vascular health. It can be synthesised by one of three isoforms of nitric oxide synthase (NOS): endothelial (eNOS), neuronal (nNOS), and macrophage/inducible (iNOS). It is the constitutively active eNOS that is implicated in production of NO within the vascular endothelium. The amino acid L-arginine is the main substrate for synthesis with requirement of several co-factors to produce NO and L-citrulline as a by-product. Once synthesised, NO diffuses across the cell membrane of endothelial cells and enters VSMCs where activation of guanylate cyclase occurs. This catalyses conversion of guanosine triphosphate (GTP) to cyclic guanosine monophosphate (cGMP), an important secondary messenger that mediates several biological targets implicated in vascular function including smooth muscle relaxation.

Endothelial NOS expression can be regulated by multiple stimuli including insulin, shear stress and vascular endothelial growth factor (VEGF). There is continuous, basal synthesis of NO to relax VSMCs and maintain vasodilatory tone in vessels, with effects exerted predominantly in the arterial system. Pharmacological agents such as glyceryl trinitrate (GTN) and sodium nitroprusside (SNP) act via cGMP-dependent mechanisms after conversion to NO. Indeed, beneficial effects of ACE inhibitors (see Section 12.7.3) may be related, in part, to amplification of the actions of bradykinin which potentiates NO release. Beyond vasomotor function, NO also has inhibitory effects on platelet adhesion and aggregation, local inflammatory responses and mitogenesis. Hence, NO participates heavily in the provision of an anti-atherogenic and anti-thrombotic environment overall within the vasculature to preserve physiological equilibrium.

8.4.4 Atrial Natriuretic Peptide (ANP)

Atrial natriuretic peptide is synthesised directly by atrial myocytes in response to chamber distension and hormones such as adrenaline and ADH. It directly relaxes VSMCs and inhibits renin, therefore having an overall natriuretic effect to reduce BP. No direct inotropic or chronotropic effects have been reported.

8.5 Local Autoregulation

Some vascular beds have the ability to regulate blood flow locally in a phenomenon termed **autoregulation** (see Figure 8.5). This occurs predominantly in arterioles of the heart, kidneys, and brain, and to a lesser extent in skin and lungs. It describes a negative feedback mechanism that preserves perfusion despite changes in arterial BP. In the absence of autoregulation, a linear relationship exists between pressure and flow. Vasodilation and vasoconstriction allow a constant flow to be achieved despite alterations in BP. This response is greatest in organs with the lowest neurogenic tone and is largely intrinsic, with myogenic mechanisms predominant and only marginal influence from neural and humoral mediators. In clinical contexts such as malignant hypertension, for example close assessment and regulation of BP are paramount to ensure preservation of cerebral autoregulatory mechanisms and avoidance of linearity in pressure–flow dynamics.

8.6 Functional Hyperaemia

There are certain clinical states in which metabolic demand of end organs is enhanced. This occurs commonly in skeletal muscle during exercise or in the myocardium during periods of tachycardia. In response, there is demonstrable enhancement of perfusion via arteriolar dilatation and one that is independent of perfusion pressure. This is known as **functional hyperaemia** and represents an eloquent system whereby metabolic need is coupled with perfusion. Accumulation of metabolic by-products such as carbon dioxide (CO_2) and lactic acid leads directly to VSMC relaxation in arterioles. Tissues vary in the extent of this hyperaemic response. The myocardium shows a classically large response. For instance, when there is a sudden, significant interruption of blood flow in the context of a coronary thrombus resulting in ischaemia, immediate perfusion post-intervention is transiently higher than at baseline, although this is strictly defined as 'reactive hyperaemia' as opposed to functional or active hyperaemia.

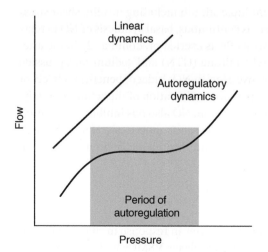

Figure 8.5 Pressure–flow dynamics in autoregulation.

Hot Points

- The CCC has two major subdivisions: the cardiac control centre (stimulatory and inhibitory) and the vasomotor centre (vasoconstrictor and vasodilator).
- The cardiostimulatory, cardioinhibitory and vasoconstrictor areas are tonically active.
- Vasomotor tone refers to summation of muscular forces intrinsic to the vessel that oppose vessel dilatation. It is mediated by VSMCs and influenced by the ANS and humoral agents.
- The CCC modulates the ANS, which itself is composed of two opposing systems: sympathetic and parasympathetic.
- Arterial baroreceptors and chemoreceptors affect intrinsic reflexes and play a significant role in circulatory regulation. Extrinsic reflexes are less impactful.
- The RAA system is critical in enabling humoral regulation of BP during periods of hypovolaemia or impaired output.

8.7 Self-assessment Questions

1 Which of these statements is correct?
   A The adrenal medulla releases cortisol.
   B Angiotensin II acts on the loop of Henle.
   C ADH induces translocation of aquaporin channels in collecting ducts to enhance free water resorption.
   D Nitric oxide is synthesised from L-citrulline.
   E ANP reduces blood pressure and increases myocardial contractility.

2 With regard to the sympathetic nervous system, which of the following is incorrect?
   A Preganglionic nerve fibres release acetylcholine.
   B It stimulates β_1-adrenergic fibres in the heart.
   C Heart rate responds more gradually to the sympathetic than parasympathetic nervous system.
   D In the peripheral circulation, its distribution is far exceeded by the PNS.
   E Normal basal sympathetic activity maintains cardiac contractility 20% higher than a denervated heart.

3 Which of the following is a feature of the Cushing reflex?
   A Excess activation of parasympathetic nervous system.
   B Hypotension.
   C Tachycardia.
   D Secondary to intoxication with narcotics.
   E Related to raised intracranial pressure.

4 Which of the following statements is correct?
  A The cardiovascular control centres are located in the prefrontal cortex.
  B The cardiostimulatory centre increases HR and reduces BP.
  C The vasomotor centre has separate vasoconstrictor and vasodilator centres.
  D The vascular smooth muscle cells are located in the adventitial layer.
  E Basal vasomotor tone is mediated by low-level continuous parasympathetic activity.

5 Which of the following organs does not show local autoregulation?
  A Heart.
  B Liver.
  C Kidneys.
  D Skin.
  E Brain.

Further Reading

Atochin, D.N. and Huang, P.L. (2011). Role of endothelial nitric oxide in cerebrovascular regulation. *Curr. Pharm. Biotechnol.* 12 (9): 1334–1342.

Chopra, S., Baby, C., and Jacob, J.J. (2011). Neuro-endocrine regulation of blood pressure. *Indian J. Endocrinol. Metab.* 15 (Suppl 4): S281–S288.

He, F.J. and MacGregor, G.A. (2003). Salt, blood pressure and the renin-angiotensin system. *J. Renin Angiotensin Aldosterone Syst.* 4 (1): 11–16.

Raven, P.B. and Chapleau, M.W. (2014). Blood pressure regulation XI: overview and future research directions. *Eur. J. Appl. Physiol.* 114 (3): 579–586.

Thomas, G.D. (2011). Neural control of the circulation. *Adv. Physiol. Educ.* 35 (1): 28–32.

9

Coronary Vasculature

CHAPTER MENU

9.1   Learning Objectives

- Arterial supply to the heart including branches.
- Clinical contexts that precipitate formation of collaterals.
- Venous drainage of the heart including greater cardiac veins and Thebesian vessels.
- Coronary microcirculation and its function.
- Mechanical, metabolic and neural factors that regulate blood flow.

9.2   Overview

The heart is unique as an organ in its need to provide blood flow to all systems and generate its own perfusion pressures. This results in substantial metabolic needs that are subject to extravascular forces which differ in their impact on blood flow depending on period of the cardiac cycle. The myocardium is almost exclusively reliant on aerobic metabolism of glucose and fatty acids which prohibits oxygen debt to be accumulated to any significant extent. In normal physiology, myocardial oxygen consumption is tightly matched with coronary perfusion to meet tissue requirements. This chapter provides an overview of coronary arterial and venous anatomy and regulatory factors.

Cardiology at its Core, First Edition. Peysh A. Patel.
© 2023 John Wiley & Sons Ltd. Published 2023 by John Wiley & Sons Ltd.

9.3 Arterial System

The initial portion of the aortic root houses leaflets of the aortic valves (see Section 13.3). It is occupied distally by the sinuses of Valsalva from which the coronary vessels arise (see Figure 9.1). Left coronary vessel originates as the left main stem (LMS) and branches into left anterior descending (LAD) and circumflex (Cx) arteries. The LAD artery travels along the anterior interventricular groove and provides septal and diagonal branches. Traditionally, the first septal distinguishes proximal from mid segment whilst the second diagonal differentiates mid from distal region Cx artery traverses along the left atrioventricular groove and provides obtuse marginal (OM) and posterolateral branches. The right coronary artery (RCA) is situated along the atrioventricular groove on the right and supplies an acute marginal artery which travels anteriorly along the lateral wall of right ventricle (RV). The main artery continues towards the crux where, in the majority of cases, it provides the posterior descending artery (PDA) that continues along the posterior interventricular groove and a posterolateral branch. **Dominance** conventionally refers to the vessel providing the PDA and perfusing the inferior wall of left ventricle and atrioventricular node (AVN). Right-sided dominance is seen in the majority of cases (~ 85%).

Branches originating from these larger arteries penetrate perpendicularly into the myocardium and divide into extensive networks (plexuses) to generate a capillary bed. Some branches are predominantly in the subepicardium while others impregnate deeply to form a subendocardial network. Vasomotor function varies between these two types and enables local alteration in distribution of transmural flow. Collateral vessels are anastomotic channels that form pre-existing connections without intervening capillaries. These may occur between main coronary arteries (intercoronary) or between branches of the same coronary artery (intracoronary). They originate from pre-existing arterioles that undergo vascular regeneration, termed angiogenesis, via proliferation of endothelial cells and VSMCs. Broadly speaking, they arise in two clinical contexts: (i) chronic ischaemia resulting in hypoxia and inflammation, and (ii) increased flow velocity proximal to vessel occlusion resulting in physical endothelial stress. Collaterals play a role in supporting hibernating myocardium although their presence may be insufficient to maintain normal contractile function.

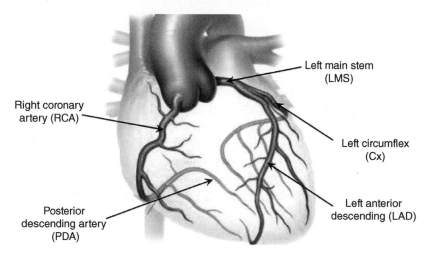

Figure 9.1 Coronary arterial anatomy.

9.4 Venous System

The low-resistance venous system drains blood from the myocardium and returns it to the right atrium for oxygenation in the lungs. It can be considered as two subgroups: **smaller** and **greater** cardiac veins (see Figure 9.2).

The smaller cardiac veins are known as Thebesian vessels and carry around 5% of total venous blood. They drain directly into their respective chambers, mainly the right ventricle. The greater cardiac veins are composed of the coronary sinus, its tributaries and drainage vessels. The coronary sinus is located in the right atrioventricular groove with its origin typically defined at the valve of Vieussens. It drains directly into the right atrium (RA) at the crux cordis, located inferiorly on the RA septum between inferior vena cava (IVC) and tricuspid valve. Its orifice can be obscured by a Thebesian valve although there is heterogeneity in anatomy. The great cardiac vein commences at the apex and travels superiorly in the anterior interventricular septum before continuing in the left atrioventricular groove and draining into the coronary sinus, demarcated by the valve of Vieussens. The middle cardiac vein also originates near the apex but traverses in the posterior interventricular groove before draining into the sinus or directly into the RA. The small cardiac vein drains the inferolateral region of right ventricle. It originates in the inferior region of the coronary sinus and parallels the RCA before emptying into the sinus, middle cardiac vein or directly into the RA. It is not always present. Lastly, Marshall's vein drains blood from the inferolateral regions of left atrium to the atrioventricular groove and into the sinus.

Venous architecture is of direct importance when exploring technical suitability for biventricular pacing via cardiac resynchronisation therapy (CRT). This is usually performed in the context of congestive heart failure (CHF) with refractory symptoms and broadened QRS duration (see Section 12.7.12.2).

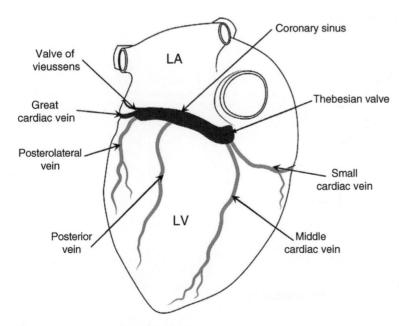

Figure 9.2 Coronary venous anatomy.

9.5 Regulation of Flow

9.5.1 Mechanical

Coronary arterial flow is phasic due to extravascular compression from the contracting myocardium during systole (see Figure 9.3). Thus, 80% of arterial flow occurs during diastole. Indeed, transmitted forces are such that in the early phase of systole, left coronary blood flow is briefly reversed. This effect is accentuated in the context of tachycardia when systole occupies a greater proportion of the cardiac cycle. The relatively lower pressures generated in the RV compared with the let ventricle (LV) permit a proportionately greater systolic flow. In all instances, however, compression propagates blood downstream which explains why, in contrast, venous flow is almost entirely during systole.

Extrinsic compression has an additional effect on intramyocardial flow distribution. As the LV contracts, intramyocardial pressure may exceed intraventricular pressure. This generated force is graded and at its peak near the endocardium and weakest in epicardial regions. Despite this, in normal physiology, subendocardial and subepicardial flow is reasonably equivalent as increased flow to the epicardium during systole is compensated by increase in endocardial flow during diastole. This disparity becomes more clinically relevant in low diastolic pressure states such as aortic regurgitation (see Section 13.5) and septic shock. In these situations, subendocardial flow is more significantly reduced and the region becomes more susceptible to ischaemia.

Coronary vasculature can demonstrate elements of **autoregulation** as indicated in Chapter 8. This ensures that coronary perfusion remains relatively constant between diastolic pressures of 60–180 mmHg. The notion of predominant diastolic coronary flow can also be applied to augment myocardial perfusion in the context of cardiogenic shock. As outlined separately in Section 11.9.2.2, intra-aortic balloon pump (IABP) counterpulsation operates via inflation in diastole and deflation in

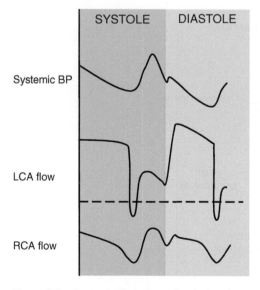

Figure 9.3 Coronary flow dynamics during the cardiac cycle.

systole. Hence, IABP raises diastolic pressure and coronary blood flow at a time when extravascular compressive effects of the myocardium are at their lowest. This is often seen with severely diseased coronary vasculature where autoregulatory mechanisms have also been obliterated.

9.5.2 Metabolic

The coupling between metabolic need and coronary blood flow is well established. Any situation that increases requirements, such as exercise, sympathetic stimulation or inotropic therapy, will result in accompanying vasodilation to enhance flow. The precise mechanism is not fully elucidated but hypoxia (i.e. reduced partial pressure of oxygen [PaO_2]) is the primary determinant. Adenosine, lactic acid, pH, partial pressure of carbon dioxide ($PaCO_2$) and NO levels are also likely to contribute. Tachycardia has a dual effect on coronary blood flow. As outlined, the relative proportion of time spent in diastole decreases but this is counteracted by coronary dilatation associated with increased metabolic activity.

9.5.3 Neural

Sympathetic α-adrenergic activation (α_1 in large vessels, α_2 in smaller vessels) has vasoconstrictive effects whilst parasympathetic, vasodilatory effects are determined by acetylcholine (Ach)-mediated release of NO. Indeed, direct stimulation of VSMCs by the sympathetic system in the context of endothelial dysfunction may result in coronary artery vasospasm and mimic acute coronary syndrome (see Chapter 11). Beyond direct neural effects on coronary vasculature, sequelae that arise from myocardial stimulation are also relevant. For instance, sympathetic activation will increase oxygen demand and local accumulation of metabolites. This will produce secondary vasodilation of coronary vasculature, as described earlier.

Hot Points

- Coronary arterial vasculature originates from the sinuses of Valsalva immediately distal to the aortic valve.
- Dominance typically refers to the vessel providing PDA and is right-sided in 85% of cases.
- The venous system can be subcategorised as smaller (Thebesian) and greater cardiac veins. The latter is composed of the coronary sinus and its tributaries, and drains into the right atrium.
- Arterial flow predominates in diastole due to extravascular compression during systole. This results in downstream propagation of flow and explains why venous perfusion is almost entirely during systole.
- Intramyocardial flow distribution in normal physiology is reasonably equivalent but abnormalities may manifest in diseased states such as aortic stenosis and septic shock.
- Coronary vasculature is regulated by metabolic need with additional neural influence via the ANS.

9.6 Self-assessment Questions

1 In relation to the coronary arterial system, select the incorrect statement.
   A The LMS bifurcates into LAD and Cx arteries.
   B The LAD provides diagonal branches.
   C The Cx provides septal branches.
   D The RCA supplies an acute marginal branch.
   E In majority of cases, the RCA bifurcates into a PDA and posterolateral branch.

2 In relation to the coronary arterial system, select the correct statement.
   A Coronary vessels originate from the sinuses of Valsalva immediately proximal to aortic valve at the root.
   B LAD artery travels along the anterior interventricular groove.
   C Cx artery traverses along the right atrioventricular groove.
   D Collateral vessels are anastomotic channels which arise in the setting of acute ischaemia.
   E Collateral vessels cannot form between branches of the same coronary artery.

3 In relation to the coronary venous system, select the incorrect statement.
   A The coronary sinus is located in the right atrioventricular groove and drains into RA.
   B The coronary sinus is supplied by the great cardiac vein, middle cardiac vein and small cardiac vein.
   C Marshall's vein drains blood from the inferolateral region of the LA to the atrioventricular groove and into the sinus.
   D The smaller cardiac veins are known as Thebesian vessels and carry around 5% of total venous blood.
   E The coronary sinus is situated on the anterior surface of the heart.

4 In relation to regulation of coronary flow, select the correct statement.
   A Coronary arterial flow is linear throughout systole and diastole.
   B During tachycardia, systole occupies a greater proportion of the cardiac cycle and therefore reduces time for diastolic coronary perfusion.
   C Extrinsic compression has minimal effect on intramyocardial flow distribution.
   D Coronary perfusion pressure varies significantly depending on loading conditions.
   E IABP counterpulsation raises systolic blood pressure and augments coronary perfusion.

5 In relation to regulation of coronary flow, select the incorrect statement.
   A During exercise, increased metabolic demand results in coronary arterial vasodilation to enhance flow.
   B Tachycardia has dual effects on coronary blood flow with decrease in relative proportion of time spent in diastole counteracted by coronary dilatation.
   C Parasympathetic, vasodilatory effects in the coronary vasculature are determined by Ach-mediated release of NO.
   D Hypercapnia is the primary determinant of coronary arterial vasodilation in the context of increased metabolic need.

E Coronary arterial spasm may be caused by direct stimulation of VSMCs in the setting of endothelial dysfunction, and can cause symptoms that may mimic myocardial infarction.

Further Reading

Duncker, D.J., Koller, A., Merkus, D., and Canty, J.M. Jr. (2015). Regulation of coronary blood flow in health and ischemic heart disease. *Prog. Cardiovasc. Dis.* 57 (5): 409–422.

Feigl, E.O. (1983). Coronary physiology. *Physiol. Rev.* 63 (1): 1–205.

Loukas, M., Groat, C., Khangura, R. et al. (2009). The normal and abnormal anatomy of the coronary arteries. *Clin. Anat.* 22 (1): 114–128.

Schelbert, H.R. (2010). Anatomy and physiology of coronary blood flow. *J. Nucl. Cardiol.* 17 (4): 545–554.

Tomanek, R.J. (1996). Formation of the coronary vasculature: a brief review. *Cardiovasc. Res.* 31: Spec No: E46–E51.

10

Stable Angina and Non-invasive Testing

10.1   Learning Objectives

- Risk stratification for stable angina.
- The ischaemic cascade.
- Comparison of hibernating, stunned and scarred myocardium.
- Anatomical assessment via CT angiography.
- Commonly utilised stress protocols.
- Exploration and comparison of non-invasive testing, including nuclear cardiology (SPECT and PET), cardiac MRI and stress echocardiography.

Cardiology at its Core, First Edition. Peysh A. Patel.
© 2023 John Wiley & Sons Ltd. Published 2023 by John Wiley & Sons Ltd.

10.2   Risk Stratification

Patients are defined as having **stable angina** if they have pain that is cardiac in nature, consistently brought on by exertion and alleviated by rest or glyceryl trinitrate (GTN) spray within five minutes. They can be considered a low event group; hence management is management is distinct from related entities such as unstable angina, crescendo angina and decubitus angina which require more prompt consideration of revascularisation. In patients with stable angina, first-line approach remains medical with conventional anti-anginals advocated in preference to revascularisation strategies for symptomatic relief [1]. This may include consideration of beta-blockers, non-dihydropyridine calcium-channel blockers or vasodilators such as isosorbide mononitrate (ISMN) and nicorandil. For those with refractory symptoms, adjunct therapy with ivabradine if in normal sinus rhythm (NSR) and/or ranolazine may be considered. In all patients diagnosed with stable angina, the implication is that atherosclerotic disease secondary to endothelial dysfunction exists, and therefore, aspirin and low-dose statin are indicated. In addition, close scrutiny and management of modifiable risk factors is of paramount importance.

Patients also require screening to determine clinical likelihood of significant coronary disease. If there is low suspicion or there is no prior history and image quality is likely to be adequate, computed tomography coronary angiography (CTCA) should be considered. In those with high probability, refractory anginal symptoms or occurring at low workload with concurrent ventricular dysfunction, invasive coronary angiography is recommended. In the remainder, including those with non-diagnostic or unclear CTCA, a non-invasive test to detect inducible ischaemia is preferentially advocated.

If there is stable angina and documented ischaemia on imaging or a haemodynamically significant lesion (fractional flow reserve [FFR] ≤ 0.80 or instantaneous wave-free ratio [iFR] ≤ 0.89; see Section 11.7), revascularisation is broadly considered if there is symptom persistence despite antianginals. It may separately be offered on prognostic grounds such as significant left main stem (LMS) or proximal triple-vessel disease. However, incremental benefit of invasive angiography and revascularisation on top of medical therapy in those with stable angina and inducible ischaemia has recently been questioned. A randomised controlled trial (RCT) showed that an invasive approach was non-superior in diminishing risk of ischaemic cardiac events or all-cause mortality [2]. These findings, notably, are not applicable to those with acute coronary syndrome (ACS) (see Chapter 11), significant LMS disease, poor left ventricular ejection fraction (LVEF – see Chapter 12), advanced CHF (i.e. New York Heart Association class III/IV) or refractory symptoms as these subcohorts were excluded from enrolment.

Various non-invasive imaging modalities are now accessible to provide both anatomical and functional assessment prior to consideration of invasive angiography. The most commonly used techniques shall be explored in the remainder of this chapter. As with all tests, there are pros and cons with additional variations in specificity, sensitivity, and predictive value. Use will also be determined by local resources, expertise and presence of contraindications. Of note, exercise treadmill testing (ETT) is an alternative approach in select patients to assess functional capacity, symptoms, dysrhythmias and event risk (namely cardiovascular mortality >3% per annum). However, the remainder of this chapter shall focus on application of imaging strategies only.

10.3   The Ischaemic Cascade

Anginal symptoms arise from mismatch between myocardial oxygen demand and supply (ischaemia) – see Figure 10.1. Initial features relate to impaired perfusion reserve due to maldistribution of blood flow, which is detectable with modalities such as cardiac magnetic resonance imaging (MRI) and nuclear imaging. This results in a cascade of downstream sequelae including metabolic perturbations. Eventually, it manifests as regional wall motion abnormalities (RWMAs) with dysfunction of diastole preceding that of systole. This tends to occur prior to ECG changes with or without accompanying cardiac symptoms. As a consequence, RWMAs are less sensitive but more specific for significant coronary stenoses. Exceptions to this progressive cascade do exist, however, such as when ECG changes occur in combination with ischaemic symptoms but without RWMAs ('alternative ischaemic cascade').

   Five broad outcomes may arise in the myocardium from coronary occlusion: preserved structure and function, ischaemia, stunning, hibernation and infarction. The subendocardium is the region that is most metabolically active but also has the lowest perfusion reverse. It is therefore most susceptible to insult. Ischaemia starts in this region and may be contained in close vicinity (nontransmural) or extend to involve the whole myocardial layer (transmural).

10.4   Nomenclature

Viability describes the absence of necrosis. It should be considered as an umbrella term encompassing both normal myocardium and that which is dysfunctional (i.e. hibernating or stunned – see Table 10.1).

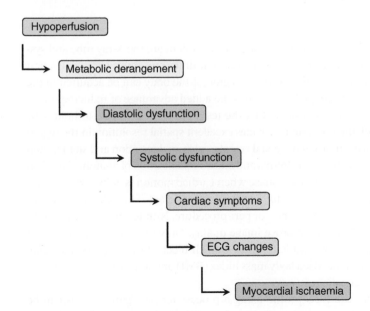

Figure 10.1   The ischaemic cascade.

Table 10.1 Summary of abnormal myocardial states.

Condition	Contractile activity	Metabolic activity	Contractile reserve	Myocardial perfusion	Recovery
Hibernating	Reduced	Preserved	+	Reduced	+
Stunned	Reduced	Preserved	++	Preserved	++
Scarred	Reduced	Absent	−	Reduced	−

Hibernating myocardium refers to the phenomenon whereby regions of dysfunctional myocardium at rest recover contractile function following revascularisation. These areas have preserved but downregulated metabolic activity. This contradicts a previously conceived notion that absence of contractility reflects irreversible myocyte necrosis. Resting perfusion to hibernating areas may be mildly reduced due to lower oxygen requirements.

Stunned myocardium is a separate entity where there is transient and spontaneously reversible contractile dysfunction following acute ischaemia. From a pathophysiological perspective, this phenomenon may arise with both stable angina and ACS (see Chapter 11). However, it is postulated that hibernating myocardium occurs due to repeated episodes of stunning. Recovery appears to be faster in stunned than in hibernating myocardium.

Scarred myocardium describes non-viable, necrotic tissue that is dysfunctional due to absent metabolic activity. No evidence of contractile reserve or recovery is present.

10.5 CT Coronary Angiography

10.5.1 Basic Principles

The most important components of a computed tomography (CT) system are the X-ray tube and system of detectors, with the latest generation providing fast rotation times and multi-slice acquisition (64–320 multi-detector scanners). Consequently, a broader region of the body can be acquired in the same time frame and with improved image quality. This has the added advantage of reducing procedure duration which is relevant when one considers that the test requires individuals to hold their breath to eliminate artefact. Overall, the CT system provides excellent spatial resolution in the region of 0.5 mm and enables visualisation of small calibre distal vessels, calcium deposition and stent lumen diameters. Temporal resolution is in the region of 165 ms and allows visualisation of anatomy based on cardiac cycle. Analysis is performed in the diastolic phase when cardiac motion is at its lowest. Heart rate (HR) should ideally be < 70 beats min^{-1} (bpm) to reduce motion artefact. This often necessitates beta-blocker therapy with intravenous metoprolol pre- or peri-procedure. Nitrates may also be administered to promote coronary vasodilation and improve image quality. Only those with slight rhythm irregularities such as atrial fibrillation (AF) and left bundle branch block (LBBB) can be included. Similarly, extensive coronary calcification, raised body mass index (BMI) or inability to breath hold are generally prohibitive and impair diagnostic accuracy.

Cardiac CT is synchronised with the ECG profile using a process termed 'gating'. This can be retrospective, based on continuous X-ray exposure and a subsequent decision to clarify the phase of diastole that warrants reconstruction. In prospective gating, the phase is decided prior to commencement and radiation is only delivered during this period. This has inevitably resulted in significant reduction in exposure to around 1–4 mSv.

10.5.2 Clinical Use

In patients with low index of suspicion, CTCA has been shown to demonstrate high sensitivity (100%), specificity (93%) and negative predictive value (NPV; 100%) for detection of stenoses [3]. It is particularly useful in those with typical symptoms where risk of significant disease is low or in atypical presentations where reassurance is sought. A negative CT scan in these cohorts should obviate the need for further testing. In individuals with previous coronary artery bypass graft (CABG), assessment for graft stenosis is proven to be accurate (see Figure 10.2) but imaging of native vasculature is less informative. Imaging of coronary stents is generally unreliable as dense metal can result in significant artefact and impede interpretation.

Computed tomography has added potential in characterising both calcific and non-calcific non-stenotic plaques, although in the case of the latter, its detection accuracy is lower compared with intravascular ultrasound (IVUS). The **Agatson score** can be calculated to quantify calcific volume in coronary vasculature (area and density). With the exception of renal failure, coronary calcification is indicative of atherosclerotic plaque and correlates broadly with overall plaque burden. However, calcium score is not a direct substitute for atherosclerotic disease and provides no indication of plaque stability. Extensive calcification can also degrade image quality and limit interpretation by increasing false-positives. Thus, calcium detection via CT is not recommended in isolation to identify those with obstructive coronary disease. Findings on CTCA may warrant or require further assessment either through functional testing (as detailed below) or direct invasive angiography if findings are suggestive of high event risk.

Of note, CTCA provides anatomical assessment but no routine data on functional significance of stenoses unless it is combined with fractional flow reserve (FFR_{CT}). This is an emerging

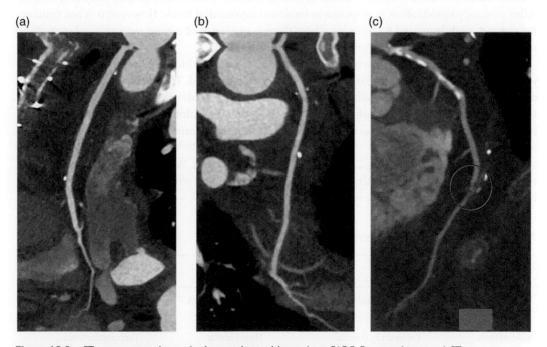

(a)   (b)   (c)

Figure 10.2 CT coronary angiography in a patient with previous CABG. Prospective gated CT at 80 kV. Saphenous vein graft to posterior descending artery (a) and first obtuse marginal artery (b) widely patent. Left internal mammary artery (LIMA) graft to LAD small but patent (c), with moderate stenosis observed at the anastomosis site (circled).

physiological simulation technique that uses generated images with a remote computational fluid dynamics model to evaluate lesion-specific ischaemia and detail haemodynamic significance [4]. FFR is defined as the ratio of flow through a coronary stenosis (Q_s) compared with flow without stenosis (Q_n). By application of **Poiseuille's law,** laminar blood flow (Q) can be equated to driving pressure divided by resistance to flow. Assuming that a) collateral flow is minimal, and b) in the context of a maximal hyperaemic state venous pressure (P_v) is significantly lower than both pressure immediately distal to stenosis (P_d) and arterial pressure upstream of stenosis (P_a), FFR can be defined as follows:

$$\text{FFR} = \left(Q_s \div Q_n\right) = \left(P_d \div P_a\right)$$

Although it cannot currently be used in vein grafts, FFR_{CT} requires no additional imaging and has been validated against stress nuclear testing. It also appears to have higher specificity and positive predictive value (PPV) compared with visual analysis of CTCA stenoses, when using invasive FFR during angiography as the gold standard [5]. Potential application of machine learning to FFR_{CT} analysis may broaden applicability in the future and reduce healthcare cost burden in the longer term.

10.6 Stress Protocols

Functional, non-invasive imaging incorporates use of stress protocols. Its general principle is to augment myocardial oxygen demand to assess whether functionally significant coronary stenoses are present. An overview of the profiles of commonly used stress agents is detailed in Table 10.2.

Exercise can be used with both treadmill testing and stress echocardiography (SE). It results in reflex coronary vasodilation in response to increased myocardial work. However, it is not suitable for patients with impaired mobility or where there is existence of severe left ventricular outflow tract obstruction (LVOTO) and/or triple-vessel disease.

Adenosine administration directly stimulates A2 receptors, which leads to coronary arteriolar vasodilation and increases myocardial perfusion three- to five-fold. This response is less marked in diseased vessels with endothelial dysfunction and enables detection of perfusion defects. Intravenous aminophylline should be readily available as an antidote. Regadenoson is an alternative adenosine analogue that has a longer half-life (around two minutes) but greater A2 receptor selectivity.

Dobutamine functions via β_1-, β_2-, and α_1-adrenergic agonism. At low dose, it has positive inotropic and chronotropic effects that increase myocardial demand with secondary coronary vasodilation. At higher dose, it directly results in vasodilation.

Table 10.2 Summary of common stress agents.

	Exercise	Adenosine	Dobutamine
Regime	Bruce or modified Bruce	$140\ \mu g\,kg^{-1}\,min^{-1}$	$5–40\ \mu g\,kg^{-1}\,min^{-1}$
Half-life	–	15 s	120 s
Side-effects	Tachyarrhythmia, ischaemia, hypotension	Heart block, bronchospasm	Tachyarrhythmia, ischaemia, hypotension
Main contraindications	Impaired mobility, severe LVOTO, triple-vessel disease	Severe asthma, high-grade AV block	Severe LVOTO, triple-vessel disease

10.7 Nuclear Cardiology (SPECT and PET)

10.7.1 Basic Principles

Nuclear cardiology relies on assessment via myocardial perfusion imaging (MPI). **Single photon emission computed tomography (SPECT)** is performed using a multi-detector gamma camera that rotates around the chest to obtain images of single emitted photons from myocardial tracers. ECG-gated acquisition of perfusion studies has become standard practice as it allows quantitative assessment of left ventricular (LV) function and volume in addition to evaluation of regional wall motion. It also improves diagnostic accuracy in the context of attenuation artefacts. This can depend on various parameters such as tissue density and compensatory correction is routinely performed to account for this. **Positron emission tomography (PET)** scanners have a different geometry and detection principle from that of SPECT. The primary aim is to produce a three-dimensional image that provides an accurate map of tracer distribution.

10.7.2 Clinical Uses

SPECT can be used to provide assessment of myocardial perfusion and function (see Figure 10.3). For perfusion imaging, technetium (^{99m}Tc) is the most common radionuclide tracer currently in use. Following intravenous injection of thallium (Tl), first-pass extraction by the myocardium is 88% with uptake occurring predominantly via sodium–potassium ATPase. This has a proportional

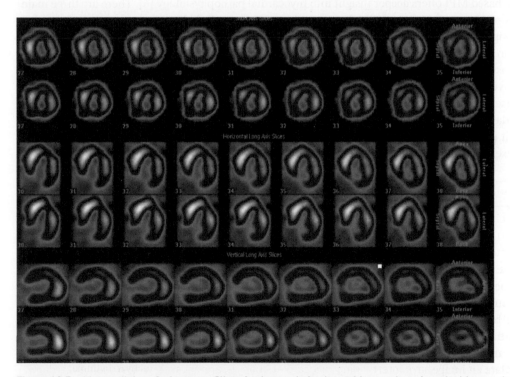

Figure 10.3 Myocardial perfusion scan. Slices in short axis, horizontal long axis and vertical long axis are demonstrated. Imaging has been performed at stress (upper panel) and rest (lower panel). There is reduction in uptake inferiorly both at stress and rest, indicative of non-viability in the right coronary artery (RCA) territory.

relationship with perfusion. It redistributes over two to four hours, allowing acquisition of delayed scans that reflect baseline perfusion and tissue viability. Comparison of stress and baseline images allows identification of regional areas of inducible ischaemia, whilst fixed areas are indicative of non-viable scar tissue. For improved assessment of viability, nitrate administration can help to avoid under-estimation. In the case of Tc injections, higher energy permits better image quality and its shorter half-life restricts radiation exposure. However, splanchnic uptake and excretion are higher than for Tl and complicates assessment of the inferior wall. Additionally, this tracer remains within myocytes and does not redistribute; hence, separate injections on the same day or over two days are required to obtain stress and imaging.

SPECT is suited to detect impaired perfusion reserve even before RWMAs and/or ECG changes are manifest. Its role in risk stratification has therefore been extensively explored. A normal scan predicts low likelihood (< 1%) of future cardiac events. Nonetheless, this demonstrates absence of functionally significant disease and not necessarily atherosclerosis entirely. It is clinically indicated in those with symptoms and intermediate index of suspicion or in those who have equivocal or uninterpretable findings from CTCA. An area of ischaemia > 10% of LV myocardium was historically deemed to be functionally significant and warrant invasive assessment although this notion is refuted by results of the ISCHAEMIA trial (as detailed earlier) if symptoms are absent. In those with established coronary disease, SPECT is relevant to define territory involvement in cases where symptoms recur after revascularisation. However, there are instances where the risk of false-negatives is higher, such as in the elderly, those with diabetes mellitus and patients with undiagnosed triple-vessel disease.

PET based MPI offers deeper insight into myocardial pathophysiology [6]. There are three main perfusion tracers: rubidium (^{82}Rb), N-ammonia and O-water. Rubidium is most commonly used as it has significant advantages including lower radiation exposure. It has a half-life of 78 s, extraction fraction of around 60% and results in average scan duration of 6 minutes. It results in superior diagnostic accuracy due to higher temporal and spatial resolution compared with SPECT; moreover, higher photon energy of the tracer results in less scatter and non-uniform attenuation. CT-based attenuation is also more readily available in PET-based MPI and circumvents image degradation arising from non-uniform attenuation due to excess body habitus. Lastly, it has added benefit in assessment of myocardial viability and blood flow quantification. Significant hardware expense limits broader clinical applicability at present.

10.8 Cardiac MRI

10.8.1 Basic Principles

Cardiac MRI is able to provide relevant information on most aspects of the heart including anatomy, perfusion and viability. This is achieved with a scan that is typically performed within 20 minutes. The principle of MRI relies upon physical properties of hydrogen nuclei (protons). These have an intrinsic 'spin', but alignment occurs when brought in proximity with a high-strength magnetic field. Application of a radiofrequency pulse can excite the spins, affect alignment and create signals while returning to their resting state (relaxation) which is used to formulate an image.

Signal magnitude arising from the tissue is influenced by two independent relaxation times, T1 (longitudinal magnetisation to baseline) and T2 (transverse magnetisation to baseline), proton density and proton movement (blood flow). Fat has short T1 and T2 times whereas water has long

T1 and T2 times. Image formation also requires comprehension of signal origin within a patient, with encoding performed using a process termed Fourier transformation. As with other imaging modalities, data is synchronised to cardiac motion using the ECG. Typically, it is performed using a retrospective approach.

First-pass perfusion imaging with gadolinium is the standard procedure for assessing myocardial perfusion with MRI. It is performed at rest and during pharmacological stress, typically with adenosine/regadenoson or dobutamine. The optimal dose of gadolinium is 0.03–0.10 mM kgW^{-1}, injected via a brachial vein. Perfusion defects are defined as regions of non-enhancing myocardium. In addition to this, assessment for early gadolinium enhancement (EGE) and **late gadolinium enhancement (LGE)** is routinely performed with a time interval of around five minutes. It crucially provides assessment of viability by establishing presence of infarcted tissue (see Figure 10.4). In acute infarcts, it is thought that myocardial cell membrane rupture allows diffusion of gadolinium from

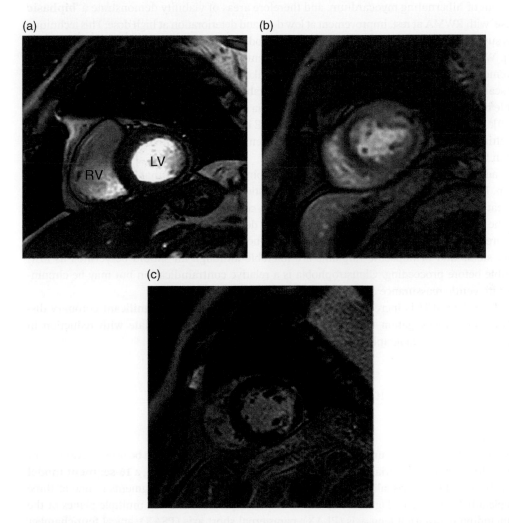

Figure 10.4 Cardiac MRI. a) PSAX view with rest perfusion showing defect in basal-mid anterolateral and inferolateral segments. (b) First-pass perfusion during stress indicating fixed perfusion defect in these regions. (c) LGE showing subendocardial hyper-enhancement (< 50% transmurality) that co-localises.

extracellular to intracellular spaces with subsequent hyper-enhancement ('bright signal'). In chronic infarcts, the mechanism may relate to increased interstitial space between collagen fibres combined with slower in/out kinetics. Velocity-encoded cardiac MRI can also be performed to establish blood flow. It is based on the principle that as 'spins' flow along the magnetic field gradient, a shift in transverse magnetisation occurs which can be used to derive flow velocities. This is of benefit in quantification of stroke volumes, valvular disease and septal defects.

10.8.2 Clinical Uses

Similar to nuclear imaging, use is generally advocated in those with symptoms and intermediate index of suspicion or in those who have equivocal or uninterpretable findings from CTCA. In addition to ischaemia assessment, low-dose dobutamine-MRI with gadolinium offers a particular means to detect viable myocardium which may benefit from targeted revascularisation. It stimulates recruitment of hibernating myocardium, and therefore areas of viability demonstrate a **'biphasic response'** with RWMA at rest, improvement at low dose and deterioration at high dose. This technique appears superior to scar imaging in predicting likelihood of functional recovery after revascularisation [7]. When transmural scar is identified, the extent of involvement is relevant as functional improvement after revascularisation is deemed more likely if there is ≤50% mural involvement [8]. Infarct scar size (i.e. area and mass) may be of comparable relevance in helping to correlate risk of inducible dysrhythmias such as ventricular tachycardia (VT) and associated sudden cardiac death (SCD) [9]. However, it should be accentuated that LGE is not specific for infarction as it can occur in the setting of myocarditis and cardiomyopathies. Hence, pattern of enhancement is particularly helpful in formulating the correct diagnosis.

A key advantage of cardiac MRI over CT angiography and SPECT is that it avoids exposure to radiation. It also becomes possible to perform diagnostic imaging in those who are unable to hold their breath or with irregular rhythms. The primary consideration relates to presence of metal within the patient, such as those with pacemakers or defibrillators. Nonetheless, MR-compatible devices are now being implanted with prominent frequency. Most sternal wires, prosthetic valves, coronary stents and orthopaedic implants are tolerable although all should be verified as MR-compatible before proceeding. Claustrophobia is a relative contraindication but may be circumvented with gentle reassurance or oral sedation.

Overall, cardiac MRI is incredibly robust in identifying presence of significant coronary disease [10]. Initial investigation using this modality also appears to correlate with reduction in unnecessary invasive angiography within 12 months [11].

10.9 Stress Echocardiography

10.9.1 Basic Principles

Echocardiography at rest and during stress, using exercise or dobutamine, can be used to evaluate for RWMAs. Although there is variability in coronary supply to the myocardium, a **16-segment model** (or 17 if the apical cap is visualised and included) is used to assign wall segments to one of three major epicardial vessels (see Figure 10.5). Confirmation is performed using multiple planes of the heart, including parasternal long axis (PLAX), parasternal short axis (PSAX), apical four-chamber and two-chamber views. A detailed exploration of image projections is beyond the scope of this chapter but referencing is provided below for further reading.

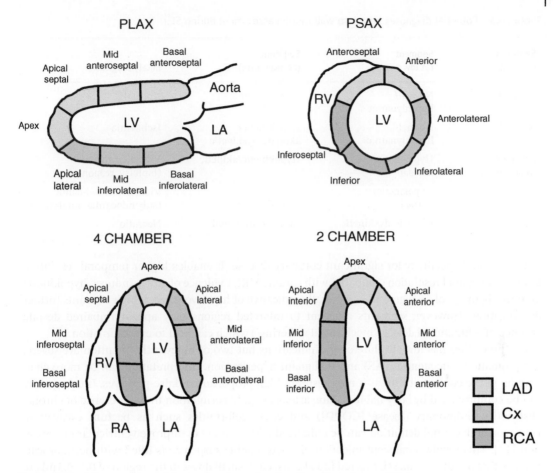

Figure 10.5 17-segment model to assess for regional wall motion abnormalities.

Regional wall motion abnormalities at rest may indicate scar tissue, hibernation or stunned myocardium (see Table 10.3). Ischaemic regions may have preserved or abnormal function at rest with manifestation of RWMAs during stress. Both wall motion and thickness are scored on a numerical scale (1, normal; 2, mild hypokinesia; 2.5, severe hypokinesia; 3, akinesia; 4, dyskinesia [outward as opposed to inward motion]; 5, aneurysmal). Crucially, akinetic and dyskinetic segments may be viable or necrotic and assessing response to stress permits clarification. If a segment is necrotic, it will be akinetic/dyskinetic at rest and during stress. In the context of hibernating myocardium, wall motion will demonstrate a biphasic response as described (i.e. improve at low dose with impairment at high dose). If there is stunned myocardium, wall motion will demonstrate sustained improvement at low and high doses. As function in the presence of hibernating myocardium improves after revascularisation, it is relevant to distinguish this entity from myocardial stunning which typically resolves spontaneously.

10.9.2 Clinical Uses

Generally, stress echocardiography is well tolerated and benefits from avoidance of radiation and ionising agents. It is also widely available, cost-effective and comparable to SPECT in terms of

Table 10.3 Potential diagnoses based on wall motion assessment during SE.

Segment (at rest)	Segment (at low dose)	Segment (at high dose)	Likely diagnosis
Normal	Normal/ hyperdynamic	Hyperdynamic	Normal
Normal	Normal/ hyperdynamic	Hypokinetic/ akinetic/dyskinetic	Ischaemia
Akinetic/ hypokinetic	Hypokinetic/ normal	Hypokinetic/akinetic	Viable, ischaemic (biphasic response)
Hypokinetic/ akinetic	Hypokinetic/ normal	Normal/ hyperdynamic	Viable, non-ischaemic (subendocardial infarction)
Akinetic	Akinetic/dyskinetic	Akinetic/dyskinetic	Necrotic

sensitivity and specificity for significant coronary disease. It enables higher temporal resolution but inferior spatial resolution compared with cardiac MRI. Evidence of stress-induced hypokinesia or akinesia in ≥ 3 of 16 segments is generally indicative of high event risk which warrants further investigation. However, segments adjacent to infarcted regions may appear impaired despite absence of a functional defect ('mechanical tethering') which can lead to overestimation.

The procedure has few absolute contraindications but two of noteworthy mention are severe, symptomatic aortic stenosis (AS) and malignant hypertension. Interpretation can be more challenging in the context of BBB as it may result in high proportion of false-positives. Image quality can be compromised by body habitus, lung artefact (e.g. hyperinflation in the presence of chronic obstructive pulmonary disease [COPD]) and chest deformities such as pectum excavatum. However, endocardial definition can be enhanced with contrast to improve ventricular opacification [12]. This involves transient injection of micro-bubble suspensions filled with perfluorocarbon gas that are of the same size as red blood cells. Only small doses in the region of 0.1–0.3 ml are required prior to image acquisition (see Figure 10.6).

(a) (b)

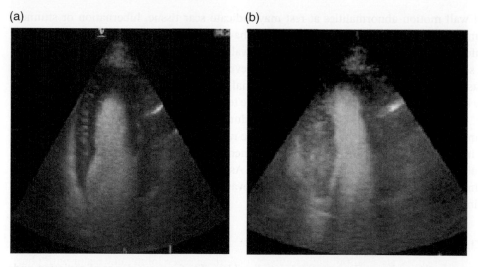

Figure 10.6 Contrast echocardiogram (4 chamber view) with normal wall thickness at rest (a) and apical hypokinesia at peak stress (b), suggestive of inducible ischaemia.

10.10 Comparison of Techniques

A comparative summary of the main non-invasive imaging modalities for assessment of stable angina is provided in Table 10.4. This is a generalised overview and inevitably cannot fully reflect geographical variations and disparities in service commissioning, access and local policies.

Table 10.4 Comparison of non-invasive imaging modalities.

	CTCA	Nuclear cardiology	Cardiac MRI	SE
Availability	++	+	+	+++
Cost	+	++	+++	+
Image degradation due to BMI	+	++	+	+++
Radiation exposure	+	++	−	−
Option of exercise stress	−	−	−	+
Potential CI if claustrophobia	+	+	+++	−
Potential CI if device present	−	−	+	−

Abbreviation: CI, contraindication.

Hot Points

- Stable angina is defined as cardiac chest pain that is typically precipitated by exertion and alleviated by rest or GTN spray within five minutes.
- CTCA provides anatomical assessment of coronary disease and has excellent NPV.
- Functional, non-invasive imaging modalities include nuclear cardiology (SPECT/PET), cardiac MRI and stress echocardiography.
- Typical stressors used for imaging protocols include exercise, adenosine and dobutamine.
- Selection depends on local resource availability, patient preference and presence of contraindications.

10.11 Self-assessment Questions

1 In relation to the ischaemic cascade, select the correct order.
   A Hypoperfusion → diastolic dysfunction → systolic dysfunction → cardiac symptoms → ECG changes.
   B Hypoperfusion → systolic dysfunction → diastolic dysfunction → cardiac symptoms → ECG changes.
   C Hypoperfusion → diastolic dysfunction → systolic dysfunction → ECG changes → cardiac symptoms.
   D Hypoperfusion → cardiac symptoms → ECG changes → diastolic dysfunction → systolic dysfunction.
   E Hypoperfusion → cardiac symptoms → ECG changes → systolic dysfunction → diastolic dysfunction.

2   In relation to abnormal myocardial states, select the incorrect statement.
   A The term 'hibernating' refers to regions of dysfunctional myocardium at rest which can recover contractile function following revascularisation.
   B Hibernating myocardium has preserved but downregulated metabolic activity and may lead to reduction in resting perfusion.
   C Stunned myocardium occurs in the context of acute ischaemia and is often associated with irreversible dysfunction.
   D It is postulated that hibernating myocardium may arise from repeated episodes of stunning.
   E The term 'scarred myocardium' describes necrotic tissue which does not benefit from revascularisation.

3   In relation to CT coronary angiography, select the correct statement.
   A The main limitation of CTCA is poor spatial resolution that limits ability to visualise small vessels.
   B Beta-blockers such as metoprolol can be used to reduce resting HR and reduce motion artefacts.
   C In comparison to retrospective gating, prospective gating allows for significant reduction in radiation exposure.
   D Studies have shown CTCA to exhibit excellent sensitivity and specificity, but at the cost of poor negative predictive value.
   E Coronary calcification poorly correlates with overall plaque burden.

4   In relation to functional stress testing, select the incorrect statement.
   A The general principle of stress testing is to augment myocardial oxygen demand to assess whether functionally significant coronary stenoses are present.
   B Commonly used stress protocols can be split into physiological and pharmacological groups, with the former including exercise and latter including administration of adenosine or dobutamine.
   C Technetium-99m (Tc) is the most common radionuclide tracer currently in use for SPECT imaging.
   D A key advantage of cardiac MRI over SPECT is avoidance of exposure to radiation.
   E In stress echocardiography, a 20-segment model is used to assign wall segments to one of three major epicardial vessels.

5   In relation to cardiac MRI, select the correct statement.
   A LGE provides viability assessment by establishing presence of infarcted tissue.
   B In acute infarcts, it is thought that myocardial cell membrane rupture allows diffusion of gadolinium from intracellular to extracellular spaces with subsequent hyper-enhancement.
   C Following LGE, functional improvement from revascularisation would be deemed more likely if 75% mural involvement was seen.
   D Hyper-enhancement with LGE can only be seen in the context of infarction whereas EGE is seen with cardiomyopathies and myocarditis.
   E Low-dose dobutamine-MRI is particularly useful for viability assessment in those where LGE imaging demonstrates $\leq 50\%$ transmural involvement in order to assess for contractile reserve.

References

1 Boden, W.E., O'Rourke, R.A., Teo, K.K. et al. (2007). Optimal medical therapy with or without PCI for stable coronary disease. *N. Engl. J. Med.* 356 (15): 1503–1516.

2 Maron, D.J., Hochman, J.S., Reynolds, H.R. et al. (2020). Initial invasive or conservative strategy for stable coronary disease. *N. Engl. J. Med.* 382 (15): 1395–1407.

3 Meijboom, W.B., van Mieghem, C.A., Mollet, N.R. et al. (2007). 64-slice computed tomography coronary angiography in patients with high, intermediate, or low pretest probability of significant coronary artery disease. *J. Am. Coll. Cardiol.* 50 (15): 1469–1475.

4 Taylor, C.A., Fonte, T.A., and Min, J.K. (2013). Computational fluid dynamics applied to cardiac computed tomography for noninvasive quantification of fractional flow reserve: scientific basis. *J. Am. Coll. Cardiol.* 61 (22): 2233–2241.

5 Zhuang, B., Wang, S., Zhao, S., and Lu, M. (2020). Computed tomography angiography-derived fractional flow reserve (CT-FFR) for the detection of myocardial ischemia with invasive fractional flow reserve as reference: systematic review and meta-analysis. *Eur. Radiol.* 30 (2): 712–725.

6 Chen, K., Miller, E.J., and Sadeghi, M.M. (2019). PET-based imaging of ischemic heart disease. *PET Clin.* 14 (2): 211–221.

7 Wellnhofer, E., Olariu, A., Klein, C. et al. (2004). Magnetic resonance low-dose dobutamine test is superior to SCAR quantification for the prediction of functional recovery. *Circulation* 109 (18): 2172–2174.

8 Kim, R.J., Wu, E., Rafael, A. et al. (2000). The use of contrast-enhanced magnetic resonance imaging to identify reversible myocardial dysfunction. *N. Engl. J. Med.* 343 (20): 1445–1453.

9 Bello, D., Fieno, D.S., Kim, R.J. et al. (2005). Infarct morphology identifies patients with substrate for sustained ventricular tachycardia. *J. Am. Coll. Cardiol.* 45 (7): 1104–1108.

10 Greenwood, J.P., Maredia, N., Younger, J.F. et al. (2012). Cardiovascular magnetic resonance and single-photon emission computed tomography for diagnosis of coronary heart disease (CE-MARC): a prospective trial. *Lancet* 379 (9814): 453–460.

11 Greenwood, J.P., Ripley, D.P., Berry, C. et al. (2016). Effect of care guided by cardiovascular magnetic resonance, myocardial perfusion scintigraphy, or NICE guidelines on subsequent unnecessary angiography rates: the CE-MARC 2 randomized clinical trial. *JAMA* 316 (10): 1051–1060.

12 Plana, J.C., Mikati, I.A., Dokainish, H. et al. (2008). A randomized cross-over study for evaluation of the effect of image optimization with contrast on the diagnostic accuracy of dobutamine echocardiography in coronary artery disease the OPTIMIZE trial. *JACC Cardiovasc. Imaging* 1 (2): 145–152.

Further Reading

Camici, P.G., Prasad, S.K., and Rimoldi, O.E. (2008). Stunning, hibernation, and assessment of myocardial viability. *Circulation* 117 (1): 103–114.

Danad, I., Szymonifka, J., Twisk, J.W.R. et al. (2017). Diagnostic performance of cardiac imaging methods to diagnose ischaemia-causing coronary artery disease when directly compared with fractional flow reserve as a reference standard: a meta-analysis. *Eur. Heart J.* 38 (13): 991–998.

Douglas, P.S., Pontone, G., Hlatky, M.A. et al. (2015). Clinical outcomes of fractional flow reserve by computed tomographic angiography-guided diagnostic strategies vs. usual care in patients with suspected coronary artery disease: the prospective longitudinal trial of FFR(CT): outcome and resource impacts study. *Eur. Heart J.* 36 (47): 3359–3367.

Husain, S.S. (2007). Myocardial perfusion imaging protocols: is there an ideal protocol? *J. Nucl. Med. Technol.* 35 (1): 3–9.

Knuuti, J., Wijns, W., Saraste, A. et al. (2020). 2019 ESC guidelines for the diagnosis and management of chronic coronary syndromes (published correction appears in Eur. Heart J. 2020 November 21;41(44): 4242). *Eur. Heart J.* 41 (3): 407–477.

11

Ischaemic Heart Disease

11.1 Learning Objectives

- Nomenclature.
- Pathophysiology of atherosclerosis and atherothrombosis.
- Associated ECG changes.

Cardiology at its Core, First Edition. Peysh A. Patel.
© 2023 John Wiley & Sons Ltd. Published 2023 by John Wiley & Sons Ltd.

- Risk scoring systems to guide management strategy.
- Revascularisation options.
- Pharmacotherapy for secondary prevention.
- Complications post-infarction, including acute pulmonary oedema, cardiogenic shock, dysrhythmias and mechanical rupture.
- Differential diagnoses.

11.2 Nomenclature

Ischaemic heart disease (IHD) is an umbrella term that encompasses disease states resulting from myocardial ischaemia due to perfusion–demand mismatch. It is often considered interchangeable with acute coronary syndrome (ACS), but strictly speaking, stable angina is an example of IHD but not ACS. This is because the majority of ACS presentations arise from progressive atherosclerosis and atherothrombosis within the coronary vasculature. They can therefore encompass ST elevation myocardial infarction (STEMI), non-ST elevation myocardial infarction (NSTEMI) and unstable angina. STEMI and NSTEMI are associated with myocardial necrosis secondary to ischaemia and result in cardiac troponin level above the 99th percentile together with significant rise and/or fall. Unstable angina occurs due to ischaemia from atherothrombosis; however, myocardial necrosis does not ensue and troponin levels do not fulfil above criteria for myocardial infarction (MI). A formal diagnosis of IHD should not be based on results of blood profiling in isolation. Rather, it ought to be placed in the context of presenting symptoms and/or associated dynamic ECG changes.

Myocardial infarction with non-obstructive coronary arteries (MINOCA) describes dynamic rise in troponin with corroborative clinical evidence of infarction, such as ECG changes or new regional wall motion abnormality (RWMA), but with non-obstructive coronaries (typically luminal stenosis $\leq 50\%$) when assessed via invasive angiography and with no reasonable alternate diagnosis. MINOCA has overlap with IHD and may be attributed to a range of pathologies including spontaneous coronary artery dissection (SCAD), microvascular disease, coronary embolus and spasm.

For the remainder of this chapter, discussion will centre around STEMI and NSTEMI as subtypes of IHD.

11.3 Pathophysiology

As alluded to, natural progression of coronary disease involves distinct processes of atherosclerosis and atherothrombosis. **Atherosclerosis** describes gradual luminal narrowing over a period of decades and predominates in patients with chronic, stable angina. **Atherothrombosis** refers to sudden vessel occlusion from thrombosis (or vasospasm) and constitutes the critical lesion typically implicated in ACS subtypes. In some cases, however, it may also be triggered by intimal erosion or by a calcified nodule.

The first macroscopic appearance in atherosclerosis begins in the early 20s as fatty streaks (see Figure 11.1). The key initiator is endothelial dysfunction which results in recruitment of inflammatory leucocytes (i.e. monocytes and T cells) and deposition of extracellular lipid within the intima as lipoproteins. Diseased states such as diabetes mellitus and dyslipidaemia confer a pro-inflammatory milieu which has initiating and potentiating effects. Recruited monocytes differentiate into

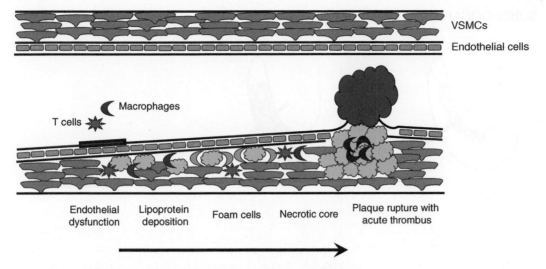

Figure 11.1 Sequence involved in atherogenesis and atherothrombosis.

macrophages which engulf lipoproteins via scavenger receptors and oxidise to become foam cells. The leucocytes and vascular smooth muscle cells (VSMCs) secrete pro-inflammatory cytokines and growth factors that amplify the process and result in smooth muscle cell migration and proliferation in addition to fibroblast-derived collagen accumulation. Thus, the fibrofatty lesion can evolve into an advanced and potentially calcified plaque with fibrous cap and necrotic core. This can cause significant luminal stenosis and anginal symptoms. However, many of these plaques are undetectable angiographically because of positive vascular remodelling.

In the context of ACS, expression of matrix metalloproteinases (MMPs) results in sudden rupture of the fibrous cap. This can occur spontaneously but may equally be triggered by physical exertion, stress, infection or drug use. The ruptured cap results in exposure of a thrombogenic and necrotic lipid core to blood coagulation factors. There is also platelet adhesion and secondary aggregation mediated by production of thromboxane A2 and adenosine diphosphate (ADP), and changes in expression of glycoprotein IIb/IIIa receptors. This results in acute thrombus at the site of plaque rupture. There is local release of vasoconstrictors such as endothelin-1 and thromboxane A2 in addition to reduced NO bioavailability, which otherwise confers vasodilatory, anti-proliferative and anti-inflammatory effects. Hence, these vessels have inherent predisposition to vasospasm which can exacerbate ischaemia.

11.4 ECG Changes

11.4.1 ST Segment Deviation

Assessment of the ECG is a critical requirement to enable correct diagnosis. Features may vary depending on duration (acute vs chronic), extent of culprit vessel occlusion (i.e. complete vs partial), topography and presence of associated abnormalities such as conduction disease.

The earliest and most consistent ECG finding during acute ischaemia is deviation of the ST segment. Under normal conditions, the ST segment is invariably isoelectric. Ischaemia can reduce resting membrane potential, shorten action potential duration and decrease rate and amplitude of phase 0. This results in a voltage gradient between ischaemic and non-ischaemic regions and flows

SUBENDOCARDIAL

TRANSMURAL

Figure 11.2 Vector shifts with corresponding ST segment changes.

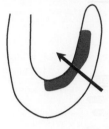
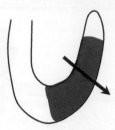

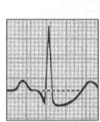
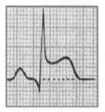

of current which are reflected on the ECG as ST segment changes. When acute ischaemia is of full thickness, i.e. transmural, overall ST vector is usually shifted in the direction of the epicardial layers (subepicardial) and ST segment elevation is produced over the ischaemic zone (see Figure 11.2). Reciprocal changes can manifest on the contralateral surface of the heart. By contrast, subendocardial ischaemia results in an overall vector that typically shifts towards the inner ventricular layer and cavity such that overlying leads demonstrate ST depression. These patterns should not be considered as absolute and universal, however, as subtle or absent ST-T changes may still be associated with significant ischaemia.

ECG changes can indicative likely coronary involvement (see Figure 11.3). Acute plaque rupture in the left anterior descending artery (LAD) territory typically presents with anterior ST elevation (V1–V4). Inferior ACS in the context of dominant right coronary artery (RCA) occlusion results in inferior ST elevation (II, III, aVF), whereas lateral ST elevation (I, aVL, V5–V6) is suggestive of circumflex artery (Cx) or diagonal territory involvement. ST elevation in aVR is strongly indicative of left main stem (LMS) or three-vessel involvement and may be accompanied by diffuse ST depression in other chest and limb leads. The presence of anterior ST depression accompanied by prominent R waves warrant assessment for posterior ST elevation using posterior leads (V7–V9) as this fulfils criteria for urgent revascularisation (see Section 11.7).

11.4.2 Q Waves and T Wave Inversion

Necrosis of sufficient myocardium can lead to persistent Q waves in one or more leads and its genesis may be explained by the theory of **electrical window of Wilson**. This describes the necrotic zone to be an electrical window that allows intraventricular normal QRS morphology to be recorded from the opposing necrotic wall of the left ventricle (LV). The lead facing the necrotic myocardium 'looks' into the cavity of the LV. Q waves were once considered markers of completed transmural infarcts and used to guide decision-making. However, it is now apparent that there is not always direct correlation, and as such, identification of Q waves in a patient with typical chest pain should be considered in addition to overall presentation rather than as an independent determinant for

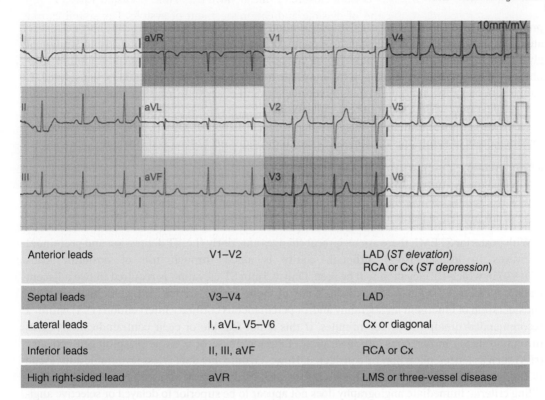

Anterior leads	V1–V2	LAD (*ST elevation*) RCA or Cx (*ST depression*)
Septal leads	V3–V4	LAD
Lateral leads	I, aVL, V5–V6	Cx or diagonal
Inferior leads	II, III, aVF	RCA or Cx
High right-sided lead	aVR	LMS or three-vessel disease

Figure 11.3 ECG territories in STEMI and associated coronary territories.

revascularisation. Q waves are considered pathological if > 1 mm width, > 2 mm amplitude, or > 25% depth of the QRS complex. Lead III often shows Q waves but this is concerning if found in isolation without changes in leads II and aVF. Complete normalisation following Q wave infarcts is uncommon but may occur if there is prompt, spontaneous recanalisation or establishment of good collaterals. It is generally associated with better prognosis. By comparison, persistent Q waves or ST segment elevation usually indicates that the involved region is severely hypokinetic, akinetic or aneurysmal.

Progressive evolution of ischaemia can result in T wave inversion within a period of hours to days. Unlike Q waves, these T wave changes can often resolve entirely. It is important to consider that there are multiple causes of T wave inversion aside from ischaemia, including ventricular hypertrophy, digoxin toxicity and electrolyte imbalance. It is also a normal variant in V1–V2 (if young) and V3 (if Afro-Caribbean).

11.5 Acute Management

Patients with suspected IHD require initial assessment using a conventional ABCDE approach. Unless there are absolute contraindications, all patients should be administered oral aspirin, a second anti-platelet (usually ticagrelor, prasugrel or clopidogrel) and subcutaneous fondaparinux (latter withheld in the context of STEMI or if estimated glomerular filtration rate [eGFR] < 20 ml min^{-1}). Fondaparinux is now favoured over low-molecular-weight heparin (LMWH) in view of similar efficacy but reduced occurrence of bleeding, long-term morbidity and mortality [1]. Conventional guidelines now advocate oxygen therapy only if saturations are not preserved at ≥94% due to potential risk of vasoconstriction and increased infarct burden associated with over-oxygenation. Alleviation of pain is of paramount importance and administration of glyceryl trinitrate (GTN) spray ought to be considered. Otherwise, titrated prescription of morphine or a long-acting nitrate (such as isosorbide mononitrate [ISMN]) should be considered. If pain is refractory, further options include commencement of a nitrate infusion and/or urgent coronary angiography with or without revascularisation.

There are certain situations in which immediate reperfusion for STEMI should be considered if maximal onset of symptoms is within 12 hours. Indications on 12-lead ECG include:

- ST elevation ≥2 mm in two adjacent chest leads;
- ST elevation ≥1 mm in two adjacent limb leads;
- new left bundle branch block (LBBB – indicative of proximal LAD disease);
- posterior infarction (anterior ST depression +/− prominent R waves).

With posterior STEMI, there are reciprocal changes anteriorly (i.e. ST depression and prominent R waves in leads V1–V2) although clarity is aided through use of posterior leads (V7–V9) in which ST elevation will be seen. Only 0.5 mm ST elevation is required in two adjacent leads for a formal diagnosis to be made. If any of these criteria are fulfilled, guidelines advocate consideration of emergent angiography and/or percutaneous coronary intervention (PCI) within a recommended timeframe of 120 minutes. If this is not feasible or clear contraindications exist, thrombolysis via intravenous administration of streptokinase or a tissue plasminogen activator (tPA) such as tenecteplase may be considered. However, outcome data is less favourable and rescue PCI may still be needed. In patients with resuscitated cardiac arrest and without ST elevation fulfilling criteria, immediate angiography does not appear to be superior to delayed or selective angiography in terms of survival at one month [2]. However, it may be considered on an individualised basis if there are concerns regarding ongoing ischaemia.

With NSTEMI presentations, there are specific subcohorts that are deemed very high-risk and warrant an immediate invasive strategy. This includes those with cardiogenic shock or haemodynamic instability, chest pain that is resistant to pharmacotherapy, life-threatening dysrhythmias, mechanical complications post-infarct, acute heart failure or ST depression >1 mm in more than six leads with ST elevation in aVR and/or V1 (indicative of LMS or three-vessel disease).

When there is a suggestive history but no ECG or clinical criteria for immediate reperfusion, troponin levels help with diagnosis and guide further management. This was conventionally performed 12 hours after the onset of maximal chest pain but newer assays are now available that facilitate earlier interpretation within three hours in the emergency department (ED) setting to enable discharge planning. A raised troponin suggests MI in the context of NSTEMI if there are no specific ECG features whereas normal troponin may imply unstable angina (i.e. plaque rupture without myocardial necrosis), stable angina or a non-cardiac cause such as musculoskeletal pain or gastro-oesophageal reflux disease (GORD). Hence, the need to seek a clear history and characterise the nature of chest pain and accompanying symptoms cannot be understated.

11.6 Risk Stratification

Once a formal diagnosis of IHD is made, it is pertinent to stratify risk so that management strategy can be guided. The **TIMI** risk score for STEMI is a prognostication scheme which includes physiological parameters such as heart rate (HR), blood pressure (BP) and weight in addition to

ECG changes (STEMI or LBBB) and time to intervention. Overall, it provides absolute risk of 30-day mortality [3]. The scoring tool for NSTEMI depends on age, cardiovascular risk factors, coronary anatomy, symptoms, ECG changes and biochemical markers. It predicts risk of all-cause mortality, new or recurrent infarction or ischaemia requiring urgent revascularisation at 14 days [4]. The **GRACE** risk score was derived from an unselected registry population of IHD presentations [5]. Eight independent variables were found to predict in-hospital mortality or further infarction or mortality within six months of discharge. These were age, HR, systolic BP, creatinine, Killip class, cardiac arrest at admission, elevated cardiac markers and ST segment changes. A risk score > 140 is suggestive of high risk and warrants early invasive strategy within 24 hours.

11.7 Revascularisation

As inferred, invasive coronary angiography is the gold standard in providing anatomical assessment for presence and extent of coronary lesions, with further intervention guided by location and distribution of 'significant' disease. This is usually defined as $\geq 50\%$ luminal involvement in the LMS or $\geq 70\%$ in one of the major epicardial arteries. There is a growing body of evidence that lesions that do not visually appear to be flow-limiting can be physiologically significant and hence may benefit from revascularisation. These are best defined by intracoronary physiological measurements that include fractional flow reserve (FFR; ≤ 0.80 deemed abnormal) and instantaneous wave-free ratio (iFR; ≤ 0.89 considered abnormal). Advocacy for use of adjunct intracoronary imaging such as intravascular ultrasound (IVUS) and optical coherence tomography (OCT) also exists based upon measurement of minimal luminal area, but this is more contentious and less used in routine clinical practice. OCT confers better spatial resolution than IVUS due to utilisation of light rather than sound energy, which has shorter wavelength. It is generally preferred for visualisation of luminal thrombus and stents but has worse penetration and requires clearing of blood, making it less favourable for ostial LMS lesions.

Radial arterial access is preferred to femoral as default approach in view of lower rates of infection, access site complication and major bleeding [6]. It also enables patients to mobilise sooner post-procedure which facilitates timely discharge. In STEMI presentations, it is usually only the culprit lesion that is intervened upon. Multi-vessel PCI is generally not explored, even in those with concurrent cardiogenic shock. However, a recent study has recognised the potential benefit of additional, preventive PCI in non-infarct coronary arteries with significant disease to reduce adverse cardiovascular events. It is therefore conventional in most centres to treat significant residual disease identified on acute angiography during their inpatient stay or in the outpatient setting within 45 days [7].

If there is evidence of three-vessel disease in the context of diabetes mellitus of any severity, clinical outcome data favours coronary artery bypass grafting (CABG) compared with PCI [8]. Infarction and all-cause mortality rate is reduced albeit with higher risk of cerebrovascular events. In the absence of diabetes mellitus, CABG is generally preferred if technically appropriate, although PCI can be considered if anatomical complexity is low (defined by angiographic-based SYNTAX score ≤ 22). Significant LMS stenosis is associated with worse prognosis. CABG has traditionally been considered standard of care for these cohorts as it provides survival benefit compared with standard medical therapy [9]. This is particularly relevant with distal LMS involvement which is technically more challenging. However, more recent randomised trials suggest non-inferiority of PCI compared with CABG [10], which has been corroborated at five years, and it may therefore be considered a suitable option in those with low SYNTAX score irrespective of glycaemic status.

A holistic approach is imperative when defining whether a patient is best served by PCI or CABG. Technical aspects that support the first approach include low SYNTAX score, severe chest deformation (e.g. scoliosis) or porcelain aorta. Drug-eluting stents (DES) with durable polymer coatings have revolutionised PCI procedures. They reduce late lumen loss and rates of lesion re-stenosis when compared with preceding bare metal stents (BMS) by more effective suppression of intimal hyperplasia. However, first-generation stents were associated with increased risk of late stent thrombosis, partly attributed to polymer hypersensitivity reaction. Contemporary practice involves use of biocompatible or biodegradable DES, or polymer-free DES that provide similar efficacy to polymer DES and comparable safety profile to BMS as the polymer coating degrades over two to nine months. CABG, on the other hand, is generally favoured if there is concurrent significant LV dysfunction, recurrent diffuse in-stent re-stenosis or established contraindication to dual antiplatelets. It may also be explored if PCI is unlikely to result in adequate and complete revascularisation or if there is a separate need for surgical intervention such as valve or aortic disease.

11.8 Secondary Prevention

11.8.1 Anti-platelets

Platelets play a crucial role in maintaining vascular integrity through the process of haemostasis. However, an exaggerated response is detrimental if there is platelet-dependent thrombosis induced by plaque rupture. For this reason, anti-platelets play a crucial role in secondary prevention post-infarction (STEMI or NSTEMI) to reduce the risk of future coronary events.

Aspirin works by inhibiting cyclo-oxygenase (COX) 1 and 2, thus preventing production of thromboxane A2 (see Figure 11.4). Lifelong therapy with low-dose aspirin is indicated to reduce risk of recurrent events and mortality [11]. As it is a relatively weak agent in isolation, synergistic effects from dual therapy are preferred to monotherapy. This is typically for a duration of 12 months after an event and roughly correlates with the time required for re-endothelialisation after insertion of DES. The second anti-platelet functions via P2Y12 ADP receptor antagonism and includes irreversible thienopyridines such as **clopidogrel** [12] and **prasugrel** [13]. These are

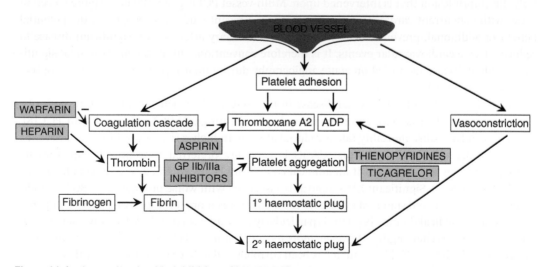

Figure 11.4 Agents involved in inhibition of haemostasis.

prodrugs and require hepatic metabolism to exert their effect. Compared with aspirin monotherapy, they are associated with reduced rate of ischaemic events and mortality, though increased risk of bleeding. More recently, reversible P2Y12 ADP receptor inhibitors such as **ticagrelor** have become available. These have more rapid onset of action, do not require hepatic metabolism and result in more pronounced platelet inhibition compared with clopidogrel. It has been shown to significantly reduce rate of ischaemic events without increase in burden of overall major bleeding, although with higher occurrence of non-procedure-related bleeding [14]. Indeed, recent trials have also advocated a potential role for long-term therapy beyond 12 months [15], although clarification is lacking on the subcohorts that are best suited for this strategy. Its main documented side-effect is the sensation of dyspnoea at rest which is potentially mediated via ADP inhibition on sensory neurons. However, symptoms are often short-lived, self-limiting and drug discontinuation is infrequent.

11.8.2 Beta-blockers

Beta-blockers are proven to reduce mortality and recurrent events after MI [16]. Evidence is largely from trials conducted in the era before reperfusion. Hence, whether beta-blockers confer long-term benefit in those with preserved LV function beyond one year in the post-reperfusion era is less apparent. Their broad mechanism of action is by competitive inhibition of β_1-adrenoceptors. Lowering of HR reduces myocardial oxygen requirement and provides symptomatic relief. Coronary blood flow is also enhanced due to greater diastolic filling of ventricles. BP is decreased primarily via reductions in HR (negative chronotropy) and stroke volume (SV; negative inotropy) rather than impact on total peripheral resistance (TPR).

Agents commonly used in clinical practice include bisoprolol (longest half-life), atenolol and metoprolol (shortest half-life). All are reasonably cardioselective, i.e. target β_1 as opposed to β_2 receptors, and are therefore less implicated with adverse effects such as bronchospasm and hypoglycaemia in the context of diabetes mellitus. They are not absolutely contraindicated in those with emphysema, asthma or peripheral vascular disease but should be used with caution and ideally initiated under specialist monitoring. A potential alternative is nebivolol which is shown to be up to 3.5 times more cardioselective than bisoprolol in pharmacological studies.

11.8.3 RAA System Inhibitors

The role of renin–angiotensin–aldosterone (RAA) system inhibitors is to attenuate neurohumoral activation and ventricular remodelling that occurs after MI. Angiotensin-converting enzyme (ACE) inhibitor therapy is associated with reduction in hospitalisation for congestive heart failure (CHF) and confers mortality benefit that is present even when ventricular dysfunction is absent (ramipril [17], perindopril [18]). This has been replicated by several agents suggestive of a class effect. The most common reason for discontinuation is bradykinin-mediated cough, and if this arises, therapy with an angiotensin II receptor blocker (ARB) appears to have comparable effectiveness in patients post-MI with evidence of severe ventricular dysfunction [19]. Aldosterone antagonists are not routinely licenced for use but eplerenone can be considered in those with left ventricular dysfunction (EF≤40%) and clinical evidence of heart failure if administered within 10–14 days of the acute event [20].

11.8.4 Statins

Increased total cholesterol and low-density lipoprotein (LDL) levels are associated with coronary disease burden and there is convincing evidence for lifelong high-dose statin therapy to reduce morbidity and mortality [21]. Statins competitively inhibit 3-hydroxy-3-methyl-glutaryl-coenzyme A (HMG-CoA) reductase, the rate-limiting enzyme of hepatic cholesterol biosynthesis. In addition, statins reduce C-reactive protein (CRP) levels via modulation of the inflammatory response and are therefore likely to play a role in abrogating plaque formation and progression. Its main side-effect is myopathy which results in muscle ache and can cause rhabdomyolysis in severe instances. Statins can also be associated with deranged liver function, usually alanine transaminase (ALT), and can enhance risk of developing diabetes. For those unable to tolerate atorvastatin or simvastatin, rosuvastatin is an alternative that has lower propensity for side-effects. In patients post-MI, target levels are LDL $\leq 1.4\,mmol\,l^{-1}$ (and 50% reduction from baseline), non-HDL $< 2.2\,mmol\,l^{-1}$ and apolipoprotein B $< 65\,mg\,dl^{-1}$.

11.8.5 Nitrate-based Vasodilators

Nitrate-based vasodilators are indicated to confer symptomatic relief but they have no mortality benefit. These agents work by being denitrated in VSMCs to produce NO (see Section 8.4.3). Subsequent activation of guanylate cyclase to convert GTP into cGMP triggers VSMC relaxation and other anti-atherothrombotic effects. This is evident in systemic arteries, including coronaries, and veins but most marked in the venous circulation. The venodilator effect reduces preload and myocardial oxygen demand. There is subsequent increase in exercise capacity and a greater total body workload can be achieved before the threshold for angina is reached. In coronary vasculature, smooth muscle relaxation can reduce resistance and enhance flow. As outlined previously, it can also alleviate local vasoconstriction caused by endothelial dysfunction in the context of atherosclerosis. Increased flow in collaterals can redistribute blood to ischaemic segments. Additionally, decrease in LV diastolic pressure through reduced preload reduces subendocardial compression of penetrating coronary branches and augments blood flow. Enhanced NO production also has anti-thrombotic, anti-inflammatory and anti-apoptotic effects.

The most commonly used vasodilator preparation is ISMN, which does not undergo first-pass hepatic metabolism and has a half-life of a few minutes. The modified release preparation provides a 'nitrate-free window', which is critical in avoiding endothelial tolerance that develops due to production of free radicals such as superoxide. Notably, these agents are contraindicated if there is significant afterload such as severe aortic stenosis and hypertrophic obstructive cardiomyopathy (HOCM).

11.8.6 Intensive Glucose Management

Patients with diabetes develop IHD 15 years earlier than the general population and mortality rates post-MI are doubled. This unfavourable prognosis has prompted studies to assess benefits of intensive glucose management in the immediate post-event phase. A landmark study suggested that initial intravenous insulin-glucose regimen followed by a multi-dose, subcutaneous insulin regimen for ≥ 3 months improved long-term prognosis compared with conventional therapy [22]. However, sample size was small and the study lacked robustness. It has since been superseded by a study that showed comparable outcome with intensive and conventional glycaemic management, although interpretation is hampered by the failure to achieve different glycaemic controls (as measured by HbA1c) between groups [23]. Nonetheless, epidemiological analysis implies that glucose levels are an independent predictor of mortality, and in view of this, close monitoring through conventional strategies are broadly advocated as initial management.

11.8.7 Lifestyle Modifications

Beyond pharmacotherapy, there is a clear need to address lifestyle modifications as an aspect of secondary prevention. Particular focus ought to be placed on modifiable risk factors such as weight, diet, exercise, BP and smoking intake. Input from the cardiac rehabilitation team plays a pivotal role both in the immediate phase and post-discharge, to ensure that recovery is optimised and risk factors are rigorously assessed.

11.9 Clinical Sequelae

The risk of developing complications post-MI is dependent upon acuity of presentation, infarct size, site and fractional thickness of involved myocardium. It is most frequently observed after late-presentation STEMI and nature is time-dependent. An overview of potential sequelae is provided in Figure 11.5.

11.9.1 Pulmonary Oedema

If the burden of myocardial involvement is extensive, as typically seen with anterior infarction, there is the risk of developing pulmonary oedema secondary to acute left ventricular failure (LVF). If this occurs, an ABCDE approach is adopted with management options that include furosemide, GTN infusion and/or continuous positive airway pressure (CPAP) treatment if there is persistent hypoxia despite high-flow oxygen.

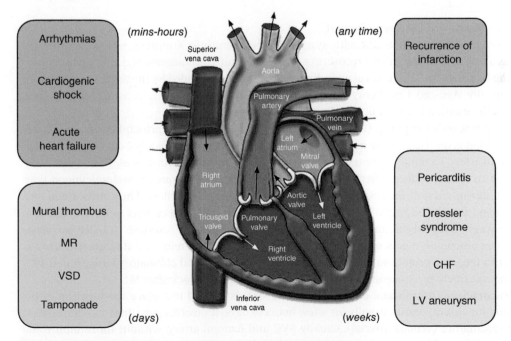

Figure 11.5 Potential clinical sequelae after myocardial infarction.

11.9.2 Cardiogenic Shock

A severe manifestation of LVF is cardiogenic shock with impaired cardiac output (CO) associated with systemic hypotension and organ hypoperfusion (e.g. oliguria). This occurs most commonly with anterior infarcts but urgent echocardiography is essential to exclude anatomical sequelae such as ventricular septal defect (VSD) and acute mitral regurgitation (MR) (see later). It is also crucial to distinguish LVF from right ventricular failure (RVF) secondary to inferior infarct. In the latter, intravascular volume augmentation via fluids is critical to maintain preload and right ventricular filling.

11.9.2.1 Inotropes and Vasopressors

Management of cardiogenic shock secondary to anterior infarct may require aggressive pharmacotherapy in the form of β-adrenergic agonists such as **dobutamine** and/or **dopamine**. The potentially detrimental α-adrenergic vasoconstrictor effects of dopamine only occur at higher dose. When administered at lower dose, it results in positive inotropy, positive chronotropy and vasodilation of renal and splanchnic vessels. This enhances CO and end-organ perfusion. Dobutamine also has positive inotropic effects comparable to dopamine but with slightly less chronotropic and vasoconstrictor potential. Of note, chronotropy increases myocardial oxygen burden and can therefore exacerbate ischaemic symptoms. As a result, continuous ECG monitoring is required with dose reduction or cessation if there is profound sinus tachycardia, supraventricular or ventricular tachycardias and/or ST segment deviation. An alternative agent that can be considered is **milrinone**. It is a phosphodiesterase inhibitor that elevates cyclic adenosine monophosphate (cAMP) levels and contrasts with other catecholamines as effects are not mediated via β-adrenergic stimulation. Hence, tachyphylaxis is not usually a clinical concern. It has inotropic and vasodilatory properties and its main side-effect is hypotension, which is compounded by its relatively prolonged half-life (one to three hours) and renal clearance.

11.9.2.2 Mechanical Circulatory Support

If hypotension remains resistant with systolic BP persistently < 90 mmHg, several devices can serve as a bridge until the patient recovers or receives definitive management, i.e. heart transplant or a long-term device. This requires an individualised approach guided by Interagency Registry for Mechanically Assisted Circulatory Support (INTERMACS) score, with consideration of local provision in addition to anatomical and physiological characteristics.

Intra-aortic balloon pump (IABP) counterpulsation describes the principle whereby a cylindrical balloon is inserted via the femoral artery into the aorta, approximately 2 cm distal to the left subclavian artery. It counter-pulsates, i.e. deflates in systole and inflates in diastole (see Figure 11.6). Deflation in systole reduces afterload via the vacuum effect and improves systemic blood flow. Inflation during diastole improves coronary perfusion via retrograde flow. Thus, myocardial oxygen demand is reduced and supply is increased. Absolute contraindications to device insertion include severe aortic regurgitation and aortic dissection. Although response to IABP correlates with better outcomes, it does not improve overall survival. It is therefore most frequently used as an interim measure prior to surgical intervention or for mechanical circulatory support peri-PCI, but is not routinely recommended in the context of cardiogenic shock after MI.

Extracorporeal membrane oxygenation (ECMO) is utilised to replace the function of the heart and lungs temporarily, usually for a few hours to days. It involves percutaneous cannulation of the vasculature (venous–arterial), usually SVC and femoral artery, without thoracotomy and allows pumping of blood from the patient to an artificial lung (oxygenator) which is then returned

Figure 11.6 Mechanisms underpinning IABP counterpulsation.

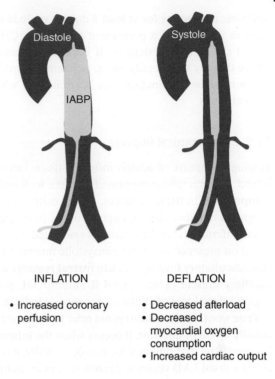

Diastole   Systole

IABP

INFLATION   DEFLATION

- Increased coronary perfusion
- Decreased afterload
- Decreased myocardial oxygen consumption
- Increased cardiac output

via a pump with retrograde flow to vital organs. It is the only percutaneous option for biventricular support and offers the option of rapid placement and haemodynamic resuscitation. However, it is non-physiological and a major drawback is its inability to provide left ventricular unloading resulting in high afterload and impaired coronary perfusion. Hence, concurrent IABP or Impella support is usually required. Other endemic complications include bleeding, renal failure, infection, leg ischaemia and cerebrovascular events.

If longer-term support is warranted, placement of an **Impella** device through a retrograde aortic approach, i.e. transfemoral, can be considered via fluoroscopic or echocardiographic guidance. It comprises a miniature rotary blood pump which is haemocompatible and allows early extubation and ambulation. It actively 'unloads' the LV by pulling blood and releasing into the aorta, which reduces myocardial oxygen demand and improves end-organ perfusion. Use also informs assessment of RV tolerance; however, there is no trial evidence of benefit.

A more advanced strategy involves use of **left ventricular assist device (LVAD)**, either as a long-term strategy or as bridge to **cardiac transplantation** (see Section 12.7.15).

11.9.3 Dysrhythmias

A broad range of dysrhythmias may occur post-MI. Narrow complex tachycardias such as sinus tachycardia, atrial fibrillation, atrial flutter and re-entry tachycardias are reasonably prevalent and managed as per conventional guidance. Broad complex tachycardias encompass a progressive spectrum from simple ectopy and non-sustained ventricular tachycardia to ventricular tachycardia (VT) with haemodynamic compromise. Management of these rhythms has been explored in earlier chapters. Conduction disease via ischaemia or infarction of the atrioventricular node can result in complete heart block (CHB). In the context of inferior MI, this is often transient and it is advisable to monitor for at least 5 days to exclude reversible precipitants and confirm persistence prior to insertion of a permanent pacemaker. CHB in the context of anterior MI suggests that infarct size is more extensive. It is generally associated with poor prognosis and threshold for device therapy is generally lower. Ischaemia or infarction of the sinoatrial node can equally result in sinus node dysfunction (see Section 5.3), which may manifest as a multitude of clinical presentations.

11.9.4 Mechanical Rupture

Tearing or rupture of acutely infarcted tissue can result in dramatic complications. A transmural infarct can precipitate rupture of the free wall and may lead to haemopericardium and **cardiac tamponade**. In these instances, urgent echocardiography with pericardiocentesis is required but prognosis remains dismal. Rupture of the interventricular septum may be apical (anterior MI) or basal (inferior MI) and the latter is associated with worse prognosis. It may be suspected clinically based on presence of a new, pansystolic murmur, often with associated thrill. The differential for this auscultatory finding is **acute mitral regurgitation** secondary to partial or total rupture of the papillary muscle (anterolateral if anterior MI, posteromedial if inferior MI). Once confirmed, urgent referral to a cardiothoracic centre is indicated to explore candidacy for valve replacement.

 True ventricular aneurysms refer to a discrete, thinned, dyskinetic region of the LV which is usually apical or anterior. It occurs when the infarcted myocardium is stretched with formation of fibrous tissue that bulges with systole. Usually, it is the consequence of total occlusion of a poorly collateralised LAD vessel and rarely occurs in multi-vessel disease where collateralisation is better established. Aneurysms can impair stroke volume although remaining segments often compensate via hyperkinesia. Nonetheless, there is increased predilection for rhythm perturbations and blood stasis within the non-contracting region can result in thrombus formation with associated embolic risk. True aneurysms rarely rupture. By contrast, **pseudoaneurysms** occur when there is contained myocardial rupture. They are often sited posteriorly and result in a narrow base. Organising thrombus and haematoma, together with pericardium, seal the site of rupture and hence, unlike with true aneurysms, the wall lacks any elements of the original myocardium. They pose an inherent high risk for rupture and cardiac tamponade.

11.9.5 Miscellaneous

Left ventricular **mural thrombus** is a recognised complication and occurrence is influenced by location and magnitude of the infarction. It is often seen in the presence of a LV aneurysm. Identification is typically with echocardiography with or without contrast, and once confirmed, formal anticoagulation is required to reduce risk of systemic embolisation. Infarction can also result in inflammation of the surrounding pericardium and cause **pericarditis**. Patients may present with chest pain that is often mistaken for recurrent angina. This pain, however, is typically stabbing in nature and alleviated by sitting forwards. It may be associated with pyrexia and raised inflammatory markers. ECG classically shows diffuse, saddle-shaped ST elevation with PR segment depression, although appearance may be obscured by infarct changes. Treatment is targeted at alleviation of pain using aspirin or non-steroidal anti-inflammatory drugs (NSAIDs) until symptom resolution, with addition of colchicine for up to six months. However, NSAIDs should be used cautiously as they can interfere with myocardial healing. Pericarditis may be associated with a pericardial effusion without features of tamponade and echocardiography can be used for confirmation. Resolution of this effusion may take several months. **Dressler syndrome** occurs one to eight weeks after infarction and is thought to be immune-mediated. It describes the association of pleurisy, pericarditis, pyrexia and raised inflammatory markers such as CRP. The condition is self-limiting and often resolves with aspirin monotherapy.

11.10 Differential Diagnoses

The differential diagnoses for patients presenting with raised troponin are broad and it is therefore imperative to consider results of biochemical profiling in the context of symptoms and ECG changes. Various clinical disorders can mimic IHD, including aortic dissection, pulmonary embolus and pneumonia. In addition, there are certain conditions that are important to consider in specific circumstances.

11.10.1 Type II Myocardial Infarction

Type II MI refers to raised troponin secondary to ischaemia due to increased oxygen demand or decreased supply. Some of the associated clinical disorders are outlined in Table 11.1. It is often the case that myocardial injury occurs in the context of pre-existent coronary disease and that ischaemia is worsened by the underlying disorder. Unlike the ACS subtype, it is without acute plaque rupture. There are no established guidelines for the management of these cohorts but conventional pharmacological agents are generally not applicable. Instead, the primary goal is to treat any underlying conditions that may have precipitated or exacerbated supply–demand mismatch.

11.10.2 Takotsubo Cardiomyopathy

This is characterised by chest pain, typical ST changes and moderate troponin rise in the setting of transient/reversible left ventricular systolic dysfunction (LVSD). Coronary angiography is unremarkable. Echocardiography and/or left ventriculography are diagnostic, however, with a typical appearance of RWMA at the LV apex with a ballooned segment ('octopus pot') (see Figure 11.7). It is often reported in the setting of severe physical or emotional stress and usually relates to sudden catecholamine surge with neurogenic myocardial damage. A higher concentration of β-receptors at the apex may be implicated in the observed phenotype. Appearances are entirely reversible although there is 10–15% risk of recurrence.

Table 11.1 Potential causes of type II myocardial infarction.

Causes of type II MI
Anaemia
Sepsis
Dysrhythmias
Hypoxia
Hypertension/hypotension
Post-cardiac surgery
Coronary vasospasm
Coronary embolism
Spontaneous coronary artery dissection

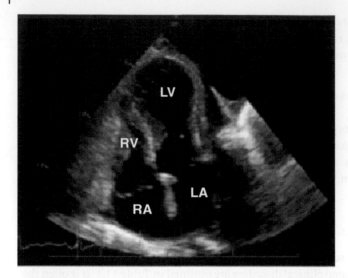

Figure 11.7 Four-chamber echocardiogram showing apical ballooning ('octopus pot').

Hot Points

- IHD encompasses disease states arising from myocardial ischaemia due to perfusion–demand mismatch.
- A subtype of IHD is ACS, which refers predominantly to atherosclerosis with acute plaque rupture. It may result in STEMI, NSTEMI, and unstable angina.
- There are specific 12-lead ECG criteria in the context of STEMI that warrant immediate coronary angiography (+/– revascularisation).
- Risk stratification can be achieved using prognostication schemes such as TIMI or GRACE risk scores.
- Pharmacotherapy for secondary prevention post-MI includes dual anti-platelets, beta-blockers, ACE inhibitors and statins. Vasodilators can be considered for symptomatic relief.
- Clinical sequelae post-MI include acute pulmonary oedema, cardiogenic shock, dysrhythmias and mechanical rupture (resulting in tamponade, acute mitral regurgitation or pseudoaneurysm formation).
- Type II MI is a mimic of ACS and refers to elevated troponin in the absence of acute plaque rupture. Potential causes include anaemia, sepsis, dysrhythmias, coronary vasospasm/embolism and SCAD.

11.11 Self-assessment Questions

1 In relation to pathophysiology of atherosclerosis, identify the correct statement.
 A The first macroscopic appearance of atherosclerosis begins in the early 50s as fatty streaks.
 B Disease states such as diabetes mellitus and hypercholesterolaemia result in anti-inflammatory milieu.
 C Recruited monocytes differentiate into macrophages which engulf lipoproteins and become oxidised foam cells.

D Positive vascular remodelling means that significant atherosclerotic plaque is always evident on coronary angiography.

E In acute coronary syndrome, progressive atherosclerosis causes progressive stenosis which ultimately results in vessel occlusion.

2   In relation to dynamic ECG changes, identify the incorrect statement.

A Transmural infarction is associated with ST segment elevation.

B Acute plaque rupture in LAD is generally associated with ST segment change in leads VI–V4.

C Acute plaque rupture in RCA is generally associated with ST segment change in leads II, III, and aVF.

D Complete ECG resolution following a transmural infarct is not possible.

E Persistent ST segment elevation may be indicative of left ventricular aneurysm formation within the affected myocardial segment.

3   Regarding acute management of STEMI, identify the incorrect statement.

A Fondaparinux is preferred to enoxaparin in view of similar efficacy but reduced incidence of bleeding, long-term morbidity and mortality.

B Patients should be given 15 l of oxygen via non-rebreathe mask.

C Glycoprotein IIb/IIIa inhibitors should not be used as first-line treatment for patients with refractory pain.

D In those who fulfil the criteria for emergency reperfusion, primary PCI is the gold standard of care.

E Analgesia is an important consideration and patients may require titrated doses of opiate.

4   With regard to revascularisation in the context of ACS, identify the correct statement.

A Significant lesions on angiography are defined as those that result in ≥ 50% stenoses in the LMS or a major epicardial vessel.

B Access via femoral artery is preferred to radial artery in view of lower rates of infection, access site complications and major bleeding.

C Adjunct techniques such as FFR or IVUS can help in decision-making for borderline angiographic lesions.

D PCI is preferred to CABG in multivessel disease particularly in the context of concomitant diabetes mellitus.

E BMS provide significant advancement over preceding DES with lower rates of in-stent restenosis.

5   With regard to secondary prevention, identify the incorrect statement.

A Aspirin functions by inhibiting COX 1 and 2, thus preventing production of thromboxane A2. Lifelong use is indicated following MI to reduce risk of recurrent events and mortality.

B Second anti-platelet agents which operate through P2Y12 ADP receptor antagonism are associated with reduced rate of ischaemic events and mortality, but with increased risk of major bleeding.

C Beta-blockers lower heart rate and reduce myocardial oxygen requirement. Coronary blood flow is also enhanced due to greater diastolic filling.

 D The most common reason for discontinuation of ACE inhibitors is bradykinin-induced cough.

 E Statins competitively inhibit HMG-CoA reductase but have the adverse effect of increasing CRP levels via modulation of the inflammatory response.

References

1 Fifth Organization to Assess Strategies in Acute Ischemic Syndromes Investigators, Yusuf, S., Mehta, S.R. et al. (2006). Comparison of fondaparinux and enoxaparin in acute coronary syndromes. *N. Engl. J. Med.* 354 (14): 1464–1476.

2 Desch, S., Freund, A., Akin, I. et al. (2021). Angiography after out-of-hospital cardiac arrest without ST-segment elevation. *N. Engl. J. Med.* 385 (27): 2544–2553.

3 Morrow, D.A., Antman, E.M., Charlesworth, A. et al. (2000). TIMI risk score for ST-elevation myocardial infarction: a convenient, bedside, clinical score for risk assessment at presentation: an intravenous nPA for treatment of infarcting myocardium early II trial substudy. *Circulation* 102 (17): 2031–2037.

4 Antman, E.M., Cohen, M., Bernink, P.J. et al. (2000). The TIMI risk score for unstable angina/non-ST elevation MI: a method for prognostication and therapeutic decision making. *JAMA* 284 (7): 835–842.

5 Granger, C.B., Goldberg, R.J., Dabbous, O. et al. (2003). Predictors of hospital mortality in the global registry of acute coronary events. *Arch. Intern. Med.* 163 (19): 2345–2353.

6 Jolly, S.S., Yusuf, S., Cairns, J. et al. (2011). Radial versus femoral access for coronary angiography and intervention in patients with acute coronary syndromes (RIVAL): a randomised, parallel group, multicentre trial (published correction appears in *Lancet*. 2011 April 23;377(9775):1408) (published correction appears in *Lancet*. 2011 July 2;378(9785):30). *Lancet* 377 (9775): 1409–1420.

7 Mehta, S.R., Wood, D.A., Storey, R.F. et al. (2019). Complete revascularization with multivessel PCI for myocardial infarction. *N. Engl. J. Med.* 381 (15): 1411–1421.

8 Farkouh, M.E., Domanski, M., Sleeper, L.A. et al. (2012). Strategies for multivessel revascularization in patients with diabetes. *N. Engl. J. Med.* 367 (25): 2375–2384.

9 Caracciolo, E.A., Davis, K.B., Sopko, G. et al. (1995). Comparison of surgical and medical group survival in patients with left main equivalent coronary artery disease. Long-term CASS experience. *Circulation* 91 (9): 2335–2344.

10 Stone, G.W., Sabik, J.F., Serruys, P.W. et al. (2016). Everolimus-eluting stents or bypass surgery for left main coronary artery disease (published correction appears in *N. Engl. J. Med.* 2019 October 31;381(18):1789). *N. Engl. J. Med.* 375 (23): 2223–2235.

11 Antiplatelet Trialists' Collaboration (1994). Collaborative overview of randomised trials of antiplatelet therapy-II: maintenance of vascular graft or arterial patency by antiplatelet therapy. *Br. Med. J.* 308 (6922): 159–168.

12 Mehta, S.R., Yusuf, S., and Clopidogrel in Unstable Angina to Prevent Recurrent Events (CURE) Study Investigators (2000). The Clopidogrel in Unstable angina to prevent Recurrent Events (CURE) trial programme; rationale, design and baseline characteristics including a meta-analysis of the effects of thienopyridines in vascular disease. *Eur. Heart J.* 21 (24): 2033–2041.

13 Wiviott, S.D., Braunwald, E., McCabe, C.H. et al. (2007). Prasugrel versus clopidogrel in patients with acute coronary syndromes. *N. Engl. J. Med.* 357 (20): 2001–2015.

14 Wallentin, L., Becker, R.C., Budaj, A. et al. (2009). Ticagrelor versus clopidogrel in patients with acute coronary syndromes. *N. Engl. J. Med.* 361 (11): 1045–1057.

15 Bonaca, M.P., Bhatt, D.L., Cohen, M. et al. (2015). Long-term use of ticagrelor in patients with prior myocardial infarction. *N. Engl. J. Med.* 372 (19): 1791–1800.

16 Freemantle, N., Cleland, J., Young, P. et al. (1999). Beta blockade after myocardial infarction: systematic review and meta regression analysis. *Br. Med. J.* 318 (7200): 1730–1737.

17 Sleight, P. (2000). The HOPE study (heart outcomes prevention evaluation). *J. Renin Angiotensin Aldosterone Syst.* 1 (1): 18–20.

18 Fox, K.M. (2003). EURopean trial on reduction of cardiac events with perindopril in stable coronary artery disease investigators. Efficacy of perindopril in reduction of cardiovascular events among patients with stable coronary artery disease: randomised, double-blind, placebo-controlled, multicentre trial (the EUROPA study). *Lancet* 362 (9386): 782–788.

19 Pfeffer, M.A., McMurray, J.J., Velazquez, E.J. et al. (2003). Valsartan, captopril, or both in myocardial infarction complicated by heart failure, left ventricular dysfunction, or both (published correction appears in *N. Engl. J. Med.* 2004 January 8;350(2):203). *N. Engl. J. Med.* 349 (20): 1893–1906.

20 Pitt, B., Williams, G., Remme, W. et al. (2001). The EPHESUS trial: eplerenone in patients with heart failure due to systolic dysfunction complicating acute myocardial infarction. Eplerenone post-AMI heart failure efficacy and survival study. *Cardiovasc. Drugs Ther.* 15 (1): 79–87.

21 Cannon, C.P., Braunwald, E., McCabe, C.H. et al. (2004). Intensive versus moderate lipid lowering with statins after acute coronary syndromes (published correction appears in *N. Engl. J. Med.* 2006 February 16;354(7):778). *N. Engl. J. Med.* 350 (15): 1495–1504.

22 Malmberg, K., Rydén, L., Efendic, S. et al. (1995). Randomized trial of insulin-glucose infusion followed by subcutaneous insulin treatment in diabetic patients with acute myocardial infarction (DIGAMI study): effects on mortality at 1 year. *J. Am. Coll. Cardiol.* 26 (1): 57–65.

23 Malmberg, K., Rydén, L., Wedel, H. et al. (2005). Intense metabolic control by means of insulin in patients with diabetes mellitus and acute myocardial infarction (DIGAMI 2): effects on mortality and morbidity. *Eur. Heart J.* 26 (7): 650–661.

Further Reading

Burkhoff, D., Sayer, G., Doshi, D., and Uriel, N. (2015). Hemodynamics of mechanical circulatory support. *J. Am. Coll. Cardiol.* 66 (23): 2663–2674.

Collet, J.P., Thiele, H., Barbato, E. et al. (2021). 2020 ESC guidelines for the management of acute coronary syndromes in patients presenting without persistent ST-segment elevation (published correction appears in *Eur. Heart J.* 2021 May 14;42(19):1908) (published correction appears in *Eur. Heart J.* 2021 May 14;42(19):1925) (published correction appears in *Eur. Heart J.* 2021 May 13). *Eur. Heart J.* 42 (14): 1289–1367.

Ibanez, B., James, S., Agewall, S. et al. (2018). 2017 ESC guidelines for the management of acute myocardial infarction in patients presenting with ST-segment elevation: the Task Force for the Management of Acute Myocardial Infarction in Patients Presenting with ST-segment Elevation of the European Society of Cardiology (ESC). *Eur. Heart J.* 39 (2): 119–177.

12

Congestive Heart Failure

CHAPTER MENU

Cardiology at its Core, First Edition. Peysh A. Patel.
© 2023 John Wiley & Sons Ltd. Published 2023 by John Wiley & Sons Ltd.

12.1   Learning Objectives

- Low vs high-output heart failure.
- Underlying aetiologies.
- Pathophysiology of systolic dysfunction.
- Categorisation.
- Diagnostic strategies.
- Management options including pharmacological agents and device therapy (ICD/CRT).
- Mechanisms, investigation and treatment of heart failure with preserved ejection fraction (HFpEF).

12.2   Low vs High-output Failure

Broadly speaking, congestive heart failure (CHF) refers to failure of the myocardial pump to provide adequate perfusion to end-organs. It is useful to define this more precisely as **low-output** heart failure, and the rest of the chapter deals with this. It should be differentiated from high-output states such as anaemia, pregnancy, thyrotoxicosis and Paget's disease, where the pump is intrinsically preserved but insufficient in the context of increased metabolic need. These underlying disorders can result in peripheral vasodilation and/or arteriovenous shunting that reduce total peripheral resistance (TPR) and systemic blood pressure (BP). There is compensatory activation of the renin–angiotensin–aldosterone (RAA) system and sympathetic outflow which results in ventricular remodelling and features of CHF.

12.3   Aetiology

There is no uniform classification to describe underlying causes of CHF. In developed countries, ischaemic heart disease (IHD) is most strongly attributable in addition to systemic hypertension. Structural disease of the mitral valve (MV) and aortic valve (AV) can also be implicated. Cardiomyopathy refers to intrinsic disease of the myocardium; hence infarction could be labelled as type of ischaemic cardiomyopathy. However, the term is conventionally used to describe hypertrophic, dilated or restrictive cardiomyopathy that may be of genetic inheritance (see Chapter 14). Of these, dilated cardiomyopathy (DCM) is most frequently encountered with infection (e.g. prior myocarditis), alcohol excess, chemotherapy (particularly anthracyclines), pregnancy and genetic predisposition all implicated in addition to true idiopathic cases. The contribution of diabetes mellitus is not entirely understood but is strongly associated with hypertension and coronary disease in addition to potentially direct glucotoxic effects on the myocardium. As outlined in Chapter 2, atrial fibrillation (AF) with persistently fast ventricular response can contribute to tachycardiomyopathy. Indeed, both disorders commonly coexist and this makes it challenging to ascertain which of the two was the precipitant. Much rarer causes of CHF to consider in specific contexts include Loeffler endocarditis, endomyocardial fibrosis, septal defects and conduction disorders.

12.4 Pathophysiology

Systolic dysfunction describes an inability of the ventricle to contract adequately, whilst diastolic dysfunction refers to a disorder of ventricular filling. In reality, these two often coexist with diastolic dysfunction preceding systolic dysfunction.

In the initial phase, there is sodium and water retention (see Figure 12.1). This increase in preload is a compensatory response to augment stroke volume (SV) via the Frank–Starling mechanism. Additionally, retention leads to arterial constriction and stiffening which heightens afterload. The heart compensates for increased preload and afterload by undergoing myocyte hypertrophy (pressure overload resulting in thickening) and dilatation (volume overload resulting in elongation). These compensatory mechanisms are a short-term solution and ultimately fail. Ventricular dilatation may stretch the mitral annulus and result in secondary functional regurgitation which perpetuates disease progression. Eventually, there is myocyte necrosis and replacement fibrosis. A reduction in sarcomere shortening also occurs and causes increased end-systole volume (ESV) and impaired SV.

The neurohumoral response in CHF is complex. Enhanced sympathetic activity in the acute setting has chronotropic and inotropic effects which augment cardiac output (CO). It also activates the RAA system via promotion of renin release which enhances preload. However, it is clear that sustained activation is detrimental, or maladaptive, with altered myocardial metabolism and direct toxic effects mediated in part by the production of angiotensin II. Endothelial dysfunction is a pathological hallmark of chronic conditions related to CHF and resultant reduction in NO bioavailability causes blunted vasodilation of coronary and peripheral vasculature. It also contributes to impaired functional hyperaemia in vascular beds that further impacts tissue perfusion.

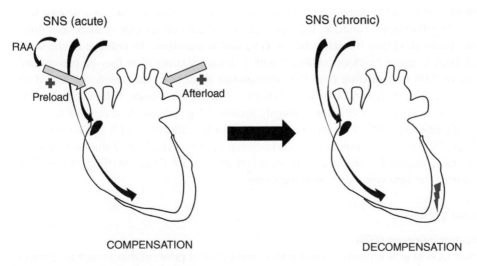

Figure 12.1 Pathophysiology of CHF.

12.5 Categorisation

Congestive heart failure is typically subcategorised based upon severity of ventricular dysfunction as quantified by ejection fraction (EF). Importantly, EF is often erroneously assumed to be a marker of myocardial contractility or CO, but in pure terms, it can only be considered as a characterisation of proportional change in chamber volume:

$$EF(\%) = \left[\left(EDV - ESV \right) \div EDV \right] \times 100$$

Heart failure with reduced ejection fraction (HFrEF) refers to typical symptoms and/or signs with EF ≤ 40%. However, there has been a recent paradigm shift in our understanding of the condition, triggered by the observation that similar clinical presentations can also occur in those whose EF is mid-range (41–49%), coined heart failure with mildly reduced EF (HFmrEF), and also those with preserved systolic function due to EF ≥ 50% (HFpEF).

12.6 Diagnosis

12.6.1 History

Breathlessness is the primary symptom and is incorporated within New York Heart Association (NYHA) classification to stratify severity based on functional capacity (class I – no limitation in ordinary activities, class IV – breathlessness at rest). There may be associated breathlessness on lying flat (orthopnoea) or bending down (bendopnea). Paroxysmal nocturnal dyspnoea (PND) can also occur where patients are awoken at night due to breathlessness. A history of 'cardiac wheeze' may be provided and must be distinguished from respiratory causes. Patients may report abdominal bloating due to ascites or leg swelling. An exploration of symptom profile and review of past medical history is paramount to clarify potential aetiology.

12.6.2 Examination

Auscultation may confirm the presence of sinus tachycardia or concurrent valvular disease (see Chapter 13). A S3 gallop may be audible. This results from sudden deceleration of blood as it flows from the left atrium (LA) into the left ventricle (LV) and is analogous to cadence of the word 'Kentucky'. Bilateral, coarse crackles consistent with pulmonary congestion may be present and occur because of fluid transudation from the intravascular space into the alveoli. Decreased air entry may be indicative of pleural effusions. Features of right ventricular failure may include raised jugular venous pressure (JVP), hepatomegaly, ascites or leg oedema. In severe left ventricular systolic dysfunction (LVSD), there may be evidence of pulsus alternans with alternating weak and strong beats. Ventricular dysfunction results in elevated left ventricular end-diastolic pressure (LVEDP) and as myocardial fibres are more stretched due to the Frank–Starling mechanism, contraction during the next systolic phase is increased.

12.6.3 Investigations

12.6.3.1 Electrocardiogram (ECG)

Resting 12-lead ECG may be entirely normal or show indicators of prior infarction such as Q waves or T wave inversion. Notably, T wave changes may equally be associated with LV hypertrophy secondary to systemic hypertension. There may be sinus tachycardia, AF or evidence of conduction disease which may demystify underlying pathophysiology. In the context of pulsus alternans,

Figure 12.2 Chest radiograph depicting CHF. Typical features are demonstrated, including cardiomegaly (although projection is anteroposterior), interstitial and alveolar oedema, upper lobe diversion and bilateral pleural effusions.

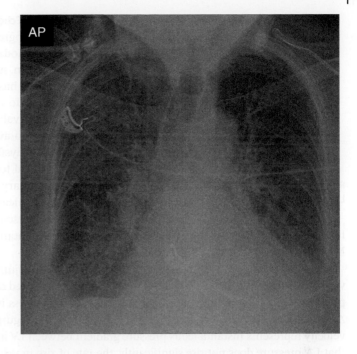

the ECG will demonstrate consecutive QRS complexes that are conducted normally but alternate in amplitude. A close assessment of QRS interval is important as presence of bundle branch block (BBB) morphology suggests more diffuse myocardial involvement and is a poor prognostic marker. As discussed later (see Section 12.7.12), it also determines suitability for cardiac resynchronisation therapy (CRT).

12.6.3.2 Chest Radiograph

A chest radiograph is useful in establishing cardiomegaly, defined as occupying > 50% of chest film in posteroanterior (PA) projection (see Figure 12.2). This will only occur in chronically diseased states as a consequence of hypertrophy or dilatation. There may be additional features including Kerley B lines (interstitial oedema), bat wing shadowing (alveolar oedema), upper lobe venous diversion (because of raised left atrial pressure) or pleural effusions. However, the absence of any of these features does not necessarily exclude the diagnosis of CHF.

12.6.3.3 Blood Profiling

Biochemical assessment should include full blood count (FBC), urea and electrolytes (U&Es), and liver function tests (LFTs). Troponin is useful if infarction is suspected as a precipitant but should not be performed routinely as troponin leak secondary to myocardial necrosis in the context of CHF is common. The use of B-type natriuretic peptide (BNP) has been advocated for screening in primary care. It is a 32-amino-acid polypeptide which is released by ventricles in response to excessive stretching of myocytes. It has excellent negative predictive value (NPV; i.e. detection of true negatives) but lacks sensitivity. In other words, it is useful as a 'rule out' test and obviates need for further testing. However, it can be raised in a variety of diseased states such as AF, valvular disease, anaemia and renal impairment. A BNP $\geq 35\,\text{pg}\,\text{ml}^{-1}$ or non-active prohormone N-terminal proBNP $\geq 125\,\text{pg}\,\text{ml}^{-1}$ with clinical symptoms and signs suggestive of CHF merits referral for echocardiography to establish whether ventricular dysfunction is present. It is of less use in the context of diastolic dysfunction and can be falsely low if body mass index (BMI) is raised.

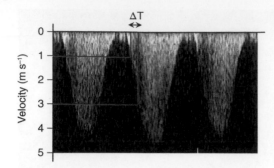

Figure 12.3 Calculation of dP/dt for assessment of LV function.

12.6.3.4 Echocardiography

Echocardiography is the most readily available imaging modality for assessment of ventricular function. A comparison with other imaging modalities has been provided in Chapter 10. It will provide anatomical assessment of atria, ventricles, valves, and pericardium. Functional data is also available to exclude diastolic and systolic dysfunction, significant valvular disease and to provide an indirect assessment of pulmonary artery pressure (PAP). Features of mechanical dyssynchrony reflecting LBBB may be present and include late septal stretch, late lateral wall shortening, late apical wall clockwise rotation ('septal flash') and delayed MV opening.

Mitral regurgitation, if present, is of particular use as an adjunct measure for assessment of left ventricular systolic function (LVSF). It involves indices obtained during the isovolumic contraction phase of ventricular systole (non-ejection) and is therefore less influenced by loading conditions. A pulsed-wave (PW) Doppler signal is obtained from the regurgitant jet and the corresponding velocity represents instantaneous pressure gradient between LV and LA in early systole. Assuming that LA pressure does not rise significantly, the rate of rise in velocity is reflective of rate in rise of LV pressure (see Figure 12.3). This can be used to calculate dP/dt using the following formula:

$$dP \,/\, dt = 32\,\text{mmHg} \div \Delta t \left(\text{between 1 and 3 m s}^{-1} \right)$$

A normal dP/dt is $> 1200\,\text{mmHg}\,\text{s}^{-1}$ and LVSD is indicated by values $< 800\,\text{mmHg}\,\text{s}^{-1}$. However, there are caveats that limit interpretation. One of the underlying assumptions is that LA pressure is insignificant during the pre-ejection period and that the atrium is compliant, which is not the case in acute mitral regurgitation. Eccentric jets may impair correct alignment of Doppler signal and similarly underestimate intensity. In patients with ventricular hypertrophy due to increased afterload, such as systemic hypertension or aortic stenosis, dP/dt may be normal even in the presence of LVSD. It should be noted that the principle of dP/dt calculation can also be extended to assessment of right ventricular systolic function (RVSF) using the tricuspid regurgitation signal, although in contrast, a pressure difference of 16 mmHg (i.e. 0–2 m s^{-1}) is measured.

12.6.3.5 Adjunct Investigations

Although echocardiography can be very informative, further investigation with cardiac MRI may be appropriate to provide more detailed tissue characterisation and aetiological evaluation through detection of myocardial oedema (e.g. active myocarditis) and classification of late gadolinium enhancement (LGE) distribution. If there is concurrent chronotropic incompetence (see Section 5.3.6), ambulatory ECG monitoring is useful. In situations where there is ambiguity about cause of breathlessness, objective lung function assessment using spirometry or cardiopulmonary exercise testing (CPEX) can be considered. Indeed, maximal oxygen consumption (VO$_{2\,\text{max}}$) is deemed a reliable indicator of cardiac dysfunction and prognosis in patients with advanced CHF [1]. However, respiratory and cardiac disease commonly coexist which makes delineation challenging. When there is suspicion of an ischaemic cause, adjunct stress imaging (see Chapter 10) or invasive coronary angiography may be considered. Cardiac biopsy is usually reserved for challenging cases where clinical uncertainty exists or where a formal diagnosis is relevant for cascade screening of first-degree relatives. Biopsy findings are particularly relevant in suspected giant cell myocarditis, eosinophilic myocarditis or sarcoidosis (see Section 14.5.3) where findings carry clear implications for treatment.

12.7 Management Strategies

12.7.1 Overview

An overview of pharmacological therapies for HFrEF is provided (see Figure 12.4) with exploration of agents that confer symptomatic and/or prognostic benefit. Angiotensin-converting enzyme (ACE) inhibitors and beta-blockers are advocated in all patients irrespective of symptoms. Adjunct treatment with aldosterone antagonist, switch from ACE inhibitor to sacubitril/valsartan and/or SGLT2 inhibitor (SGLT2 i) is advocated in those with persistent symptoms (NYHA class II or worse) and reflects contemporary foundational therapies for CHF. Treatment of HFmrEF is more contentious due to limited evidence base. As phenotype more closely resembles HFrEF than HFpEF, diuretics are indicated to alleviate congestion (class I indication) and agents such as ACE inhibitors/angiotensin receptor blockers (ARBs) and beta-blockers may be considered in symptomatic cases (class IIb indication) to reduce risk of HF hospitalisation and death. HFpEF is discussed separately in Section 12.8.

Effective management of HFrEF also requires consideration of adjunct strategies based upon individual context, including optimisation of comorbidities, rate or rhythm control of coexistent AF (if present), coronary revascularisation, exercise rehabilitation, family/genetic screening and intravenous ferric carboxymaltose.

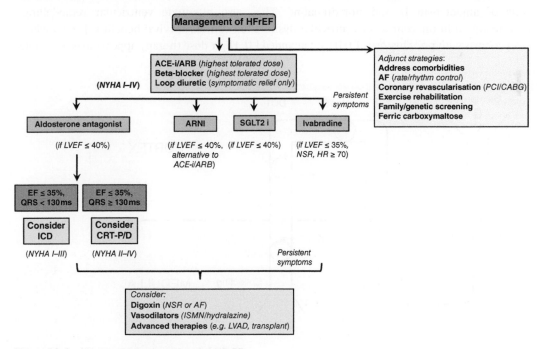

Figure 12.4 Management algorithm for HFrEF.

12.7.2 Diuretics

These primarily work by reducing fluid retention, plasma volume and preload. Hence, they can be considered for short-term, symptomatic relief rather than for prognostic benefit. Different agents vary in their targets on the renal tubular system (see Figure 12.5). Loop diuretics such as furosemide act on sodium/potassium/chloride transporters in the ascending limb of the loop of Henle. The net effect is enhanced sodium and water excretion. Oral absorption of furosemide is usually around 50% and a useful alternative is bumetanide which has better oral bioavailability (80–100%). Thiazides such as bendroflumethiazide target sodium/chloride transporters in the distal convoluted tubule (DCT). Potassium-sparing diuretics such as triamterene and amiloride target sodium–potassium exchangers in the DCT. Metolazone is a thiazide-like diuretic which acts on similar targets to conventional thiazides. Lastly, aldosterone antagonists such as spironolactone and eplerenone operate primarily on sodium–potassium transporters in the collecting ducts and, unlike other diuretics, also have prognostic benefit (see Section 12.7.5).

In the long term, diuretics may be reduced if fluid status reaches clinical euvolaemia. Indeed, chronic use is of potential detriment as it can result in the phenomenon of diuretic resistance. This relates to a failure to increase fluid and sodium excretion sufficiently to relieve volume overload, oedema or congestion despite full dosing. It can occur due to hypertrophy of tubular cells. However, the most common cause is renal venous congestion and this justifies impetus to be more aggressive with diuretic dosing when there is deteriorating renal function. Higher diuretic doses in CHF are broadly associated with worse outcomes although they may simply be a marker of more advanced disease.

12.7.3 ACE Inhibitors/ARB

The benefit of ACE inhibitors is deemed to relate to neurohumoral blockade with reduction in levels of angiotensin II and noradrenaline. They also attenuate ventricular remodelling. Administration in the context of ventricular dysfunction confers survival benefit [2], even when select cohorts with prior history of IHD are included [3]. High-dose therapy appears to be tolerable

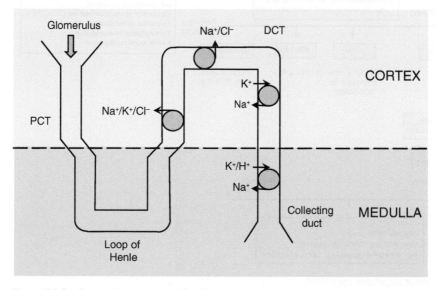

Figure 12.5 Target sites of action for diuretics.

and associated with comparable benefit on morbidity and mortality [4]. Hence, broad consensus is to uptitrate to the highest tolerated dose used in clinical trials with long-term maintenance. The primary side-effect is bradykinin-mediated cough. In those with true intolerance, an ARB can be initiated instead with comparable clinical effectiveness [5] although impact on mortality has been inconsistent.

12.7.4 Beta-blockers

As described in the context of IHD, beta-blockers have beneficial effects on chronotropy in relation to myocardial oxygen consumption. However, the coupled negative inotropy can be detrimental in the setting of acute decompensated heart failure where there is dependence on elevated sympathetic drive to maintain CO. It is generally advised that low-dose beta-blocker therapy is commenced once the acute phase has resolved and this enables positive impact on metabolism without compromising systemic circulation. Conventional beta-blockers antagonise β_1 receptors in the heart although carvedilol is a non-selective agent that also results in α_1 blockade. Beyond benefits to haemodynamic profile, beta-blockers suppress propensity for dysrhythmias such as ventricular ectopy. Hence, there is convincing evidence that long-term administration improves morbidity and survival [6, 7, 8].

12.7.5 Aldosterone Antagonists

As explored in Section 8.4.2, aldosterone is critical in mediating sodium and water retention, sympathetic activation and direct consequences such as myocardial and vascular fibrosis. When this is considered, there is a clear indication for aldosterone antagonism as adjunct therapy in combination with conventional pharmacotherapy as described earlier. Beyond diuresis, they provide neuroendocrine modulation and are associated with long-term improvement in morbidity and mortality [9, 10]. Currently, they are licensed for use in the context of CHF with left ventricular ejection fraction (LVEF) ≤40% when symptoms persist despite therapy with ACE inhibitor/ARB and beta-blocker. Eplerenone is often preferred to spironolactone as it has weaker affinity for androgen and progesterone receptors and is less likely to cause endocrine side-effects such as gynaecomastia.

12.7.6 Angiotensin receptor-neprilysin inhibitor (ARNI)

ACE inhibitors are the cornerstone of treatment for CHF with use of ARBs in those with intolerable side-effects. Contemporary research has identified a novel role for the use of combined ACE and neprilysin inhibition (ARNI) as an alternative to isolated ACE inhibitor or ARB therapy when symptoms persist and renal function allows. Neprilysin is an endopeptidase which degrades various peptides including natriuretic peptides and bradykinin. Increased levels via neprilysin inhibition counteracts the neurohumoral activation that propagates pathophysiology in CHF. Compared with enalapril, combination of valsartan and sacubitril appears to reduce hospitalisation and mortality in those with severe LVSD and NYHA class II–IV symptoms [11]. Although major guidelines identify eligibility based on LVEF ≤40%, some have adjusted criteria of ≤35%. This is because the PARADIGM-HF trial was subject to a protocol amendment one year after study commencement to optimise event rate and ensure that the study was adequately powered. Initiation ought to occur only after a washout period of ≥36 hours in those receiving ACE inhibitor. There is also emerging data to suggest adequate safety profile when initiated during inpatient stay after decompensated CHF, of which around 50% were ACE inhibitor/ARB-naïve [12]. This *de novo* initiation is yet to be incorporated into definitive guidance but can be considered (class IIb recommendation). Its main side-effect is symptomatic hypotension albeit with reduced incidence of renal dysfunction and electrolyte imbalance.

12.7.7 Sodium–Glucose Cotransporter 2 (SGLT2) Inhibitors

Dapagliflozin and empagliflozin are reversible inhibitors of sodium–glucose cotransporter 2 (SGLT2) situated in the proximal convoluted tubule (PCT). Beyond promotion of natriuresis without sympathetic nervous system (SNS) activation, they result in glycosuria, ketogenesis, erythropoiesis and exert anti-hypertrophic and anti-fibrotic properties. In patients with LVEF ≤40%, persistent symptoms (NYHA class II or worse) and adequate renal function, SGLT2 inhibitors have shown convincing benefit in reducing CHF hospitalisation and cardiovascular mortality [13, 14]. Impressively, this impact is conferred irrespective of diabetic status and across the full spectrum of glycaemic status. They may also be nephroprotective with the observation that a small initial deterioration may occur. Its side-effect profile is excellent albeit with slightly higher risk of genital infection and Fournier's gangrene. They are not currently licensed for use in those with concurrent type I diabetes mellitus.

12.7.8 Ivabradine

Ivabradine is an agent that specifically inhibits hyperpolarisation-activated cyclic nucleotide-gated (HCN) channels, thereby decreasing pacemaker current (I_f) in the sinoatrial node. It reduces heart rate (HR) without modifying inotropy, lusitropy and intracardiac conduction. Indeed, tolerability is enhanced by a compensatory increase in SV which preserves BP. It is licensed as add-on therapy in patients with severe LVSD (EF ≤35%), standard medical therapy and normal sinus rhythm (NSR) with resting HR ≥ 70 bpm [15]. It is also indicated in those who have a true contraindication or intolerance to conventional beta-blockers if HR profile allows.

12.7.9 Vasodilators

As detailed in Section 11.8.5, these agents are denitrated in vascular smooth muscle cells to produce NO and have vasodilatory effects. **Isosorbide mononitrate (ISMN)** dilates venous capacitance vessels and reduces preload. In the context of ischaemic cardiomyopathy, there is additive benefit of suppressing myocardial oxygen demand. Arterial vasodilators such as **hydralazine** decrease TPR and afterload with beneficial effects on SV and CO. Vasodilators are of particular benefit in those of Afro-Caribbean descent (who are often resistant to ACE inhibitors) and in situations where pre-existent renal dysfunction precludes initiation and uptitration of traditional agents. Despite conferring symptomatic relief, however, they do not exhibit prognostic advantage.

12.7.10 Digoxin

Digoxin is a cardiac glycoside with positively inotropic effects. It appears to reduce morbidity from hospitalisations due to CHF but has no impact on survival [16]. A clear indication for digoxin is in the subset with symptomatic CHF and coexistent permanent AF when it may indeed be superior to beta-blockers (see Section 2.6.1). It can similarly be considered as additional treatment when there is underlying sinus rhythm although evidence is less compelling. It is eliminated exclusively by the kidneys and this warrants close monitoring of renal function once loaded. Potassium competitively binds with digoxin for its receptor, and therefore, those with hypokalaemia are at particular risk of digoxin toxicity.

12.7.11 Ferric Carboxymaltose

Coexistent anaemia is estimated to be present in around 33% of patients with CHF. Mechanistically, it can result from impaired erythropoiesis, iron malabsorption secondary to gut oedema or haemodilution. Blood transfusion can be considered if there is critical illness but is not recommended as long-term therapy in view of inherent risk of infection, iron/fluid overload and human leucocyte antigen (HLA) sensitisation. Ferric carboxymaltose consists of a ferric hydroxide core that is stabilised by a carbohydrate shell, allowing controlled iron deposition to target tissues. A landmark randomised control trial (RCT) explored intravenous therapy in those with CHF and LVEF ≤40% (NYHA class II) or LVEF ≤45% (class III) and iron deficiency with or without anaemia, defined as haemoglobin ranging between 95 and $135\,gl^{-1}$ and ferritin $<100\,\mu gl^{-1}$, or $100\text{–}299\,\mu gl^{-1}$ with transferrin saturation $<20\%$ [17]. Intravenous ferric carxoxymaltose was shown to improve symptoms, functional capacity and quality of life with a tolerable side-effect profile. This data has also been corroborated by two more recent RCTs (LVEF cut-off ≤45% [18] and LVEF cut-off $<50\%$ [19]). Intravenous supplementation is therefore advocated if there has been recent hospitalisation, with no evidence for concurrent use of erythropoietin-stimulating agents. The risk of hypersensitivity reactions is considered to be in the region of 0.1–0.01%, with the primary reported side-effect being hypophosphataemia. Current trials are seeking to identify whether symptom relief translates into – mortality benefit in the longer term.

12.7.12 Device Therapy

Device therapy offers a potential therapeutic and prognostic strategy in certain instances (see Figure 12.6). It is generally not considered during an acute admission with decompensated CHF, but instead after adequate offloading and medical optimisation for a minimum period of three months.

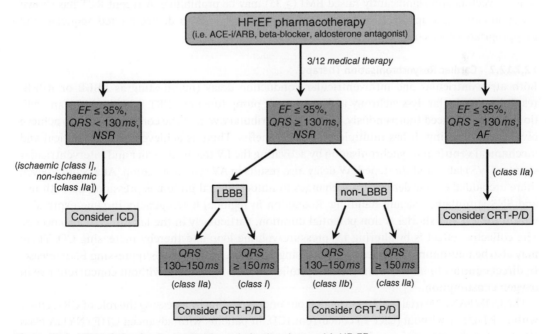

Figure 12.6 Device therapy for medically optimised patients with HFrEF.

12.7.12.1 Implantable Cardioverter–Defibrillator (ICD)

Sudden cardiac death occurs in approximately 40% of patients with CHF. Consequently, there has been extensive research to clarify added benefit of primary prevention ICD, with or without CRT. The MADIT trial [20] included those with ischaemic cardiomyopathy and severe ventricular dysfunction (EF≤40%) with non-sustained ventricular tachycardia (NSVT) and/or inducible ventricular tachycardia (VT) on electrophysiological testing. ICD significantly reduced mortality when compared with standard therapy. This was consistent with the MADIT-II trial [21] which incorporated LVEF ≤30% but no arrhythmic inclusion criteria and still demonstrated favourable outcome with ICD implant. Benefit was most pronounced in those with broadened QRS (i.e. ≥ 120 ms). Interestingly, the DANISH trial [22] showed that prophylactic ICD in patients with severe CHF of non-ischaemic aetiology (mostly diagnosed with invasive angiography) was not advantageous when compared with standard therapy, although there was age interaction with those < 59 years still likely to gain independent of CRT status.

Broadly speaking, if there is severe ventricular dysfunction (EF≤35%) despite optimised medical therapy (defined as ACE inhibitor, beta-blocker and aldosterone antagonist at highest tolerated dose), narrow QRS duration (< 130 ms) with predicted life expectancy > 1 year, candidacy for primary prevention ICD ought to be explored. This discussion is irrespective of underlying aetiology as it is superior to traditional anti-arrhythmics alone [23]. It is generally not recommended in the setting of NYHA class IV symptoms unless the patient is likely to be worked up for advanced CHF therapies (see Section 12.7.15).

Implantation can be considered via a transvenous system or using a subcutaneous approach. The latter reduces perioperative and long-term risks associated with conventional transvenous implantation, and also offers an alternative when anatomy would otherwise be prohibitive or preservation of access is required (such as in the context of haemodialysis). It can only be considered when there is no pacing indication or requirement, as in isolation, the system can only provide post-shock pacing for 30 s and is unable to deliver ATP. Eligibility requires screening for adequate sensing vectors and significantly raised BMI (≥ 35) may be prohibitive. A recent RCT has shown subcutaneous ICD approach to be non-inferior with regards to device-related sequelae and inappropriate shocks over a median follow-up of four years [24].

12.7.12.2 Cardiac Resynchronisation Therapy

Both atrioventricular and intraventricular conduction delay (manifesting as LBBB or RBBB) result in ventricular dyssynchrony and can impair pump function. CRT is achieved by an additional LV lead placed transvenously, typically in a tributary vein of the coronary sinus, to achieve biventricular pacing. It has multiple potential benefits. There is achievement of electrical and mechanical ventricular synchronisation by activating the LV free wall earlier and interventricular septum (IVS) later, and shortened AV delay also results in AV synchronisation. At a cellular level, there are added effects derived from changes in mitochondrial protein expression and both rest and SNS-stimulated calcium handling. Reduction in regional heterogeneity in gene expression within the LV and shorter action potential duration, particularly in the lateral wall, also occurs. The collective effect is by altering LV pressure/volume loop and thereby increasing CO. There may also be neurohumoral benefit by decreasing sympathetic drive and suppressing BNP release. In direct contrast to inotropes, improved systolic function is achieved without concurrent rise in oxygen consumption.

The COMPANION trial [25] has extended our understanding by assessing the role of CRT, either with (CRT-D) or without (CRT-P) concurrent ICD, in patients with advanced CHF (NYHA class III/IV) of ischaemic and non-ischaemic origin. In those with prolonged QRS, CRT decreased all-cause mortality when compared with medical therapy but no superiority of CRT-D over CRT-P was observed. More recently, the MADIT-CRT trial [26] included those with severe CHF (ischaemic and non-ischaemic), QRS duration ≥ 130 ms and milder NYHA class I/II symptoms. In comparison to ICD, CRT-D reduced morbidity from heart failure events with no disparity in mortality. This benefit was most apparent with QRS duration ≥ 150 ms. Based upon these trials, current guidelines impress that device eligibility is guided by symptom severity, QRS duration and BBB presence/morphology. In those with LBBB, a lower threshold for device implantation can be applied as the likelihood of significant remodelling is lower.

If QRS duration is < 130 ms, CRT is not indicated and may indeed be of detriment by heightening mortality risk [27]. Notably, most clinical trials exclusively included patients in sinus rhythm. The role of device therapy in the presence of concurrent persistent or permanent AF is less established though generally accepted if intrinsic QRS ≥ 130 ms with NYHA class III/IV symptoms and there is an adopted strategy to ensure adequate biventricular pacing.

Finally, if conventional criteria for CRT are fulfilled but there are anatomical restraints or inadequate response (termed 'non-responders' although this entity is not clearly defined), alternative strategies may include His pacing, left bundle branch area (LBBA) pacing and/or implantation of a surgical epicardial LV lead. Further discussion of these advanced techniques is beyond the scope of this chapter.

12.7.13 Coronary Revascularisation

Consideration for coronary revascularisation is guided primarily by symptoms and confirmation of inducible ischaemia on functional testing. If there are positive findings, it is prudent to proceed with angiography to assess extent and severity of disease. The anatomical profile determines further management with regards to PCI or CABG.

If truly asymptomatic, the historical perspective was that those with extensive areas of viable albeit dysfunctional myocardium (i.e. hibernating substrate) may benefit from intervention. In the setting of severe LVSD and known coronary disease, CABG appeared to be superior to standard therapy in reducing hospitalisation and cardiovascular mortality due to both pump failure and sudden cardiac death (SCD), although no difference in immediate all-cause mortality was observed [28]. There was apparent survival benefit with extended follow-up although only seen in specific groups such as those with three-vessel disease and aged < 60 years. A substudy analysis, however, failed to show that viability testing modulates likelihood of benefit from intervention. There has only been a single RCT exploring this notion [29], which found no difference in major adverse cardiac events (MACE) or mortality after five-year follow-up although a *post hoc* analysis suggested potential benefit in those with extensive hibernating myocardium. Coronary revascularisation also does not appear to improve LVEF to any significant extent with mean increase of only 2% at four months exhibited in the STICH trial. However, the potential for long-term recovery and its impact on survival have not been scrutinised. A recent RCT does inform present discussions by showing that in those with ischaemic cardiomyopathy (including LMS disease in around one-seventh), LVEF 35% and viability in four or more segments, revascularisation via PCI did not improve ventricular function or positively impact CHF hospitalisation or all-cause mortality [30].

Of course, mortality in patients with ischaemic cardiomyopathy may arise from aetiologies aside from isolated pump failure such as ventricular dysrhythmias. Scar tissue is a recognised substrate for arrhythmogenesis, as is the 'grey zone' between infarcted and viable myocardium due to heterogeneous conduction and differing refractoriness. It is conceptually plausible that revascularisation can modify this risk independent of improvement in contractile function, but a unifying comprehension of interplaying mechanisms is lacking.

12.7.14 Family Screening

Molecular analyses have uncovered causative mutations in genes coding for a range of proteins including those located in the sarcomere, cytoskeleton, nuclear envelope, and desmosomes. As most cases do not have distinctive phenotypic characteristics to indicate a genetic propensity, assessment of family history across at least three successive generations is paramount. The clinical presentation may also provide useful indication as atrioventricular block is implicated in *LMNA* or *SCN5A* mutations, raised ferritin/transferrin saturations with haemochromatosis and generalised muscle weakness with neuromuscular disorders (such as myotonic dystrophy). If no clear cause for DCM is elucidated (i.e. true 'idiopathic' DCM), clinical screening of first-degree relatives initially with 12-lead ECG and echocardiography may be warranted. Genetic testing is best reserved for contexts where there is clear familial involvement or where index of suspicion exists due to clinical profile. It has a variable diagnostic yield in the region of 33%. The primary implication is to facilitate mutation-specific cascade screening of family members as it does not affect treatment strategy or prognosis to any significant extent. This is with the notable exception of confirmed *LMNA* mutations when threshold for primary prevention ICD may be reduced to LVEF < 50% based on presence of concurrent risk factors such as LGE on cardiac MRI.

12.7.15 Advanced Therapies

12.7.15.1 Left Ventricular Assist Device (LVAD)

Left ventricular assist device therapy can be considered in three general contexts: (i) bridge to transplantation; (ii) bridge to transplant candidacy; and (iii) temporary support to reverse existent contraindications to transplantation, such as secondary pulmonary hypertension. The pump operates by providing non-pulsatile, continuous flow with the inflow cannula surgically implanted in the LV apex and outflow connected to ascending aorta. They also require a driveline which is tunnelled through the anterior abdominal wall and connects to the power supply and controller. A formal assessment for patient screening and selection is required; in particular, adequate RV function is crucial to achieve sufficient delivery of blood to the LV whilst preserving low venous pressures to avoid peripheral congestion. Most derive significant improvement in quality of life and functional capacity post-implant with comparable two-year survival to cardiac transplantation. However, adverse events can include bleeding, infection, cerebrovascular events, blood clots, device malfunction, progressive aortic regurgitation, and right-sided heart failure.

12.7.15.2 Cardiac Transplantation

Cardiac transplantation is a preferred treatment of choice in select patients with advanced CHF, on the premise that improved quality of life and overall survival is expected. Indications for referral with ambulatory cases include resistant symptoms despite medical optimisation, two or more hospital admission over the past year due to decompensation, deteriorating RV function, renal function or rising PAP and persistent ventricular dysrhythmias. In the context of acute admission, inpatient work-up may be indicated if there is inotrope dependence, reliance on ventilatory support for pulmonary congestion or resistant ventricular arrhythmias.

As significant mismatch between demand and supply exists, careful patient selection is imperative to maximise use of a limited donor pool. In view of this, rigorous pre-transplant screening is undertaken that includes blood profile, microbiology screen, blood group and tissue type, imaging, right heart catheterisation and functional assessment (such as via CPEX). Absolute and relative contraindications to transplantation need to be explored, including severe respiratory disease, irreversible renal impairment, active infection or malignancy and significantly raised BMI. Pulmonary hypertension *per se* does not result in ineligibility by default as reversibility may occur with pharmacological vasodilators and/or mechanical unloading with LVAD. However, if there is irreversibility despite these interventions with invasive PAP > 60 mmHg, transpulmonary gradient ≥ 15 mmHg and/or pulmonary vascular resistance (PVR) > 5 Woods units, transplantation cannot be considered.

12-month survival post-transplant is in the region of 85–90%, with median patient longevity in the region of 12–13 years. This improvement has been primarily driven by stabilisation in the immediate post-transplant phase.

12.8 Heart Failure with Preserved Ejection Fraction (HFpEF)

12.8.1 Pathophysiology

A number of mechanisms have been implicated in the development of HFpEF including impaired ventriculo-arterial coupling, chronotropic incompetence and endothelial dysfunction. The most significant contributor is deemed to be diastolic dysfunction, a feature that is typically coexistent and often precedes LVSD. Diastolic dysfunction results in elevated LVEDP and LA pressure with secondary pulmonary congestion.

Given the close relationship between HFpEF and diastolic dysfunction, a comprehension of normal diastolic physiology is critical. Diastole is typically defined as the period between closure of AV (end-systole) and MV (end-diastole) with four distinct phases: isovolumic relaxation, early rapid diastolic filling ('E wave'), diastasis and late diastolic filling ('A wave'). These periods can also be categorised into two broad groups: active myocardial relaxation which encompasse the first two, and passive ventricular filling which constitutes the final two.

As the name implies, active myocardial relaxation requires production of ATP within the myocardium. During isovolumic relaxation, LV pressure falls following AV closure but without change in volume. When pressure falls below atrial pressure, the MV opens. This defines onset of rapid diastolic filling with blood entering LA from the pulmonary veins and flowing across the valve into LV ('E wave'). The flow rate is influenced by several parameters that include pressure gradient, ventricular relaxation and ventricular compliance. Left ventricular compliance is a passive feature that is impacted by myocardial characteristics such as hypertrophy or extrinsic factors such as constrictive pericarditis. With blood flow, there is gradual pressure equalisation between atrium and ventricle resulting in a period of diastasis when there is minimal flow. This duration is longer at slower heart rates. The final phases of diastole arise as a result of atrial contraction which transiently increases LA pressure and causes a period of late diastolic filling ('A wave'). Phases of diastole in the RV are analogous to those already described, aside from shorter total duration due to longer ejection systolic period.

12.8.2 Aetiology

Systemic hypertension with secondary hypertrophy is the most discernible risk factor for development of HFpEF. Other contributors include diabetes mellitus, coronary disease, cardiomyopathies (see Chapter 14) and extrinsic factors such as constrictive pericarditis. In comparison with LVSD, patients with HFpEF tend to be older, predominantly female and with higher prevalence of noncardiac comorbidities such as renal impairment and chronic lung disease. Notably, diastolic filling can be influenced by multiple causes aside from diastolic function *per se*, such as HR, respiratory variation and coexistent disease including MV abnormalities and AF.

12.8.3 Diagnosis and Assessment

An initial strategy is to identify signs and/or symptoms of heart failure such as dyspnoea, orthopnoea and peripheral oedema. N-terminal proBNP can be used for screening, but should not be used in isolation as threshold differs in the presence of AF and can be falsely low with concurrent obesity. In view of this, evidence of preserved EF and absence of significant valvular disease must be sought. Echocardiography is the most commonly used diagnostic tool for this purpose as it is non-invasive and has the added benefit of allowing formal assessment of left ventricular diastolic function. This is done via measurement of PW Doppler flow across the MV, with particular scrutiny of early filling (E wave), late filling (A wave), rapidity of decline in flow velocity in early diastole (DT) and time for ventricular filling to begin after relaxation (IVRT).

A classification of diastolic dysfunction based upon echocardiographic parameters has been developed and broadly speaking, three grades are described (see Figure 12.7). In Grade I diastolic dysfunction, impaired ventricular relaxation results in reduced rate of decrease in ventricular pressure. This delays MV opening and reduces transmitral gradient, resulting in prolonged isovolumic relaxation time (IVRT), reduced E wave, prolonged deceleration time (DT) and increased A wave due to compensatory atrial filling. Classically, this manifests as reversed E : A ratio (i.e. height of A wave > E wave). In grade II (pseudo-normal) diastolic dysfunction, there is transition in pathophysiology from abnormal relaxation alone to an impairment of relaxation and compliance. Thus, the E velocity is normal due to concurrent increase in LA pressure which drives flow across the valve. Additionally, there is DT normalisation as decreased compliance results in rapid rise of ventricular pressure during early diastole. Detection of grade II diastolic dysfunction is via tissue Doppler imaging (TDI) to assess E : E' ratios, as well as identification of flow reversal into pulmonary veins, Valsalva manoeuvres to transiently reduce LA pressure and objective identification of ancillary findings such as LV hypertrophy or atrial dilatation. Grade III diastolic dysfunction represents restrictive filling, whereby relaxation and compliance remain impaired but compensatory increase in LA pressure masks underlying abnormalities. Thus, shortened IVRT arises due to earlier opening of MV with increased E : A and E : E' ratios, shortened DT and reduced/absent A wave with little filling because of raised LVEDP.

In cases where echocardiography is unable to provide diagnostic certainty, such as in the context of AF, invasive haemodynamic assessment via catheterisation remains the modality of choice with pulmonary capillary wedge pressure ≥ 15 mmHg (at rest, or ≥ 25 mmHg with exercise) and/or LVEDP ≥ 16 mmHg (at rest) considered diagnostic. Further testing may be needed if HFpEF is thought to be secondary to a reversible cause such as poorly controlled hypertension or myocardial ischaemia. In these circumstances, ambulatory blood pressure monitoring or coronary angiography may be of adjunct benefit.

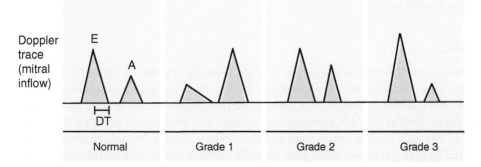

Figure 12.7 Mitral valve Doppler profiles in diastolic dysfunction.

12.8.4 Management

Evidence from clinical trials and observational studies remain limited and conflicting. This is primarily because diastolic dysfunction in isolation is rare and often coexists with other disease processes, including LVSD. Whereas a number of specific therapies are of proven mortality benefit in LVSD, the same is not true of HFpEF. ACE inhibitors, ARBs and beta-blockers have all failed to improve outcomes. Initial promise was demonstrated with use of aldosterone antagonists among patients with mild HFpEF but a subsequent trial failed to replicate this in a cohort of patients with more advanced disease [31]. Sacubitril/valsartan did not result in lowering of CHF hospitalisation or cardiovascular mortality compared with valsartan in patients with HFpEF, although inclusion criteria stipulated LVEF $\geq 45\%$ [32].

Most recently, dapagliflozin and empagliflozin have independently been shown to reduce composite outcome of CHF hospitalisation or cardiovascular mortality irrespective of diabetic status, although LVEF threshold of $> 40\%$ was used to define HFpEF [33, 34]. Current guidelines generally suggest for the primary focus to be placed on rigorous identification and treatment of underlying causes. Diuretics are indicated for symptomatic relief but caution is warranted to avoid excess lowering of preload. It is of no prognostic benefit.

Hot Points

- Low-output CHF refers to inability of the myocardial pump to provide adequate perfusion to end-organs.
- The initial response to increased preload and afterload in the context of CHF is ventricular dilatation and hypertrophy. Eventual failure of these compensatory mechanisms perpetuates pathophysiology.
- Echocardiography is the gold standard for diagnosis, with quantification of function in addition to anatomical data that may elucidate primary aetiology.
- Pharmacological options that have proven prognostic benefit include ACE-inhibitors (or ARB), beta-blockers, aldosterone antagonists, ARNIs and SGLT2 inhibitors.
- Primary prevention ICD via transvenous or subcutaneous approach should be considered if there is persistently severe ventricular dysfunction (EF $\leq 35\%$) and narrow QRS (< 130ms).
- Device therapy via CRT is indicated in those with persistent symptoms despite optimised medical therapy who have severe ventricular dysfunction (EF $\leq 35\%$) and BBB.
- HFpEF refers to patients with typical symptoms and signs of CHF and preserved systolic function. Diastolic dysfunction is deemed the primary contributor and current management relies primarily on treatment of co-morbidities.

12.9 Self-assessment Questions

1 Which of the following statements is true?
   - **A** Furosemide bioavailability is 100%.
   - **B** Metolazone acts on the loop of Henle.
   - **C** Eplerenone acts on the sodium/potassium exchanger in the distal convoluted tubule.
   - **D** Furosemide has prognostic benefit in CHF.
   - **E** Chronic diuretic use can result in resistance secondary to hypertrophy of tubular cells.

2 Which of the following statements on device therapy in heart failure is false?
 A CRT is indicated in patients with severe ventricular dysfunction despite medical optimisation and QRS duration ≥ 130ms.
 B The MADIT-II trial showed that ICDs improve survival over standard pharmacological therapy in patients with ischaemic cardiomyopathy.
 C The MADIT-CRT trial showed that in presence of prolonged QRS and severe heart failure, even those with milder symptoms (NYHA I/II) could derive morbidity benefit from CRT-D rather than ICD alone.
 D CRT is predominantly used in those admitted with acute decompensation of heart failure.
 E The COMPANION trial showed improved mortality for both CRT-D and CRT-P over standard treatment if patients had NYHA II/III symptoms and QRS duration ≥ 120 ms.

3 Which of the following is not a cause of high-output heart failure?
 A Diabetes.
 B Anaemia.
 C Thyrotoxicosis.
 D Paget's disease.
 E Pregnancy.

4 Regarding diastolic dysfunction, which of the following statements is correct?
 A Diastole is the period between mitral valve closure and aortic valve closure.
 B The 'E wave' signifies late rapid diastolic filling.
 C The 'A wave' is caused by atrial contraction.
 D Patients with HFpEF tend to be younger, female and less comorbid.
 E An 'E wave' that is greater than 'A wave' consistently rules out diastolic dysfunction.

5 Regarding low-output cardiac failure, which of the following statements is false?
 A Ischaemic heart disease and hypertension are common causes in the developed world.
 B The heart initially compensates for increased fluid retention by hypertrophy and dilatation.
 C Breathlessness at rest constitutes NYHA class II symptoms.
 D Chest radiograph may show Kerley B lines, upper lobe venous diversion, pleural effusions and cardiomegaly.
 E BNP is sensitive but not specific for diagnosis.

References

1 Lund, L.H., Aaronson, K.D., and Mancini, D.M. (2005). Validation of peak exercise oxygen consumption and the heart failure survival score for serial risk stratification in advanced heart failure. *Am. J. Cardiol.* 95 (6): 734–741.
2 CONSENSUS Trial Study Group (1987). Effects of enalapril on mortality in severe congestive heart failure. Results of the Cooperative North Scandinavian Enalapril Survival Study (CONSENSUS). *N. Engl. J. Med.* 316 (23): 1429–1435.

3 The Acute Infarction Ramipril Efficacy (AIRE) Study Investigators (1993 Oct 2). Effect of ramipril on mortality and morbidity of survivors of acute myocardial infarction with clinical evidence of heart failure. *Lancet.* 342 (8875): 821–828.

4 Packer, M., Poole-Wilson, P.A., Armstrong, P.W. et al. (1999). Comparative effects of low and high doses of the angiotensin-converting enzyme inhibitor, lisinopril, on morbidity and mortality in chronic heart failure. ATLAS Study Group. *Circulation* 100 (23): 2312–2318.

5 Granger, C.B., McMurray, J.J., Yusuf, S. et al. (2003). Effects of candesartan in patients with chronic heart failure and reduced left-ventricular systolic function intolerant to angiotensin-converting-enzyme inhibitors: the CHARM-alternative trial. *Lancet* 362 (9386): 772–776.

6 Hjalmarson, A., Goldstein, S., Fagerberg, B. et al. (1999). Effect of metoprolol CR/XL in chronic heart failure: Metoprolol CR/XL Randomised Intervention Trial in Congestive Heart Failure (MERIT-HF). *Lancet* 353 (9169): 2001–2007.

7 Packer, M., Coats, A.J., Fowler, M.B. et al. (2001). Effect of carvedilol on survival in severe chronic heart failure. *N. Engl. J. Med.* 344 (22): 1651–1658.

8 CIBIS-II Investigators and Committees (1999). The Cardiac Insufficiency Bisoprolol Study II (CIBIS-II): a randomised trial. *Lancet* 353 (9146): 9–13.

9 Pitt, B., Zannad, F., Remme, W.J. et al. (1999). The effect of spironolactone on morbidity and mortality in patients with severe heart failure. Randomized Aldactone Evaluation Study Investigators. *N. Engl. J. Med.* 341 (10): 709–717.

10 Pitt, B., Remme, W., Zannad, F. et al. (2003). Eplerenone, a selective aldosterone blocker, in patients with left ventricular dysfunction after myocardial infarction (published correction appears in *N. Engl. J. Med.* 2003 May 29; 348(22): 2271). *N. Engl. J. Med.* 348 (14): 1309–1321.

11 McMurray, J.J., Packer, M., Desai, A.S. et al. (2014). Angiotensin-neprilysin inhibition versus enalapril in heart failure. *N. Engl. J. Med.* 371 (11): 993–1004.

12 Velazquez, E.J., Morrow, D.A., DeVore, A.D. et al. (2019). Angiotensin-Neprilysin inhibition in acute decompensated heart failure (published correction appears in N. Engl. J. Med. 2019 March 14;380(11):1090). *N. Engl. J. Med.* 380 (6): 539–548.

13 McMurray, J.J.V., Solomon, S.D., Inzucchi, S.E. et al. (2019). Dapagliflozin in patients with heart failure and reduced ejection fraction. *N. Engl. J. Med.* 381 (21): 1995–2008.

14 Packer, M., Anker, S.D., Butler, J. et al. (2020). Cardiovascular and renal outcomes with Empagliflozin in heart failure. *N. Engl. J. Med.* 383 (15): 1413–1424.

15 Swedberg, K., Komajda, M., Böhm, M. et al. (2010). Ivabradine and outcomes in chronic heart failure (SHIFT): a randomised placebo-controlled study (published correction appears in Lancet 2010 December 11; 376(9757): 1988. Lajnscak, M. (corrected to Lainscak, M.); Rabanedo, I. Roldan (corrected to Rabadán, I. Roldan); Leva, M. (corrected to Ieva, M.)). *Lancet* 376 (9744): 875–885.

16 Digitalis Investigation Group (1997). The effect of digoxin on mortality and morbidity in patients with heart failure. *N. Engl. J. Med.* 336 (8): 525–533.

17 Anker, S.D., Comin Colet, J., Filippatos, G. et al. (2009). Ferric carboxymaltose in patients with heart failure and iron deficiency. *N. Engl. J. Med.* 361 (25): 2436–2448.

18 Ponikowski, P., van Veldhuisen, D.J., Comin-Colet, J. et al. (2015). Beneficial effects of long-term intravenous iron therapy with ferric carboxymaltose in patients with symptomatic heart failure and iron deficiency. *Eur. Heart J.* 36 (11): 657–668.

19 Ponikowski, P., Kirwan, B.A., Anker, S.D. et al. (2020). Ferric carboxymaltose for iron deficiency at discharge after acute heart failure: a multicentre, double-blind, randomised, controlled trial (published correction appears in *Lancet* 2021 Nov 27; 398(10315): 1964). *Lancet* 396 (10266): 1895–1904.

20 Moss, A.J., Hall, W.J., Cannom, D.S. et al. (1996). Improved survival with an implanted defibrillator in patients with coronary disease at high risk for ventricular arrhythmia. Multicenter Automatic Defibrillator Implantation Trial Investigators. *N. Engl. J. Med.* 335 (26): 1933–1940.

21 Moss, A.J., Zareba, W., Hall, W.J. et al. (2002). Prophylactic implantation of a defibrillator in patients with myocardial infarction and reduced ejection fraction. *N. Engl. J. Med.* 346 (12): 877–883.

22 Køber, L., Thune, J.J., Nielsen, J.C. et al. (2016). Defibrillator implantation in patients with nonischemic systolic heart failure. *N. Engl. J. Med.* 375 (13): 1221–1230.

23 Bardy, G.H., Lee, K.L., Mark, D.B. et al. (2005). Amiodarone or an implantable cardioverter-defibrillator for congestive heart failure (published correction appears in *N. Engl. J. Med.* 2005 May 19; 352(20): 2146). *N. Engl. J. Med.* 352 (3): 225–237.

24 Knops, R.E., Olde Nordkamp, L.R.A., Delnoy, P.H.M. et al. (2020). Subcutaneous or Transvenous defibrillator therapy. *N. Engl. J. Med.* 383 (6): 526–536.

25 Bristow, M.R., Saxon, L.A., Boehmer, J. et al. (2004). Cardiac-resynchronization therapy with or without an implantable defibrillator in advanced chronic heart failure. *N. Engl. J. Med.* 350 (21): 2140–2150.

26 Moss, A.J., Hall, W.J., Cannom, D.S. et al. (2009). Cardiac-resynchronization therapy for the prevention of heart-failure events. *N. Engl. J. Med.* 361 (14): 1329–1338.

27 Ruschitzka, F., Abraham, W.T., Singh, J.P. et al. (2013). Cardiac-resynchronization therapy in heart failure with a narrow QRS complex. *N. Engl. J. Med.* 369 (15): 1395–1405.

28 Velazquez, E.J., Lee, K.L., Deja, M.A. et al. (2011). Coronary-artery bypass surgery in patients with left ventricular dysfunction. *N. Engl. J. Med.* 364 (17): 1607–1616.

29 Beanlands, R.S., Nichol, G., Huszti, E. et al. (2007). F-18-fluorodeoxyglucose positron emission tomography imaging-assisted management of patients with severe left ventricular dysfunction and suspected coronary disease: a randomized, controlled trial (PARR-2). *J. Am. Coll. Cardiol.* 50 (20): 2002–2012.

30 Perera, D., Clayton, T., O'Kane, P.D. et al. (2022). Percutaneous revascularization for ischemic left ventricular dysfunction (published online ahead of print, 2022 Aug 27). *N. Engl. J. Med.* https://doi.org/10.1056/NEJMoa2206606.

31 Pitt, B., Pfeffer, M.A., Assmann, S.F. et al. (2014). Spironolactone for heart failure with preserved ejection fraction. *N. Engl. J. Med.* 370 (15): 1383–1392.

32 Solomon, S.D., McMurray, J.J.V., Anand, I.S. et al. (2019). Angiotensin-Neprilysin inhibition in heart failure with preserved ejection fraction. *N. Engl. J. Med.* 381 (17): 1609–1620.

33 Anker, S.D., Butler, J., Filippatos, G. et al. (2021). Empagliflozin in heart failure with a preserved ejection fraction. *N. Engl. J. Med.* 385 (16): 1451–1461.

34 Solomon S.D., McMurray J.J.V., Claggett B., et al. (2022). Dapagliflozin in Heart Failure with Mildly Reduced or Preserved Ejection Fraction. *N. Engl. J. Med.* 387 (12): 1089–1098.

Further Reading

Bhagra, S.K., Pettit, S., and Parameshwar, J. (2019). Cardiac transplantation: indications, eligibility and current outcomes. *Heart* 105 (3): 252–260.

McDonagh, T.A., Metra, M., Adamo, M. et al. (2021). 2021 ESC guidelines for the diagnosis and treatment of acute and chronic heart failure (published correction appears in Eur. Heart J. 2021 October 14). *Eur. Heart J.* 42 (36): 3599–3726.

Sharma, A., Verma, S., Bhatt, D.L. et al. (2022). Optimizing foundational therapies in patients with HFrEF: how do we translate these findings into clinical care? *JACC Basic Transl. Sci.* 7 (5): 504–517.

13

Valvular Disease

Cardiology at its Core, First Edition. Peysh A. Patel.
© 2023 John Wiley & Sons Ltd. Published 2023 by John Wiley & Sons Ltd.

13.1   Learning Objectives

- Pathophysiology of heart sounds including dynamic manoeuvres.
- Anatomy of cardiac valves.
- Causes, diagnostic criteria and treatment options for valvular disease, including aortic stenosis, aortic regurgitation, mitral stenosis, mitral regurgitation and tricuspid regurgitation.

13.2   Pathophysiology of Heart Sounds

13.2.1   S1

The first heart sound (S1) results from closure of mitral valve (MV) and tricuspid valve (TV). It therefore corresponds to the end of diastole and commencement of systole. The sound can be diminished if pliability of the valve cusps is impaired, such as in the presence of calcification. It can also be muffled if there is increased tissue between the heart and stethoscope, in the context of obesity, chronic obstructive pulmonary disease (COPD) or pericardial effusion as examples. Normally, MV closure precedes TV closure although this 'split' is often undetectable. A pronounced split may occur with early MV closure (e.g. acute aortic regurgitation [AR]) or delayed TV closure (e.g. atrial septal defect [ASD], Ebstein anomaly). Reversed split S1 occurs when TV closes before MV, such as with RV pacing or LBBB.

13.2.2   S2

The second heart sound (S2) arises from closure of aortic and pulmonary valve at the end of systole. Intensity of aortic valve (AV) closure (A2) is increased with systemic hypertension and decreased with aortic stenosis (AS). Indeed, A2 component may be completely obliterated in severe AS. The intensity of pulmonary valve (PV) closure (P2) is increased with pulmonary hypertension. Normally, AV closure precedes PV closure (see Figure 13.1). This physiological splitting is accentuated during inspiration due to increased preload and decreased pulmonary arterial resistance that delays PV closure. A **widened split S2** can result from early AV closure (e.g. mitral regurgitation [MR], VSD) or late PV closure (e.g. RBBB, LV pacing, pulmonary stenosis [PS]).

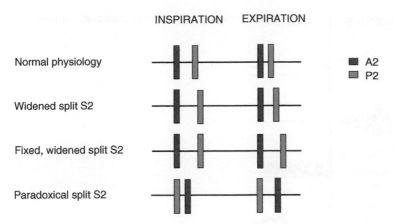

INSPIRATION   EXPIRATION

Normal physiology

Widened split S2

Fixed, widened split S2

Paradoxical split S2

■ A2
□ P2

Figure 13.1 Splitting of heart sounds.

In these contexts, respiratory variability is preserved. If there is **fixed, widened split S2**, respiratory variability is lost and this may occur in the presence of ASD. **Paradoxical split S2** occurs when PV closure precedes AV closure (i.e. reversed), such as with LBBB, RV pacing and AS. It is most evident during expiration.

13.2.3 S3 and S4

S3 is a low-pitched sound in early diastole. Its exact mechanism has not been fully elucidated but is thought to originate from sudden deceleration of blood flow from atria to ventricles once the latter reaches elastic limit. It can therefore occur in hyperdynamic or volume-overloaded states (e.g. anaemia, pregnancy, acute AR, systemic hypertension) or when there is impaired ventricular compliance such as in LV hypertrophy and diastolic dysfunction. S3 can be physiological in those aged < 40 years but is associated with a poorer prognosis when it coexists with CHF (**S3 gallop**).

S4 occurs in late diastole and corresponds with late ventricular filling due to atrial contraction. Again, mechanisms are not fully understood but the 'impact theory' proposes that it arises directly from blood flow secondary to atrial contraction that impacts with the wall of ventricular myocardium. Thus, it cannot theoretically occur in the presence of AF or flutter.

13.2.4 Dynamic Manoeuvres

A comprehension of normal valvular physiology is crucial to help identify pathological states. Murmurs result from turbulent blood flow and usually occur across valves. Evaluation relies upon correct analysis of timing, location, duration, character, configuration, radiation and response to dynamic manoeuvres. A diagrammatic overview of common cardiac murmurs based on correlation with heart sounds and cardiac cycle is provided in Figure 13.2. Inspiration leads to reduced intrathoracic pressure and increased preload. Thus, right-sided murmurs are loudest in inspiration. Expiration leads to the converse with reduced preload. Blood in the lungs is forced into the left side of the heart, and therefore, left-sided murmurs are loudest in expiration. Standing from a sitting position causes peripheral pooling and decreases venous return. Most murmurs are therefore reduced in intensity, with the notable exceptions of HOCM and mitral valve prolapse (MVP).

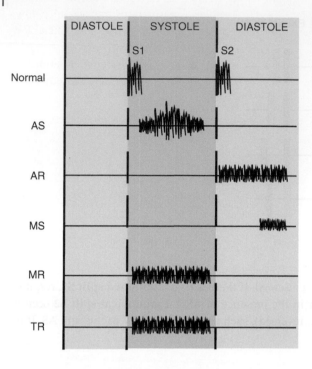

Figure 13.2 Timing of cardiac murmurs.

The opposite is true with squatting. Valsalva manoeuvres involve asking the patient to strain, which increases intrathoracic pressure and reduces preload. Hence, the majority of murmurs will diminish in magnitude.

13.3 Aortic Valve Anatomy

The AV is located between left ventricular outflow tract (LVOT) and ascending aorta. In most patients, it is composed of three cusps or leaflets (right coronary cusp [**RCC**], left coronary cusp [**LCC**] and non-coronary cusp [**NCC**]), which correspond to the sinuses that they overlie (see Figure 13.3). The right and left coronary cusps are similar in size with the non-coronary cusp typically being the largest. Each cusp has two free edges with the centre of each containing a small fibrous bulge termed the **nodule of Arantius**. The rim of each cusp is known as the lunula and is marginally thicker than its corresponding body. There is slight overlap between the lunulae of adjacent cusps and this has stabilising effects on structural integrity. Each cusp attaches to the aortic wall at a level termed the **sinotubular junction**. This also corresponds to the functional level of the valve orifice. The coronary **sinuses of Valsalva** reflect origins of the right and left coronary arteries and are located immediately proximal to this junction. The regions between each of the cusp's attachments refer to the **commissures**. Congenital cardiac anomalies can occur due to abnormal fusion of the AV during embryonic development and may result in malformations of AV leaflet anatomy. The most common form is a bicuspid AV in which only two cusps are present, typically with a conjoined area of two underdeveloped segments termed **raphe**. This is associated with aortic dilatation, coarctation of the aorta and Turner syndrome. More rarely, unicuspid AV can exist with a single, posterior commissural attachment, or quadricuspid AV with four similarly sized cusps in a X-shaped pattern.

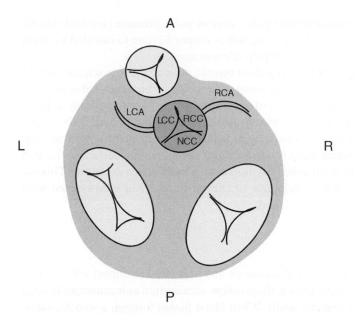

Figure 13.3 Gross anatomy of the aortic valve. LCA, left coronary artery; RCA, right coronary artery.

13.4 Aortic Stenosis

13.4.1 Aetiology

The most common cause of AS is age-related calcific degeneration of a tricuspid AV. It initially presents on echocardiography as aortic sclerosis with areas of increased echogenicity typically at the base of the cusps, but with no obstruction to outflow. This can progress and result in significant calcific disease with restricted opening of one or more cusps. Secondary calcification of a congenital bicuspid valve often results in younger symptom onset than calcific degeneration, between 45 and 65 years of age. Long-axis views may show systolic bowing with a = 'dome-like' appearance. The anterior leaflet is slightly larger than posterior leaflet although it may contain a raphe and thus appear tri-leaflet. Less commonly, rheumatic disease may be involved although it preferentially affects the MV (discussed later) and indeed may be coexistent. Imaging will classically demonstrate thickening of leaflet tips and commissural fusion resulting in a triangular orifice area.

13.4.2 Diagnosis

Symptoms tends to occur only once stenosis reaches a severe grade. There may be exertional breathlessness due to diastolic dysfunction. Other typical symptoms include exertional chest pain due to subendocardial ischaemia and/or reduced coronary perfusion, and light-headedness or syncope as a result of impaired cerebral perfusion. These symptoms may be accentuated by exercise due to peripheral vasodilation in the presence of fixed SV. If left untreated, it may progress to symptoms at rest such as orthopnoea and PND as a consequence of systolic dysfunction.

12-lead ECG may show LVH or LAD. On auscultation, AS will classically manifest as an ejection systolic murmur. This is because it results from turbulent blood flow through the narrowed valve during systole (i.e. after S1 when AV and PV open for ventricular outflow). It will typically be loudest in the aortic area with radiation to the carotids and accentuation during expiration. Features suggestive of severe disease include small volume pulse, narrow pulse pressure (reduced systolic component because of impaired SV – see Figure 13.6), soft or absent S2 (due to calcified leaflets), paradoxical splitting of S2 and/or associated thrill (palpable murmur).

There are various differential diagnoses for an ejection systolic murmur. Aortic sclerosis would not classically radiate to carotids, S2 would be normal and there would be no associated symptoms. PS would be exacerbated by dynamic manoeuvres, but in contrast to AS, it would typically be loudest during inspiration. Other pathologies relate to subvalvular disease and include HOCM and subaortic membrane, both of which are confidently excluded by echocardiography. Alternatively, supravalvular AS can occur rarely when there is narrowing of the ascending aorta and this can occur sporadically or more classically in inherited conditions such as Williams syndrome. This is a genetic disorder of AD inheritance due to deletions in chromosome 7 and is associated with developmental abnormalities and mental retardation.

13.4.3 Stratification of Severity

Proximal to a narrowed (stenotic) AV, the flow is smooth and organised (laminar) with normal velocity. Immediately adjacent to the valve orifice, there is flow acceleration as it converges to form a high-velocity jet but this region is spatially small. When blood passes through a stenotic valve, increased velocity can result in flow vortices whereby jets are generated in multiple directions in a random, chaotic manner ('turbulence'). This typically occurs when **Reynolds number**, which is influenced by flow velocity, vessel diameter, blood density and viscosity, is > 2000. Clinically, it is determined on auscultation as a harsh, raspy tone as opposed to laminar flow which is less coarse.

13.4.3.1 Pressure Gradient

An estimation of the pressure gradient across a stenotic valve is reliant upon the principle of **conservation of energy**. This stipulates that in the absence of applied forces, total energy flowing into a system equals that flowing out. It also assumes that flow acceleration can be ignored at peak velocity (as it equals 0) and that viscous friction is negligible as flow profiles within the centre of lumens are generally flat. Velocity and pressure are inversely related and their relationship can be represented by the **modified Bernoulli equation**, where ΔP is the peak pressure gradient, V_2 is peak velocity across the stenotic valve and V_1 is peak velocity immediately prior to stenotic valve (i.e. in the LVOT):

$$\Delta P = 4 \times \left(V_2^2 - V_1^2 \right)$$

This can be simplified to $\Delta P = 4V^2$ if peak velocity immediately prior to stenotic valve is less than $1.0\,\mathrm{m\,s^{-1}}$. Thus, for example, if peak velocity (V_{max}) across a stenotic AV is $4.2\,\mathrm{m\,s^{-1}}$, pressure gradient would be 71 mmHg. In a similar fashion, mean pressure gradient (V_{mean}) can be calculated as $2.4V^2$ (i.e. 42 mmHg). Conventionally, $V_{max} \geq 4.0\,\mathrm{m\,s^{-1}}$ (i.e. mean pressure gradient [MPG] $\geq$ 40 mmHg) is considered severe assuming high-flow states have been excluded (see Section 12.2), with V_{max} of 3.0–$3.9\,\mathrm{m\,s^{-1}}$ (MPG 20–39 mmHg) deemed moderate and V_{max} of 2.5–$2.9\,\mathrm{m\,s^{-1}}$ (MPG < 20 mmHg) considered mild. If $V_{max} < 4.0\,\mathrm{m\,s^{-1}}$ but with aortic valve area (AVA) $\leq 1\,\mathrm{cm^2}$ (see later), an additional calculation of stroke volume index (SVI) is beneficial in stratifying those that merit further assessment via dobutamine stress echocardiography (DSE) and/or CT calcium scoring (see Section 13.4.3.3).

There are important limitations to the ΔP equation. It should be applied with caution if there is significant flow acceleration (e.g. prosthetic valve) or proximal flow velocity (e.g. AS with high-output state or HOCM), viscous forces (e.g. muscular VSD, long coarctation) or higher blood viscosity such as with polycythaemia. Notwithstanding, the most critical limitation for accurate velocity estimation across a stenotic AV is incident angle between ultrasound beam and blood flow during echocardiography. The ultrasound beam should be as close to parallel with blood flow as possible and failure to achieve this, particularly once angle is $> 20°$, leads to underestimation of transvalvular peak velocity. It is also imperative that continuous-wave (CW) as opposed to pulsed-wave (PW) Doppler is utilised as correct placement of sample volume is difficult and may hinder interpretation if velocity exceeds the Nyquist limit (maximum Doppler shift frequency that can be measured without colour aliasing).

13.4.3.2   Valve Area
Pressure gradients in isolation have limited use in assessing severity of stenosis as they are directly influenced by SV. Calculation of AVA can be performed directly using planimetry to trace around the valve orifice. In practice, this is challenging to perform accurately and an alternative strategy relates to the continuity principle of **conservation of mass**, i.e. whatever mass flows in must also flow out. The stroke volume proximal to AV and that in the stenotic valve orifice must be equal. As flow is laminar with reasonably flat velocity profile, it can be represented by cross-sectional area (CSA)×velocity time integral (VTI). Hence,

$$CSA_{LVOT} \times VTI_{LVOT} = CSA_{AV} \times VTI_{AV}$$

$$CSA_{AV} = \left(CSA_{LVOT} \times VTI_{LVOT}\right) \div VTI_{AV}$$

Velocity time integral of the LVOT and AV can be measured by tracing Doppler profile of LVOT and AV flow, respectively. LVOT diameter is measured on parasternal long axis (PLAX) view at the level of cusp insertion and used to calculate CSA using the equation $\textbf{0.785} \times \textbf{\textit{D}}^{2}$ (where D is LVOT diameter). As SV is a measure of blood flow through a specific region with each heartbeat, CSA must be determined within the flow period (i.e. during systole for LVOT).

The above equation relies on a broad assumption that flow is occurring in a rigid, circular tube, there is uniform velocity across the vessel and CSA remains constant throughout the period of flow. However, blood vessels are elastic and annular diameter may also change throughout systole. Additionally, arrhythmias such as AF can result in varying beat-to-beat stroke volumes. Where there is discrepancy in profiling, it is best to use the average value from 5 to 10 consecutive beats to ensure accurate VTI measurement.

Overall, correct calculation of LVOT diameter is of primary importance to derive a precise assessment of AVA. Positioning of PW Doppler beam should be at the same level as measurement of LVOT diameter, i.e. 0.5 cm proximal to AV, to avoid flow acceleration immediately proximal to the orifice. Anatomically, the region of interest is junction of anterior aortic wall and interventricular septum, and junction of posterior aortic wall and AMVL. The measurement should be corrected for body surface area (BSA). Typically, calculated AVA $\leq 1 \, cm^{2}$ via planimetry or continuity equation is considered severe (see Figure 13.4).

13.4.3.3   True vs Pseudo-severe
The ventricle's response to chronic pressure overload is concentric hypertrophy. Left ventricular function tends to be preserved until late-stage disease. Accurate quantification of severity of valve stenosis is of vital importance but it becomes problematic if there is severe ventricular dysfunction. Even in the presence of severe stenosis, pressure gradients may appear normal because of low

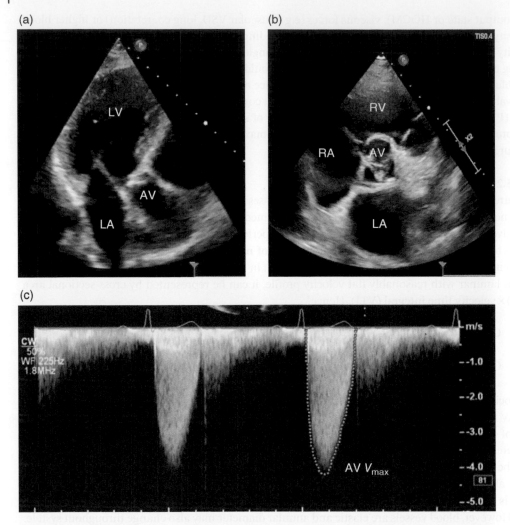

Figure 13.4 Echocardiographic features of severe aortic stenosis. (a) 3-chamber view demonstrating thickened, calcified AV cusps. (b) PSAX view showing thickened cusps with valve area of $0.92\,\text{cm}^2$ (when assessed separately by planimetry). (c) CW Doppler assessment across AV with V_{max} of $4.24\,\text{m s}^{-1}$, consistent with severe AS.

transaortic flow rate. Conversely, AVA may appear to be reduced even when stenosis is not severe due to failure of the ventricle to generate sufficient force to fully open leaflets. In these situations, assuming there is sufficient contractile reserve with LVEF $<50\%$, low-dose DSE is beneficial to 'normalise' SV and differentiate true, severe AS from pseudo-severe AS (see Figure 13.5).

In patients with true AS, this results in increased V_{max} but minimal increase in AVA ($\leq 1.0\,\text{cm}^2$). In those with pseudo-severe AS, AVA appears to improve with a relatively modest increase in V_{max}. This distinction is clinically important. Those with true valve disease may benefit from valve intervention. Those with pseudo-severe AS are unlikely to improve and effort should instead be placed on improving morbidity associated with ventricular dysfunction.

If there is preserved LV function at rest or insufficient flow reserve on DSE, dobutamine challenge is not helpful. In these circumstances, an integrated approach that includes CT calcium

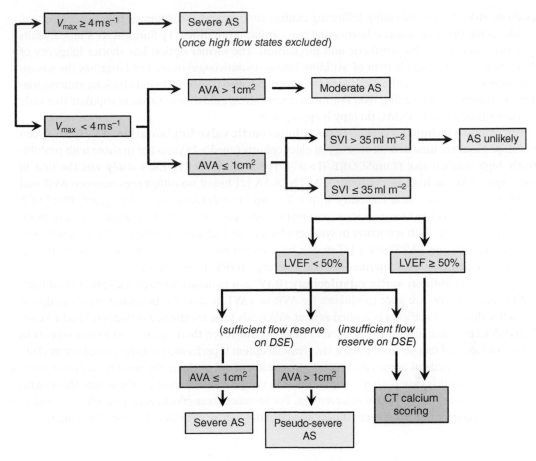

Figure 13.5 Integrated assessment of aortic stenosis severity using multi-modality imaging.

scoring is beneficial. Broadly speaking, values < 800 (females) or < 1600 (males) make severe AS unlikely whereas score > 1600 (females) or > 3000 (males) makes the diagnosis more probable.

13.4.4 Management

AS gradually progresses in severity over time and periodic surveillance is therefore essential to monitor rate of deterioration and guide management. Those with mild AS require surveillance scans every three years whereas those with asymptomatic severe AS warrant imaging every six months. Symptoms do not typically develop until AS has reached severe grading and, once it occurs, intervention ought to be considered. Similarly, surgical intervention should be offered to those with truly asymptomatic, severe AS if LVEF $< 55\%$ without alternative cause, symptoms or sustained blood pressure reduction during exercise testing, severe valve calcification with V_{max} progression $> 0.3\,cm\,s^{-1}\,yr^{-1}$, elevated B-type natriuretic peptide (BNP) ($>$ three-fold) with no other precipitant, and in those with critical AS ($V_{max} > 5\,m\,s^{-1}$, MPG $> 60\,mmHg$). Lastly, those who require another form of cardiac surgery should be considered for concurrent **surgical AV replacement (AVR)** assuming there is at least moderate stenosis.

Intervention was traditionally via surgical AVR and this remains first-line therapy in younger patients aged < 75 years with low surgical risk (EuroSCORE II $< 4\%$). This calculation is used to evaluate risk of early mortality following cardiac surgery and incorporates factors such as age, gender, renal function, cardiac history and non-cardiac morbidities [1]. Surgical AVR broadly falls into two categories – bioprosthetic and mechanical. The former option has shorter longevity of 10 years but the marked benefit of avoiding long-term anticoagulation. The latter has the advantage of potentially lasting the lifetime of the patient but also commits them to lifelong anticoagulation with associated bleeding risk. For mechanical valves, guidelines currently stipulate that only warfarin as opposed to DOAC therapy is appropriate.

Percutaneous techniques such as **transcatheter aortic valve implantation** (**TAVI**) have been developed and are now default strategy in older cohorts (aged ≥ 75 years) or in those with prohibitively high surgical risk (EuroSCORE II > 8%). The seminal PARTNER 1 study was the first to investigate TAVI in high-risk patients. PARTNER 1A [2] found no differences between AVR and TAVI in terms of all-cause mortality with follow-up for a duration up to five years. PARTNER 1B [3] showed TAVI to be superior to conservative management, including valvuloplasty, in those unsuitable for AVR with reduction in symptom burden and all-cause mortality. More recently, the PARTNER 2 [4] and PARTNER 3 [5] studies have shown non-inferiority of TAVI compared with AVR even in patients with intermediate and low surgical risk, respectively.

Percutaneous **balloon aortic valvuloplasty** (**BAV**) is a palliative therapeutic option in patients with severe AS who are poor candidates for AVR or TAVI. It can also be considered as bridge to definitive therapy. Its efficacy is limited as final AVA tends to be maximised between 0.7 and 1.1 cm^2. It also does not alter disease progression in isolation. However, there are modest improvements in valve function and can be considered a safe, feasible option if performed in experienced centres [6].

There are no medical agents that retard progression of AS or delay the need for valvular intervention. Despite this caveat, they can play a role in symptom alleviation for those subcohorts who are not candidates for definitive intervention. For instance, beta-blockers can be administered to reduce symptoms of exertional chest pain and diuretics can be considered for breathlessness.

13.5 Aortic Regurgitation

13.5.1 Aetiology

Aortic regurgitation is due to an abnormality in valve leaflets (primary AR) or disease of the aortic root (secondary AR), or a combination of both. As with AS, calcific degeneration is the commonest cause in the developed world. Other valvular causes include bicuspid aortic valve with incomplete closure lines, endocarditis which can result in leaflet destruction or perforation, rheumatic valve disease with resultant thickening and restriction, and connective tissue disorders such as rheumatoid arthritis (RA) and systemic lupus erythematosus (SLE) with consequent fibrosis and leaflet dysfunction.

Aortic root disorders can cause dilatation of the aortic annulus, thereby pulling apart otherwise anatomically normal valve leaflets and resulting in AR. Causes include systemic hypertension, aortic dissection, connective tissue disorders (such as Marfan syndrome, Ehlers–Danlos syndrome and osteogenesis imperfecta), and conditions that directly cause aortitis such as ankylosing spondylitis, giant cell arteritis, Behcet's disease and tertiary syphilis.

13.5.2 Diagnosis

Acute, severe AR occurs in a non-compensated, non-dilated LV and results in significant increase in left ventricular end-diastolic pressure with impaired cardiac output (CO). In chronic AR, the LV compensates via gradual dilatation to augment SV and thereby preserve CO in the early stage. Additional eccentric hypertrophy may occur as a response to increased afterload. These compensatory mechanisms cause AR to be largely asymptomatic until late in disease progression. When clinical manifestations occur, dyspnoea is the most common symptom although myocardial ischaemia from impaired coronary perfusion can result in angina.

On examination, there will be evidence of an early diastolic murmur (i.e. after S2 when AV has closed), which is maximal at the left sternal edge and accentuated with expiration. There may be a collapsing (water hammer) pulse if disease is severe though usually difficult to elicit. Pulse pressure will be widened (defined as severe if > 80 mmHg) due to lower diastolic pressure secondary to regurgitant flow from aorta into LV (see Figure 13.6). If there is associated hypertrophy or dilatation, the apex beat may be displaced. Rarer eponymous signs include Corrigan's (carotid artery pulsation), Rosenbach's (liver pulsation in the absence of tricuspid regurgitation [TR]) and Duroziez's (femoral murmur). In severe disease, an **Austin Flint murmur** may be heard. This is a low-pitched, mid-diastolic and presystolic murmur audible at the apex and results from regurgitant jet causing shuddering of the AMVL. ECG may show LVH with cardiomegaly often observed on radiographic imaging.

13.5.3 Stratification of Severity

Echocardiography is the gold standard for diagnosing and assessing severity. Physiological regurgitation is present in a high percentage of healthy individuals but will be spatially restricted to the area immediately adjacent to valve closure and short in duration. In PLAX and PSAX views (see Section 10.9.1), the AMVL may appear curved in diastole with region of curvature corresponding to the regurgitant jet and directed towards LA. This is termed **reversed doming** in contrast to that seen in rheumatic mitral stenosis (MS). Additionally, focal disturbance may result in an area of increased echogenicity on the leaflet termed jet lesion. The presence of severe AR will result in increased forward flow due to higher volumes, and thus, a coexistent systolic murmur is often audible and visualised on echocardiography as increased flow velocity through the valve.

When using colour Doppler, a severe jet of AR will extend to LV apex. Careful measurement of the narrowest segment of the regurgitant jet (vena contracta) is particularly useful in PLAX view (< 0.3 cm = mild; > 0.6 cm = severe; see Figure 13.7). Assessment of blood flow in the descending aorta provides extra indicators. There is normally slight reversal of flow in the first third of diastole due to elastic recoil in healthy, large arteries. If there is holodiastolic flow reversal, this is suggestive of at least moderate AR with a principle analogous to Duroziez's sign.

In addition, measurement of pressure half-time (PHT) and effective regurgitant orifice area (EROA) can be of use to clarify disease severity. An exploration of each is now provided.

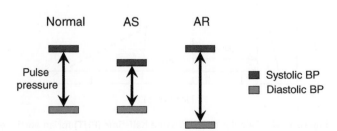

Figure 13.6 Pulse pressures in aortic stenosis and regurgitation.

(a)

(b)

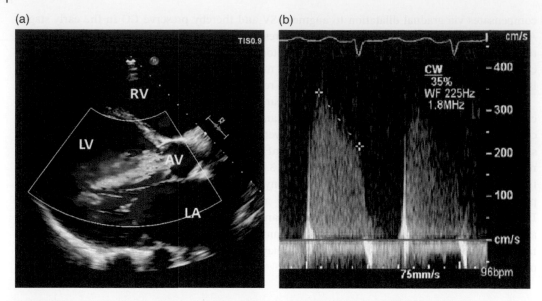

Figure 13.7 Echocardiographic features of moderate aortic regurgitation. (a) PLAX view showing jet of regurgitation extending to mid-LV cavity, with vena contracta measuring 0.34 cm. (b) CW Doppler measurement of jet with pressure half-time of 342 ms, consistent with moderate AR.

13.5.3.1 Pressure Half-time (PHT)

Pressure half-time remains relatively constant even with exercise-induced changes in flow. AR will result in a CW Doppler trace that has onset at AV closure (during isovolumic relaxation), with a rapid rise in velocity followed by gradual decline (see Figure 13.8). It then abruptly decelerates during isovolumic contraction before reaching baseline at AV opening. The shape of this trace is influenced by rapidity with which aortic and LV pressures equalise and hence provides a marker of severity. In severe AR, there is rapid decline in aortic pressure correlating with exaggerated reduction in Doppler velocity (i.e. steeper deceleration slope during diastole).

This can provide a semi-quantitative measure of severity using the following equation:

$$PHT = 0.29 \times DT$$

Categorisation of severity is as follows: PHT $> 500\,$ms (mild), 250–500 ms (moderate) and $< 250\,$ms (severe). PHT is influenced by conditions that affect LV compliance. Caution is

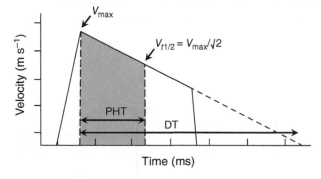

Figure 13.8 Calculation of pressure half-time (PHT) for an aortic regurgitant jet.

warranted in the presence of coexistent diastolic dysfunction or MV disease due to risk of over- or underestimating AR severity.

13.5.3.2 Effective Regurgitant Orifice Area (EROA)

This calculation is less influenced by loading conditions. It is based on colour Doppler to measure the flow convergence region proximal to regurgitant orifice, termed proximal isovelocity surface area (PISA) – see Figure 13.9. Flow acceleration occurs proximal to valve plane and leads to a high-velocity jet in regurgitant orifice. Immediately adjacent to the orifice, surfaces are small with high flow velocities. With increased distance, velocities are lower but areas are larger. First, the regurgitant volume can be calculated using the following equation:

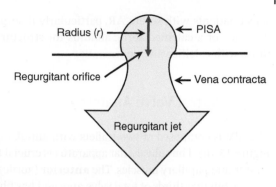

Figure 13.9 Components of EROA.

$$\text{Regurgitant volume} = \text{aliasing velocity} \times \text{PISA}$$

The aliasing velocity is determined by the Nyquist limit (i.e. red–blue interface on colour Doppler) and this can be determined using the velocity colour scale. The shape of PISA is typically hemispherical and on this assumption, PISA can be determined using the formula $\textbf{PISA} = \textbf{2}\boldsymbol{\pi}\textbf{r}^{2}$, where r is the radius of the hemisphere. Armed with this information, the regurgitant volume can be calculated with $< 30\,\text{ml}$ defined as mild and $> 60\,\text{ml}$ as severe. Using VTI of aortic regurgitant jet from CW Doppler trace (measured in cm), the maximum EROA can be determined as follows:

$$\text{EROA} = \text{regurgitant volume} \div \text{VTI}_{\text{AR}}$$

For reference purposes, $< 0.10\,\text{cm}^{2}$ is defined as mild and $> 0.30\,\text{cm}^{2}$ as severe. A primary limitation of the PISA method is that it provides an 'effective' rather than 'anatomical' orifice area and tends to therefore be relatively smaller. As inferred, it is also highly reliant on accurate measurement of the radius. It is therefore crucial that imaging is optimised by shifting colour Doppler baseline towards direction of blood flow to reduce aliasing velocity and increase radius. Lastly, valve motion that occurs during systole and diastole can impair interpretation.

13.5.4 Management

In asymptomatic individuals with chronic, severe AR, a surveillance strategy with six-monthly echocardiography is appropriate. Evidence for medical therapy is not convincing. Beta-blockers are generally avoided as augmented diastole can worsen regurgitant volumes. ACE inhibitors or dihydropyridine calcium-channel blockers such as nifedipine may provide symptomatic relief in those with severe AR who are not candidates for valvular intervention, due to vasodilation helping to alleviate afterload and regurgitant volume.

Definitive treatment involves valvular intervention which is typically in the form of surgical AVR. This is indicated in all symptomatic cases and in those who are asymptomatic but with LVEF $\leq 50\%$ or left ventricle end-systolic diameter (LVESD) $> 5\,\text{cm}$. If there is significant enlargement of ascending aorta, typically defined as $\geq 5.5\,\text{cm}$ in the absence of underlying connective tissue disease, valve surgery is indicated irrespective of regurgitant severity. TAVI can also be considered in select patients with severe AR, particularly if surgery is contraindicated. This approach relies on presence of a calcified aortic annulus for structural stability and so is generally only suitable in those with calcific valve degeneration.

13.6 Mitral Valve Anatomy

The MV is composed of two leaflets with annular attachment at the atrioventricular junction (see Figure 13.10). The subvalvular apparatus is crucial for structural integrity and comprises tendinous chords and papillary muscles. The **anterior** (aortic) leaflet constitutes one-third of annular circumference but two-thirds of total valve area and has fibrous continuity with the LCC and NCC of aortic valve. It is arbitrarily divided into three further regions, termed **A1, A2**, and **A3**. The **posterior** (mural) leaflet has indentations that form three scallops along its free edge. In normal physiology, they do not extend to the annulus. These regions are defined as **P1** (anterolateral), **P2** (central), and **P3** (posteromedial). Each leaflet is additionally described to have differing zones extending from attachment point at the annulus to its free edge. The area leaflet attachment to atrioventricular junction refers to the basal zone, with central portion being the free zone and distal region with chordal attachment corresponding to the rough zone.

The annulus is an oval-shaped fibrous ring that demarcates LA from LV. Beneath, the chordae tendinae are observed with primary, secondary and tertiary segments. It is the former that attaches to the free edge of both leaflets. These have apical attachments to two papillary muscles – anterolateral and posteromedial. Of clinical relevance, chordae arising from each muscle attach to both leaflets.

13.7 Mitral Stenosis

13.7.1 Aetiology

MS is most commonly caused by rheumatic disease. It is initiated by *Streptococcus pyogenes* infection of the throat, usually during childhood, with autoantibody production. These can target native valves and recurrent, chronic inflammation can result in characteristic abnormalities after a latent

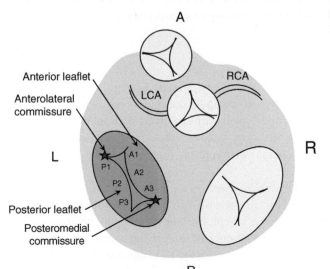

Figure 13.10 Gross anatomy of the mitral valve.

period. Degenerative and congenital MS are rarely seen. The former is associated with annular calcification too, but does not restrict leaflet mobility.

13.7.2 Diagnosis

Valve obstruction results in elevated LA pressure and pulmonary hypertension. Raised capillary pressure causes transudation from the capillaries with pulmonary oedema. In chronic states, RV failure may manifest and predominate. LV function is initially preserved due to compensatory mechanisms but eventually fails due to reduction in preload. The co-occurrence of AF secondary to LA dilatation has potentiating impact due to compromised SV mediated by loss of atrial kick.

Patients classically describe exertional dyspnoea. There may be associated haemoptysis due to rupture of bronchial veins. If there is significant LA enlargement with secondary impingement of the recurrent laryngeal nerve, a hoarse voice may be apparent (Ostner's phenomenon). They may demonstrate malar flush to their cheeks or clinically be in AF. Specific features of rheumatic disease are defined by **Jones criteria**, with major signs that include pancarditis, arthralgia, erythema marginatum, subcutaneous nodules, and Sydenham's chorea.

Auscultatory findings include a rumbling, mid-diastolic murmur after S2 and MV opening. Differential diagnoses include carcinoid disease, cor triatrium sinistrum (subdivision of LA by a thin membrane) or obstruction because of an atrial tumour (e.g. myxoma) or large vegetation. The murmur of MS is typically loudest in the apex and exaggerated during expiration. Its duration rather than amplitude correlates with severity. In significant cases, there may be an associated diastolic murmur from pulmonary regurgitation as a consequence of pulmonary hypertension (**Graham–Steele murmur**). This would correlate with loud S1 and P2. S2 may be of fixed, widened split if there is associated ASD (Lutembacher syndrome), both congenital and acquired. A tapping apex beat may be evident although invariably difficult to elicit in practice. 12-lead ECG may confirm AF and/or demonstrate P-mitrale. The latter occurs because of LA enlargement which prolongs atrial depolarisation without shift in amplitude (i.e. height of P wave is normal but duration is longer – see Section 1.5.1). Chest radiograph may confirm MV annular calcification or features of congestion.

Confirmatory diagnosis is achieved using echocardiography. Rheumatic valve disease manifests as fibrosis and thickening of leaflet tips, commissural fusion, chordal thickening and shortening/fusion with diastolic bowing or doming of valve leaflets towards LV due to relative mobility of leaflet bases in comparison with their tips (see Figure 13.11). As the disease progresses, leaflets become calcified. Unlike calcific degeneration which initially arises from leaflet base and is associated with mitral annular calcification, rheumatic MS causes calcification at the leaflet tips.

13.7.3 Stratification of Severity

Disease severity can be assessed through measurement of various parameters. Quantification of PHT and valve orifice area via planimetry is particularly useful, however, and an exploration of each is now provided.

13.7.3.1 Pressure Half-time

As explored in Section 6.4.2, there are four phases of diastole and this is reflected in PW Doppler trace across the MV. Measurement of PHT ($0.29 \times DT$) has the inherent advantage of being independent of CO or coexistence of MR. In the presence of MS, there is prolonged PHT as pressure gradient between LA and LV is increased and rate of decline is extended to allow LV filling. For

(a) (b)

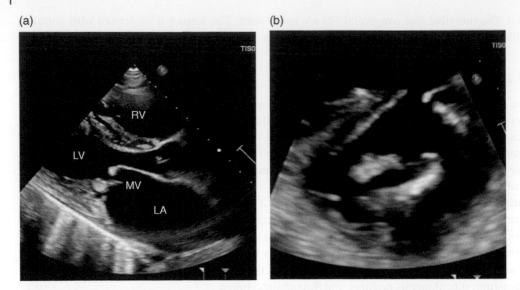

Figure 13.11 Echocardiographic features of severe mitral stenosis. (a) PLAX view demonstrating thickened anterior MV leaflet tip with diastolic doming of anterior MV leaflet. (b) PSAX view showing thickened leaflet tips and commissural fusion.

this calculation, influence of LA and LV chamber compliance is assumed to be negligible, which makes it invalid for measurements post-valvuloplasty. PHT can also be used to derive estimated mitral valve area (MVA) and is based upon the observation that PHT of 220 ms equates to MVA of $1.0 \, cm^2$. Based on this, the following formula is applied:

$$MVA = 220 / PHT$$

PHT of <71–139 ms is considered mild and one >219 ms as severe. However, generalisability may be limited by a non-linear diastolic slope, coexistent significant AR, raised LA pressure and the presence of prosthetic valves. If so, direct planimetry is advised. Lastly, it is worth remarking that MR will increase transmitral gradient but does not affect PHT.

13.7.3.2 Planimetry

Assessment of MVA using planimetry is derived using PSAX view. It is reasonably simple as the elliptical orifice is relatively constant in position during mid-diastole. This approach has been validated with regards to accuracy and appears to closely correlate with anatomical findings at surgery. As the shape of inflow is like a funnel and narrowest at its tips, it is important to work sequentially through different image planes to identify the smallest orifice. A value $<1.5 \, cm^2$ is considered haemodynamically significant as studies suggest that virtually all of these patients have reduced CO at rest. Imaging is compromised by presence of artefacts from dense fibrosis or calcification. An 'over-gained' image can also result in blooming effects.

13.7.4 Management

13.7.4.1 Medical Therapy

This can help to improve symptoms by offloading fluid. Diuretics can alleviate breathlessness, and if there is coexistent AF, anticoagulation with warfarin is advised if disease is moderate to severe. It can also be considered if patients are in sinus rhythm but with enlarged LA (> 5.0–5.5 cm) or there is evidence of spontaneous echo contrast. Invasive treatment is considered in those with severe disease based on outlined parameters, with options predicated on accurate assessment of valve morphology and function. Hence, a transoesophageal echocardiogram (TOE) is paramount to guide decision-making. Scoring systems such as **Wilkins** and **Cornier** are available and incorporate features such as valve thickening, calcification, mobility and involvement of commissures or subvalvular apparatus to guide selection.

13.7.4.2 Percutaneous Mitral Valve Commissurotomy (PMC)

Percutaneous mitral valve commissurotomy can be considered in symptomatic, severe MS, and similarly as a palliative measure to improve symptoms in instances where surgery is not appropriate. It can also be explored in asymptomatic individuals if there is high risk of embolism (e.g. previous stroke, paroxysmal AF/AF, spontaneous contrast in LA) or haemodynamic decompensation, such as desire for pregnancy, need for major non-cardiac surgery and/or systolic pulmonary artery pressure (PAP) > 50 mmHg. Additionally, symptoms on exercise testing necessitate consideration.

The procedure is performed via a trans-septal approach and usually provides > 100% increase in valve area with end dimensions of > 2 cm². This is associated with significant reduction in pulmonary pressure. It is reasonably well tolerated and without major embolic risk. However, non-commissural leaflet tearing can result in severe MR in a minority of patients (~5%). Procedural contraindications include moderate or severe MR, LA thrombus, severe or bi-commissural calcification and/or concomitant coronary or valve disease requiring surgical intervention. Long-term success rates are reasonable with functional deterioration occurring late and primarily related to re-stenosis [7]. If immediate results are unsatisfactory, surgical valve replacement should be considered.

13.7.4.3 Surgical Valve Replacement

Open-heart valve commissurotomy using bypass can be performed in certain centres and offers the added ability to correct not only commissural fusion but also chordae and papillary muscles. In young patients, long-term outcomes are promising [8]. Valve replacement involves use of predominantly prosthetic valves because of better durability and established requirement for anticoagulation. Results from surgical valve replacement are broadly equivocal to PMC and decision-making is primarily guided by anatomical and clinical features.

13.8 Mitral Regurgitation

13.8.1 Aetiology

Mitral regurgitation is typically defined as primary or secondary. In **primary MR**, there is an abnormality of one or more components of the valve apparatus, i.e. leaflets, chordae tendinae or papillary muscles, whilst secondary MR occurs due to a disease process of LV or LA, which in turn pulls apart otherwise normal valve leaflets. The main cause of primary MR is MVP as a result of myxomatous degeneration. Other aetiologies include rheumatic valve disease, endocarditis and acute papillary muscle rupture secondary to ACS. **Secondary MR** can also occur following ACS due to inferolateral RWMA that displace the posteromedial papillary muscle and tethers the posterior MV leaflet. Alternatively, it can arise due to LV or LA dilatation which can both cause annular dilatation and failure of leaflet coaptation.

13.8.2 Diagnosis

With chronic MR, a compensatory response to volume overload is ventricular dilatation. In the initial phase, LVEF is preserved due to the Frank–Starling mechanism. LA also dilates to compensate for the regurgitant volume. This may not be associated with symptoms for years until late in the disease process when dyspnoea manifests. On auscultation, MR will present classically as a pansystolic murmur, loudest in the apex and during expiration. Its peak intensity is often in early systole in the case of ischaemic MR, and late systole if due to valve prolapse. If there is LV dilatation, the apex beat may be displaced. In chronic, severe MR, there may be secondary pulmonary hypertension with loud P2. S3 gallop may be present in addition to features of right-sided failure such as raised JVP and peripheral oedema. 12-lead ECG may show evidence of AF or P-mitrale. LV enlargement may be associated with LBBB. Chest radiograph can reveal LA enlargement, cardiomegaly or features of pulmonary hypertension and, more rarely, annular calcification is visible. Nonetheless, echocardiography is required to confirm diagnosis and assess underlying pathology.

Myxomatous degeneration refers to pathological weakening of connective tissue and is characterised by thickened leaflets and chordae with excessive motion. The severity is variable and ranges from **prolapsed** leaflets, where there is bowing into LA during systole but with tips that continue to be directed towards the apex, to **flail** leaflets where there is severe involvement with tips directed away from ventricular apex. There is an association with chordal elongation which exacerbates regurgitant disease because of inadequate tensile support of leaflets in systole. **Barlow's disease** is characterised by pronounced annular dilatation, bileaflet bowing (or prolapse) and thick, spongy leaflets with or without calcification.

A RWMA may lead to tethering of valve closure and restricted motion, resulting in a tented appearance. If the RWMA is not present at rest but is inducible, MR will be intermittent. In the context of acute MI, papillary muscle or chordal rupture can occur and result in acute, severe MR as there is insufficient time for fibrous scarring which provides long-term structural support. Rupture of the posteromedial muscle occurs more frequently as it receives blood supply solely from the PDA whilst the anterolateral muscle is dually perfused from LAD and Cx territories. If there is total rupture, a mass is often seen attached to flail leaflet segments which prolapse into LA during systole.

Annular dilatation causes incomplete coaptation of leaflets with tethering secondary to papillary muscle displacement. The leaflets and chordae will be structurally normal (i.e. secondary MR). This may occur with LVSD, but volume overload secondary to chronic MR is also implicated and can trigger a vicious circle. Moreover, systolic dysfunction can decrease MV closing force. For these reasons, it can be challenging to establish whether MR is the cause or consequence of ventricular dilatation. Leaflets do have partial anatomical overlap, however, and this enables some degree of dilatation to be accommodated without compromise of function.

Rheumatic disease, as with MS, is associated with commissural fusion and leaflet tip thickening and restriction. Annular calcification impairs systolic contraction which can exacerbate regurgitation. Infective endocarditis can result in MR via leaflet destruction or perforation. Marfan syndrome is classically associated with a long, redundant anterior leaflet that sags into LA during systole. Infiltrative diseases result in irregular leaflet thickening and inadequate coaptation.

13.8.3 Stratification of Severity

Echocardiography remains the cornerstone for accurate assessment of mechanism and severity. An integrative approach using qualitative, semi-qualitative and quantitative parameters is required.

The normal MV apparatus is a saddle-shaped eclipse, and thus, its most apical points are seen in PLAX view and most basal segments in apical four-chamber view. As the MV apparatus is posteriorly placed, a low threshold for TOE exists to explore anatomy with greater clarity. In situations where surgical intervention is being considered, this is a mandatory requirement.

13.8.3.1 Gross Morphology

The Carpentier classification is useful to assess valve function based on leaflet motion:

Type 1 – normal leaflet motion: annular dilatation, leaflet perforation
Type 2 – excess leaflet motion: leaflet prolapse, papillary muscle rupture
Type 3a – restricted leaflet motion in both systole and diastole (rheumatic disease)
Type 3b – restricted leaflet motion in diastole: LV dilatation, papillary muscle dysfunction

13.8.3.2 Qualitative Assessment

Visual assessment of leaflet thickness, size and mobility together with appearance of subvalvular apparatus can elucidate underlying mechanism. Colour Doppler characteristics provide further detail regarding severity and potential aetiology. If the jet extends to posterior wall of LA, it is more likely to be severe (see Figure 13.12). However, chronic disease can cause significant LA dilatation which hinders interpretation. A restricted/tethered valve usually results in an ipsilateral regurgitant jet whilst a prolapsed or flail leaflet results in a contralateral jet. Annular dilatation differs as it tends to cause a central jet.

13.8.3.3 Semi-qualitative Assessment

As with all venous flow, pulmonary vein (PV) flow is continuous throughout the cardiac cycle (i.e. diastole and systole). An apical four-chamber view can be utilised to characterise PW Doppler flow

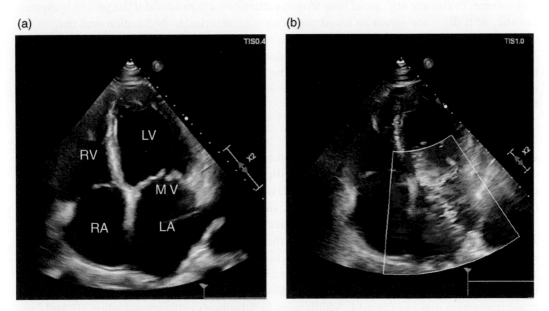

Figure 13.12 Echocardiographic features of severe mitral regurgitation. (a) Apical four-chamber view confirming significant LA dilatation when indexed to BSA. (b) Additional colour Doppler showing broad jet of regurgitation extending to the base of the LA. This was associated with systolic flow reversal in the pulmonary vein (not shown) in keeping with severe MR.

in the right inferior PV. It will ordinarily exhibit systolic forward flow (as a result of LA relaxation), diastolic forward flow (due to open conduit between PV, LA, and LV) and atrial flow reversal (as a result of atrial contraction). Systolic flow reversal may be seen with severe MR. False-negatives can occur if LA is severely dilated as the extra regurgitant volume is accommodated without displacement into the PV. False-positives may also occur if there is an eccentrically directed jet, or in the context of AF. Other physiological factors such as respiratory phase, chamber compliance and age can similarly limit interpretation and analysis should always therefore be used in conjunction with other measurements.

Vena contracta diameter relates to the narrowest segment of regurgitant jet and should be assessed. This is optimally visualised in PLAX or apical four-chamber views. The apical two-chamber view is not reliable as jet width may appear broad in this plane even when regurgitation is not severe. Generally, vena contracta ≤0.3 cm is considered mild and ≥0.7 cm deemed severe. Mitral inflow should also be measured with E-wave dominance ($> 1.2\,\mathrm{m\,s^{-1}}$) indicative of severe regurgitation.

13.8.3.4 Quantitative Assessment
Quantitative evaluation of MR provides one of the most accurate means of assessing severity but is technically challenging. It requires calculation of regurgitant volume followed by EROA (see Section 13.5.3.2). A regurgitant volume < 30 ml is thought to be mild and one > 60 ml considered severe. EROA $< 0.2\,\mathrm{cm^2}$ is deemed mild and EROA $\geq 0.4\,\mathrm{cm^2}$ labelled as severe.

13.8.4 Management

13.8.4.1 Medical Therapy
A reduction in filling pressure is favourable in acute MR. This can be achieved using diuretics and nitrates which reduce preload. Vasodilators are also beneficial in reducing afterload and regurgitant volume. In chronic MR, use of long-term vasodilators is controversial if the patient is asymptomatic, as it does not appear to retard progression of ventricular dysfunction and may mask symptoms that would otherwise lead to surgical referral [9]. In functional MR secondary to systolic dysfunction and ventricular dilatation, conventional CHF therapy remains first-line due to its beneficial impact on ventricular remodelling. The risk of thrombus is inherently lower with MR than MS because of reduced blood stasis, and in view of this, current guidelines do not advocate long-term anticoagulation.

13.8.4.2 Intervention
In patients with acute, severe MR that results in pulmonary oedema, prompt referral to explore candidacy for surgery is indicated. For those with severe, primary MR, surgery is appropriate if patients are symptomatic, or in asymptomatic individuals with (i) evidence of LV dilatation (LVESD ≥ 4 cm) or LV dysfunction (EF ≤ 60%), (ii) new onset AF, or (iii) raised systolic PAP > 50 mmHg at rest. Surgery can also be considered if there is significant LA dilatation (≥ 5.5 cm) and a high chance of durable surgical repair. In the absence of symptoms or any of the aforementioned features of adverse remodelling, serial echocardiograms every 6 months (if severe MR) or 12 months (if moderate MR) should be performed for surveillance. Treatment options in the context of secondary MR are less established. If deemed to arise because of inducible ischaemia, revascularisation may be of benefit. Additionally, in subcohorts with symptomatic CHF and prolonged QRS duration, device therapy via CRT may increase MV closing force and reduce severity.

If valve intervention is indicated, the gold standard is surgical intervention with repair preferred over replacement where anatomically feasible. If surgery is deemed prohibitively high-risk, medical therapy is first-line with consideration for percutaneous valve repair using Mitraclip if symptoms are refractory. It can be used in both degenerative (primary) and functional (secondary) MR, and involves access via the femoral vein with trans-septal puncture. A RCT comparing surgical replacement with Mitraclip repair has shown that those treated with repair more commonly required surgery to treat residual MR. However, after 12 months, there was no discernible difference in rate of re-intervention or progression of regurgitant disease and longer-term mortality rate was comparable [10]. An alternative option is annuloplasty. In degenerative MR, annuloplasty rings are used to remodel the posterior annulus to optimise surface of coaptation. With functional MR, the main technique is restrictive annuloplasty (two sizes under) to obtain a coaptation length of ≥ 8 mm. In endocarditis, the first step is to resect all infected tissue and then assess for repair.

13.9 Tricuspid Valve Anatomy

As the name suggests, the tricuspid valve (TV) has three discernible cusps: **anterior, posterior** (largest) and **septal** (smallest) (see Figure 13.13). Fibrous attachments of the septal cusp make it relatively immobile, and as a consequence, the TV operates functionally rather like a bicuspid valve with annular descent predominantly along the margins of the anterior and posterior cusps. As with MV, the subvalvular apparatus consists of papillary muscles and chordae tendinae. Typically, the septal leaflet is also supported by chordae that arise from the ventricular septum.

13.10 Tricuspid Regurgitation

13.10.1 Aetiology

TR may arise due to abnormalities in one or more components of the valve apparatus (**primary TR**). Causes include rheumatic disease (usually in conjunction with pathology involving other valves), carcinoid disease, endocarditis (e.g. in the context of intravenous drug abuse) and Ebstein's

Figure 13.13 Gross anatomy of the tricuspid valve. LCA, left coronary artery; RCA, right coronary artery.

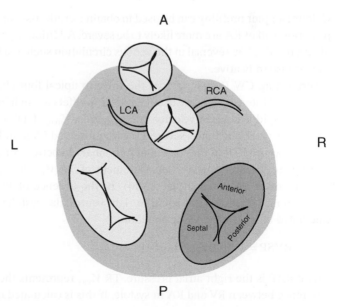

anomaly. In the vast majority of cases, it is due to annular stretch (**secondary TR**), most commonly due to pulmonary hypertension of all aetiologies that causes RV hypertrophy and dilatation before eventual right ventricular systolic dysfunction (RVSD).

13.10.2   Diagnosis

Tricuspid regurgitation is tolerated for long periods without overt symptoms. Peripheral oedema, dyspnoea and fatigue may manifest at a later stage. There is progressive RV and RA dilatation due to volume overload. This dilatation itself may act as a vicious circle by exacerbating regurgitant jets. On auscultation, TR will present as a pansystolic murmur which is loudest at the parasternal edge and amplified by inspiration. If there is evidence of pulmonary hypertension with RV hypertrophy, there may be loud P2 associated with parasternal heave. In severe disease, pulsatile JVP and/or liver may be detectable. In those with chronic, regurgitant disease, signs of RV failure may be apparent. 12-lead ECG can demonstrate P-pulmonale (see Section 1.5.1) due to LA enlargement and/or RBBB. Chest radiograph often shows cardiomegaly or features of pulmonary hypertension. However, as with other types of valvular disease, echocardiography is required for confirmatory purposes.

As alluded to, underlying rheumatic disease would usually involve multiple valves and evidence of commissural fusion may be present. Carcinoid disease is characterised by thickened, shortened and immobile leaflets, with pulmonary valves also potentially affected. Ebstein's anomaly is a congential defect in which there is displacement of one or more of the leaflets, usually septal, towards the apex which results in an 'atrialized' ventricle. The TV insertion plane is ordinarily more apical than that of MV, and therefore, the disorder should be considered when separation between both valve planes is > 1 cm. In cases of RV volume overload, a pattern of **paradoxical septal motion** may be visualised on PSAX or apical four-chamber views. This describes septal flattening in diastole due to increased filling into a dilated RV. If this is present in systole, it is indicative of RV pressure overload into a non-dilated ventricle.

13.10.3   Stratification of Severity

Colour Doppler profiling can be used to obtain a crude assessment of severity. Jets extending to the posterior wall of RA are more likely to be severe. Additionally, vena contracta > 0.7 cm is suggestive of severe TR. Flow reversal in the venous circulation such as a hepatic vein visualised on subcostal view is also indicative.

Performing CW Doppler across the valve in apical four-chamber view can provide additional data. Signal intensity relative to antegrade flow offers a rough indication. Severe disease also results in more rapid decline in velocity in late systole. V_{max} of TR jet does not always correlate directly with severity. For instance, severe TR with preserved RV systolic pressure results in a low-velocity jet whereas mild TR in the context of pulmonary hypertension causes a high-velocity jet. If there is non-severe disease, however, measurement of TR V_{max} has the specific use in providing crude assessment of PAP (see Figure 13.14). In the absence of PS or right ventricular outflow tract obstruction, systolic PAP is equal to right ventricular systolic pressure (RVSP). The latter can be calculated using the following equation:

$$RVSP = 4 \times \left(TR\,V_{max}{}^{2} \right) + RAP$$

where RAP is the right atrial pressure. TR V_{max} represents the maximum instantaneous pressure difference between RV and RA in systole. If this is calculated using the Bernouilli equation, it can

(a)

(b)

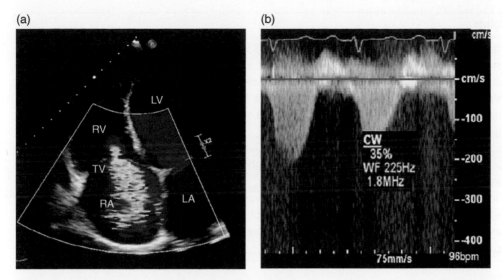

Figure 13.14 Echocardiographic features of moderate tricuspid regurgitation. (a) Apical 4-chamber view demonstrating an eccentric jet of regurgitation extending to mid-atrium, with vena contracta of 0.4 cm in keeping with moderate TR. (b) CW Doppler assessment confirmed V_{max} of 2.09 m s^{-1}, correlating with MPG of 17 mmHg. Calculated RAP (not shown) was 5 mmHg, resulting in estimated systolic PAP of 22 mmHg.

be added to an estimate of RAP to quantify systolic PAP. RAP is obtained from assessing the calibre of inferior vena cava (IVC) and extent of respiratory collapse in a subcostal view. A patient 'sniff' generates sudden decrease in intrathoracic pressure and resultant drop in IVC diameter. Corresponding estimates range from 0 to 5 mmHg (< 1.5 cm with total collapse during sniff) to > 20 mmHg (> 2.5 cm with no change during sniff). Systolic PAP > 35 mmHg at rest raises the possibility of pulmonary hypertension. This technique relies on signal optimisation and correct angulation of ultrasound beam. When there is free, voluminous flow jet of TR such as in severe disease, this estimate becomes inaccurate due to non-turbulent flow with rapid equalisation. In general, estimation of systolic PAP via echocardiogram correlates well with invasive assessment using right heart catheterisation though the former has a tendency to overestimate pressures.

13.10.4 Management

Severe functional TR may improve as RV failure subsides after treatment of the underlying cause. Pulmonary hypertension is, however, an important marker for persistent disease. Diuretics are helpful in alleviating symptoms associated with congestion. If more aggressive intervention is warranted, an individualised approach through a multidisciplinary framework is required to inform decision-making. This invariably necessitates TOE to assess anatomical lesions in greater detail.

Timing of intervention remains unclear but is generally indicated if there is prioritising need for left-sided valve surgery and presence of severe TR (primary or secondary) or mild-to-moderate TR (if secondary). If left-sided valve disease is absent, surgery can be considered if there is severe, primary TR with symptoms or progressive RV dilatation, or in the context of severe, secondary TR once severe LVSD, severe RVSD and severe PHT have been excluded. Valve intervention favours repair compared with replacement wherever feasible. Annuloplasty with selective sparing of the membranous septum is also an option with better long-term outcomes using a ring rather than stitch technique.

Hot Points

- S1 and S2 correspond to valve closure, whilst S3 and S4 refer to low-pitched sounds in diastole.
- Quantification of AS severity in the context of severe LVSD can be challenging, but dobutamine challenge is helpful in distinguishing true from pseudo-severe disease.
- Management of severe AR depends on concurrent symptoms but definitive treatment is with surgical AVR.
- The mitral valve is bicuspid with anterior (A1, A2, A3) and posterior (P1, P2, P3) leaflets. Its structural integrity is maintained by the subvalvular apparatus consisting of tendinous chords and papillary muscles.
- Definitive treatment for severe MR is surgical valve repair or replacement. Percutaneous intervention may be considered in those with prohibitive surgical risk.
- Measurement of TR jet during echocardiography (CW Doppler) can be added to RAP to calculate systolic PAP.

13.11 Self-assessment Questions

1 Which of the following statements regarding dynamic manoeuvres during auscultation for murmurs is false?
  A Right-sided murmurs are loudest in inspiration.
  B The Valsalva manoeuvre increases intensity of most murmurs.
  C Standing from a sitting position reduces intensity of most murmurs.
  D Squatting increases intensity of most murmurs.
  E Left-sided murmurs are loudest in expiration.

2 Which of the following helps differentiate true severe aortic stenosis from pseudo-severe aortic stenosis?
  A Peak pressure gradient measured across aortic valve by CW Doppler on transthoracic echocardiography.
  B Significant increase in V_{max} and minimal increase in AVA on dobutamine stress echocardiography.
  C Assessment of AVA on transthoracic echocardiography.
  D Significant increase in AVA without increase in V_{max} on dobutamine stress echocardiography.
  E Measurement of LVOT V_{max}.

3 Which of the following is not an indication for surgical AVR in aortic stenosis?
  A Symptomatic patient with peak V_{max} across the aortic valve of $5.0\,\mathrm{m\,s}^{-1}$.
  B Patient with mild aortic stenosis undergoing CABG.
  C Asymptomatic patient with severe AS and LVSD (not due to any other cause).
  D Asymptomatic patient with severe AS and symptoms on treadmill testing.
  E Symptomatic patient with AV MPG of 45 mmHg.

4 Which of the following is not a cause of primary mitral regurgitation?
  A Rheumatic disease.
  B Endocarditis.
  C Dilated cardiomyopathy.
  D Systemic lupus erythematosus.
  E Marfan syndrome.

5 Which of the following clinical signs is not a characteristic feature of aortic regurgitation?
  A Quincke's sign.
  B Rosenbach's sign.
  C Duroziez's sign.
  D Rivero-Carvallo's sign.
  E De Musset's sign.

References

1 Nashef, S.A., Roques, F., Michel, P. et al. (1999). European system for cardiac operative risk evaluation (EuroSCORE). *Eur. J. Cardiothorac. Surg.* 16 (1): 9–13.
2 Smith, C.R., Leon, M.B., Mack, M.J. et al. (2011). Transcatheter versus surgical aortic-valve replacement in high-risk patients. *N. Engl. J. Med.* 364 (23): 2187–2198.
3 Leon, M.B., Smith, C.R., Mack, M. et al. (2010). Transcatheter aortic-valve implantation for aortic stenosis in patients who cannot undergo surgery. *N. Engl. J. Med.* 363 (17): 1597–1607.
4 Leon, M.B., Smith, C.R., Mack, M.J. et al. (2016). Transcatheter or surgical aortic-valve replacement in intermediate-risk patients. *N. Engl. J. Med.* 374 (17): 1609–1620.
5 Mack, M.J., Leon, M.B., Thourani, V.H. et al. (2019). Transcatheter aortic-valve replacement with a balloon-expandable valve in low-risk patients. *N. Engl. J. Med.* 380 (18): 1695–1705.
6 Gajanana, D., Wheeler, D., Hsi, D. et al. (2016). Percutaneous balloon aortic valvuloplasty and clinical outcomes in severe aortic stenosis: correlation of procedural technique and efficacy. *J. Interv. Cardiol.* 29 (6): 612–618.
7 Iung, B., Nicoud-Houel, A., Fondard, O. et al. (2004). Temporal trends in percutaneous mitral commissurotomy over a 15-year period. *Eur. Heart J.* 25 (8): 701–707.
8 Antunes, M.J., Vieira, H., and Ferrão de Oliveira, J. (2000). Open mitral commissurotomy: the 'golden standard'. *J. Heart Valve Dis.* 9 (4): 472–477.
9 Grayburn, P.A. (2000). Vasodilator therapy for chronic aortic and mitral regurgitation. *Am. J. Med. Sci.* 320 (3): 202–208.
10 Mauri, L., Foster, E., Glower, D.D. et al. (2013). 4-year results of a randomized controlled trial of percutaneous repair versus surgery for mitral regurgitation. *J. Am. Coll. Cardiol.* 62 (4): 317–328.

Further Reading

Awtry, E. and Davidoff, R. (2011). Low-flow/low-gradient aortic stenosis. *Circulation* 124 (23): e739–e741.
Garbi, M. and Monaghan, M.J. (2015). Quantitative mitral valve anatomy and pathology. *Echo Res. Pract.* 2 (3): R63–R72.

Otto, C.M., Burwash, I.G., Legget, M.E. et al. (1997). Prospective study of asymptomatic valvular aortic stenosis. Clinical, echocardiographic, and exercise predictors of outcome. *Circulation* 95 (9): 2262–2270.

Perera, P., Lobo, V., Williams, S.R., and Gharahbaghian, L. (2014). Cardiac echocardiography. *Crit. Care Clin.* 30 (1): 47–v.

Taniguchi, T., Morimoto, T., Shiomi, H. et al. (2015). Initial surgical versus conservative strategies in patients with asymptomatic severe aortic stenosis. *J. Am. Coll. Cardiol.* 66 (25): 2827–2838.

Vahanian, A., Beyersdorf, F., Praz, F. et al. (2021). ESC/EACTS guidelines for the management of valvular heart disease (published online ahead of print, 2021 August 28). *Eur. Heart J.* 2021: ehab395.

14

Cardiomyopathies

Cardiology at its Core, First Edition. Peysh A. Patel.
© 2023 John Wiley & Sons Ltd. Published 2023 by John Wiley & Sons Ltd.

14.1 Learning Objectives

- Nomenclature of cardiomyopathies.
- Pathophysiology, diagnosis and management options for hypertrophic, dilated, restrictive and arrhythmogenic cardiomyopathy.
- Comparison of restrictive cardiomyopathies with constrictive pericarditis.
- Family screening.

14.2 Nomenclature

Conventionally, 'cardiomyopathy' is defined as primary, intrinsic disease of the myocardium which may be of genetic inheritance. The most common subtypes are hypertrophic (HCM), dilated (DCM), restrictive and arrhythmogenic (ACM). They could perhaps be best described as **primary** myocardial disease to distinguish it from **secondary** disease where there are established causes. These commonly include ischaemia, hypertension, valvular disease, alcohol excess, metabolic disorders, and peripartum cardiomyopathy. Regardless, there is a certain degree of overlap as dilated cardiomyopathy (DCM), for instance, is considered a primary cardiomyopathy but may arise as a consequence of alcohol excess. A separate category is **inflammatory** myocardial disease, namely myocarditis.

14.3 Hypertrophic Cardiomyopathy (HCM)

14.3.1 Pathophysiology

Hypertrophic cardiomyopathy (HCM) results most commonly from mutations in sarcomeric genes, such as contractile proteins actin and myosin, and result in ineffective ATP utilisation. The most common pattern of inheritance is autosomal dominant (AD) although penetrance is incomplete and age-related. An array of pathophysiological processes are implicated.

14.3.1.1 Diastolic Dysfunction and Ischaemia

HCM results in diastolic dysfunction with cellular energy deficit and altered affinity of mutant sarcomeric proteins for calcium implicated in the active ATP-consuming phase. Reduced coronary flow reserve due to systolic extravascular compression and diffuse ischaemia in the setting of left ventricular outflow tract obstruction (LVOTO) are likely to potentiate. Hypertrophy and interstitial fibrosis impair compliance and directly affects the passive phase. Restriction in diastolic filling limits capability of the left ventricle (LV) to augment stroke volume (SV) via the Frank–Starling mechanism. Nonetheless, cavity dilatation and systolic dysfunction rarely occurs ($<5\%$) and its presence is associated with poorer prognosis.

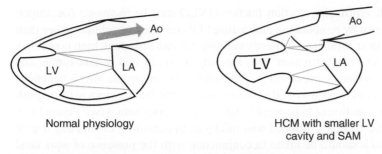

Figure 14.1 Mechanism of LVOTO in patients with HCM. Ao, aorta.

14.3.1.2 Left Ventricular Outflow Tract Obstruction

This coexists in around 25% of patients with HCM. It can occur at any level along the cavity depending on distribution of hypertrophy but subaortic obstruction is the most common (see Figure 14.1). It results from systolic anterior motion (SAM) of the anterior mitral valve leaflet (AMVL) and premature, mid-systolic aortic valve (AV) closure. Anterior haemodynamic forces because of the Venturi effect and/or flow drag effect are thought to be implicated in SAM. Premature AV closure is thought to occur because of abnormal valve apparatus with leaflet slack. Differential diagnoses for LVOTO include sub-aortic stenosis and hyperdynamic LV systolic function secondary to basal septal hypertrophy.

14.3.1.3 Abnormal BP Response to Exercise

In normal individuals, CO increases during exercise. At high heart rate (HR), diastolic filling is impaired due to reduced cycle length with compensatory augmentation through increase in venous return. This relies on sympathetic-induced venoconstriction to counteract vasodilation that ensues in skeletal muscles during exercise. Around 30% with HCM fail to increase systolic blood pressure (BP) by ≥ 25 mmHg during exercise or show paradoxical fall of ≥ 20 mmHg. This vasodilatory response has been attributed to excess stimulation of LV mechanoreceptors by abnormal wall stress, exaggerated sensitivity of arterial baroreceptors and raised levels of natriuretic peptides.

14.3.1.4 Dysrhythmias

This can be triggered by ischaemic insult secondary to LVOTO and reduced coronary flow reserve, whilst myocyte disarray and fibrosis confers additional substrate. 20% of patients with HCM have evidence of non-sustained ventricular tachycardia (NSVT) although sustained VT is less frequent. Propensity for AF is also increased because of raised LA pressure due to diastolic dysfunction.

14.3.2 Diagnosis

Patients may have a family history of the disorder. Symptoms may include reduced exercise toler-ance, chest pain, palpitations and/or syncope, often in the post-prandial setting or when they are dehydrated. Examination may reveal a jerky carotid pulse and double impulse apex beat although often difficult to elicit. If there is associated LVOTO, an ejection systolic murmur can be auscul-tated which would be accentuated with standing and Valsalva manoeuvres (i.e. dynamic) unlike fixed valvular obstructions such as aortic stenosis where murmur would diminish.

The first indication is usually a grossly abnormal 12-lead ECG with characteristic findings that include left bundle branch block (LBBB), left axis deviation (LAD), inferolateral Q waves ('dagger-shaped'), T wave inversion or ST changes. Echocardiography will allow thorough assessment of LV dimension and function. Left ventricular ejection fraction (LVEF) may be increased (i.e. 'super-normal') although usually driven by remodelling and reduced LV end-diastole volume rather than increased SV or contractility *per se*. SAM can be directly visualised, as can turbulent, high flow velocity through the LVOT suggestive of obstruction. This typically occurs in mid to late-systole and explains why systolic function is usually preserved. Adjunct imaging with cardiac MRI is beneficial in delineating morphology and scar burden as well as provision of discriminatory clues to distinguish from phenocopies based on distribution of hypertrophy and tissue characterisation (see Figure 14.2).

Although original diagnostic criteria stipulated wall thickness in diastole ≥ 15 mm, any degree and distribution may occur so it should be taken in conjunction with the presence of associated signs. In clinical practice, the challenge is to distinguish HCM from hypertensive heart disease and this may rely on historic BP trend and morphological features. It is also important to exclude athlete's heart secondary to physiological adaptation, and a comparison to aid discrimination is provided in Table 14.1.

It is also prudent to consider phenocopies of HCM aside from athlete's heart. These include Anderson–Fabry disease, caused by mutations of the X-linked *GLA* gene that results in a

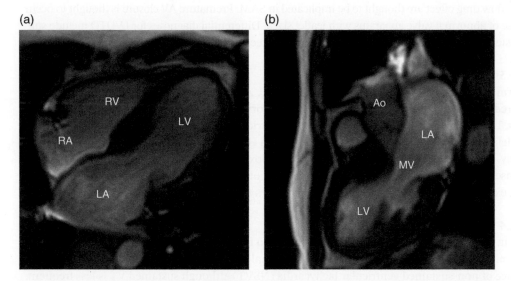

Figure 14.2 Cardiac MRI demonstrating typical features of hypertrophic obstructive cardiomyopathy. (a) 4-chamber cine view showing LVH with asymmetrical septal hypertrophy (20 mm maximum) and LA dilatation. (b) Sagittal view of LVOT with SAM of AMVL.

Table 14.1 Comparison of HCM and athlete's heart.

HCM	Athlete's heart
Small LV cavity	Normal or dilated LV cavity
Higher relative wall thickness	Lower relative wall thickness
Abnormal diastolic function	Preserved diastolic function
Dilated LA	Normal LA
Pathological ('dagger') Q waves	No pathological Q waves

deficiency of the lysosomal enzyme α-galactosidase A. It is similarly pertinent to consider amyloidosis, a systemic disorder that arises due to abnormal folding of normal soluble proteins and leads to fibril formation and amyloid deposits (see Section 14.5.2). More rarely, inherited storage disorders such as Pompe and Danon disease and mitochondrial disease arising from m.3243 A > G mutations can be implicated.

14.3.3 Management

14.3.3.1 Monitoring and Lifestyle Advice
Holter monitoring is recommended to assess for incident AF and broad complex tachycardias. This is typically performed via 48-hour ambulatory ECG monitoring every 12–24 months, or more frequently if LA size is > 4.5 cm. Cardiopulmonary exercise testing (CPEX) ought to be considered every two to three years or sooner in cases of progressive disease, with cardiac MRI every five years or sooner based on severity. Exercise and sports participation are not contraindicated but individualised exercise prescription with annual follow-up is recommended after exclusion of markers suggestive of increased risk.

14.3.3.2 Medical Therapy
Asymptomatic patients with mild left ventricular hypertrophy (LVH) should be monitored conservatively. Those with symptoms or presence of severe LVH/LVOTO (≥ 50 mmHg) ought to be initiated on a negative chronotrope such as beta-blocker or NDHP CCB. Improved diastolic filling increases LV cavity size and reduces outflow tract gradient. In those with even mild LVSD, prompt initiation of disease-modifying agents for congestive heart failure (CHF) is advocated to retard disease progression. Interestingly, beta-blockers do not appear to suppress serious ventricular dysrhythmias in HCM. On the contrary, amiodarone appears to be highly effective though data is limited and prophylactic implantable cardioverter–defibrillator (ICD) is still warranted in those at higher risk (see later). Disopyramide, an anti-arrhythmic that alters calcium kinetics, has been associated with symptom improvement and gradient reductions relating to negative inotropy and peripheral vasoconstriction. 12-lead ECG to measure QTc interval should be performed at treatment initiation for baseline purposes and after dose adjustment.

14.3.3.3 Device Therapy
Indication for primary prevention ICD depends on five-year risk of sudden cardiac death (SCD) and should be assessed at one to two-yearly intervals. It incorporates age, history of unexplained syncope, family history of SCD, LV wall thickness, LVOT gradient, LA size and presence of NSVT [1]. EP testing is not a component of risk stratification at present. Broadly speaking, risk score $\geq 6\%$ with life expectancy over one year warrants ICD implant with consideration for device therapy if 4–6%. This tool should not be used in paediatric cases aged < 16 years, elite/competitive athletes, those with secondary prevention indication and HCM that is associated with metabolic disorders. Dual-chamber pacing with shortened AV delay is postulated to reduce outflow tract gradient, with benefits relating to dyssynchronous septal contraction because of RV apical pacing. However, it is not routinely offered in clinical practice and its role in reducing propensity for VT has not been clarified. Cardiac resynchronisation therapy (CRT) can be explored as add-on therapy if LVOTO is < 30 mmHg in the presence of coexistent LBBB.

14.3.3.4 Surgery

In those with refractory, obstructive symptoms, surgery may be considered. Septal myomectomy to remove excess muscle is highly effective but ventricular remodelling can occur. It is therefore reserved for select cases and often performed in combination with MV repair if SAM is the primary cause of obstruction. Alcohol ablation of ventricular septum is an alternative with 1–3 ml of pure ethanol injected over five minutes into the first or second septal branch via echocardiographic guidance. Secondary septal hypokinesia effectively reduces outflow gradient to its entirety in 33% [2]. Procedural sequelae may include transient or permanent AV blockade in up to 20% and often limits applicability. Lastly, in those with resistant NYHA class III/IV symptoms or intractable ventricular arrhythmias, cardiac transplantation is a possibility.

14.4 Dilated Cardiomyopathy (DCM)

14.4.1 Pathophysiology

DCM is considered to be familial in around 20–35% of cases with the most common pattern of inheritance being AD. The majority of familial phenotypes are caused by variants in genes encoding proteins of the cardiac myocyte, namely filamin C, lamin A/C, and titin. Diagnosis is complicated by incomplete penetrance and variable expressivity. Secondary causes, including chemotherapy, alcohol excess, human immunodeficiency virus (HIV), thyroid dysfunction, and peripartum (within late third trimester of pregnancy or up to six months postpartum), possibly arise when incomplete penetrant genetic disease is unmasked by a triphasic model of myocardial insult followed by chronic inflammation, ventricular remodelling and dysfunction. Enterovirus and adenovirus are most strongly implicated. Indeed, polymerase chain reaction (PCR) techniques to detect viral RNA in cardiac tissue have returned positive findings in up to 35% of DCM patients [3]. A labelling of **idiopathic DCM** should only be made after confident exclusion of other subtypes.

Whatever the initial insult, secondary neurohumoral activation with pathological remodelling leads to increased wall stress. β-adrenergic system activation, production of angiotensin II and generation of inflammatory cytokines and reactive oxygen species (ROS) can result in programmed cell death ('apoptosis') of cardiomyocytes. It is therefore unsurprising that conventional agents used to treat CHF antagonise these pathways. Altered calcium handling and release of atrial and B-type natriuretic peptides are also implicated.

14.4.2 Diagnosis

A thorough exploration of family history is required but as there is high phenotypic variability, this should always be allied with clinical symptoms and signs. These are similar in presentation to conventional CHF although often less symptomatic. NT-proBNP measurement can offer useful additional information. 12-lead ECG may show evidence of AF and/or BBB morphology which guides management considerations including device resynchronisation. Holter monitoring can demonstrate reduced HR variability due to excess sympathetic drive and is associated with adverse prognosis. It can also highlight intermittent atrioventricular block, NSVT or atrial dysrhythmias indicative of underlying inherited or metabolic aetiology.

Echocardiography is mandated to formulate the correct diagnosis. In patients with DCM, LV dilatation is a hallmark with left ventricular end-diastolic diameter (LVEDD) > 5 cm (women) or 6 cm (men), although it should be indexed to body surface area (BSA). This is usually associated with impaired LVSF but may not manifest if there is early involvement. Classic DCM presents as dilatation of all four chambers with coexistent right ventricular systolic dysfunction. Secondary valvular disease due to annular dilatation, such as functional mitral or tricuspid regurgitation, can be present. CPEX testing assesses adequacy of cardiac response to exertion and is a predictor of risk [4]. Cardiac MRI provides supplementary data and more robust assessment of chamber volumes and function in those with suboptimal image quality (see Figure 14.3). It can confirm presence of myocardial fibrosis which is of diagnostic use, such as highlighting historic myocarditis (typically mid-wall) or arrhythmogenic cardiomyopathy (ACM) (typically sub-epicardial), and can be a potent guide for prognostication. Lastly, no patient should be labelled as idiopathic DCM without excluding coronary disease via anatomical/functional imaging or invasive angiography and ensuring there are no correctable metabolic triggers.

14.4.3 Management

General advice relates to avoidance of precipitants such as alcohol. Those with established peripartum cardiomyopathy have 50% chance of functional recovery. However, they should be strongly counselled regarding risk of future pregnancies and need for close surveillance within a specialised cardio-obstetrics service should they choose to proceed. Mortality risk is in the region of 1% with recovered function and significantly higher at 10% in those with persistent dysfunction.

In those without a clear cause, referral to a tertiary inherited cardiovascular conditions (ICC) centre is prudent to determine suitability for genetic testing and clinical screening of first-degree relatives. Pharmacotherapy is consistent with established guidelines for CHF with loop diuretic for

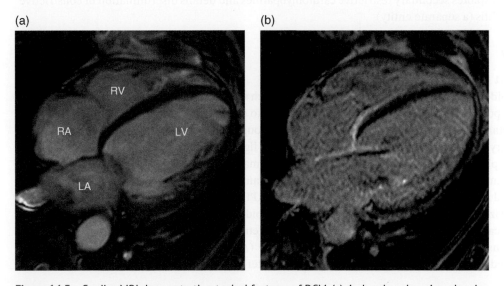

(a) (b)

Figure 14.3 Cardiac MRI demonstrating typical features of DCM. (a) 4-chamber cine view showing dilatation of all four chambers with LVEDD of 6 cm. (b) Evidence of accompanying late gadolinium enhancement (LGE) suggestive of mid-wall fibrosis in the apex extending to apicolateral and mid-lateral segments.

symptomatic benefit in addition to ACE inhibitor, beta-blocker, aldosterone antagonist, ARNI and SGLT2 inhibitor based on symptom burden and LVEF. Anticoagulation may be indicated to suppress thromboembolic risk in patients with CHF and coexistent AF based on CHA_2DS_2-VASc score.

Device therapy is often a bespoke decision. Certain metabolic and inherited causes of DCM have high propensity for bradyarrhythmias and warrant dual-chamber pacemaker implantation. As stated, CRT may be an option if there are persistent symptoms (NYHA class II or worse) despite optimal therapy and evidence of dyssynchrony, i.e. BBB pattern (see Section 12.7.12.2). Eligibility for primary prevention ICD is driven primarily by LVEF and cardiac MRI finding in addition to results of genetic screening when performed. In young patients such as those with previous myocarditis, advanced symptoms may necessitate referral to a specialist heart failure centre and workup for cardiac transplantation.

14.5 Restrictive Cardiomyopathy

14.5.1 Categorisation

Secondary restrictive cardiomyopathies can occur due to infiltrative disorders such as amyloidosis, sarcoidosis and haemochromatosis. In the latter, iron deposition is localised to the sarcoplasm and absent from interstitium and this results in a storage disorder rather than infiltration *per se*. Other causes include drugs (e.g. anti-malarials such as chloroquine and hydroxychloroquine), metastatic malignancy, radiotherapy and, infrequently, glycogen storage disorders such as Anderson–Fabry disease, Friedreich's ataxia and Danon disease where deposition is intracellular rather than within the interstitium. Primary (idiopathic) restrictive cardiomyopathy may be caused by Loeffler eosinophilic endocarditis (acute) and endomyocardial fibrosis (chronic). These are rare in the Western world but endemic in South America and Africa. The remainder of this section explores secondary restrictive cardiomyopathies and details discrimination of constrictive pericarditis (a separate entity).

14.5.2 Amyloidosis

14.5.2.1 Pathophysiology

Amyloidosis refers to a spectrum of disorders in which soluble extracellular proteins are misfolded and deposited in tissues as insoluble fibrils, leading to disruption of tissue architecture. It may be hereditary or acquired with the latter occurring through several means. In primary forms (**AL**), fibrillary proteins are composed of immunoglobulin light chains, and hence, neoplastic proliferation of plasma cells in the context of multiple myeloma is strongly associated. It can also occur in secondary forms (**AA**) due to states of chronic inflammation such as rheumatoid arthritis. **Aβ** amyloid is derived from a larger glycoprotein called APP and is found in cerebral lesions of patients with Alzheimer's disease. **β2-microglobulin** amyloidosis is a specific subset which arises as a complication of long-term dialysis. Lastly, a separate entity relates to mutations in the gene encoding transthyretin, a transport protein for thyroxine (**ATTR**). It can be both inherited (AD) or acquired (senile systemic amyloidosis) and has a better prognosis.

14.5.2.2 Diagnosis

As with all infiltrative disorders, amyloid deposition can be multi-systemic and affects the kidneys, liver, spleen, endocrine glands (e.g. pituitary, thyroid, adrenal), gastrointestinal tract and tongue. Amyloidosis may also involve the heart with deposition in the myocardium, papillary muscles, valves and vessels. It is often a diagnostic challenge but index of suspicion should be heightened in any presentation with restrictive cardiomyopathy of unclear aetiology.

12-lead ECG will classically show low-voltage complexes although varying degrees of atrioventricular block and BBB may also be present. Echocardiography often shows widespread and biventricular hypertrophy with relative sparing of apex. Interatrial septum may be thickened, atria are usually dilated and bilateral AV regurgitation can be present. A concomitant pericardial effusion is typically observed. Assessment of diastolic function demonstrates a pseudo-normal pattern (i.e. grade II as opposed to grade III – see Section 12.8.3) with associated systolic dysfunction in advanced disease. Cardiac MRI may identify pathognomonic appearances with features on tissue characterisation that include increased T1 mapping times, raised extracellular volume, inability to null myocardium and widespread fibrosis in a non-coronary distribution (see Figure 14.4). This may obviate need for histological confirmatory diagnosis in modern practice although can be obtained if needed via Congo red staining to assess for apple-green birefringence. In suspected ATTR amyloidosis, 99mTc-deoxypyridinoline (DPD) bone scintigraphy with Perugini scoring is required for formal diagnosis once plasma cell dyscrasia has been excluded [5].

14.5.2.3 Management

This is primarily targeted at the underlying cause but is often challenging to elicit. Those with systolic dysfunction should be treated as per established guidance. Digoxin has traditionally been contraindicated as it can bind to amyloid fibrils and toxicity may develop at otherwise therapeutic dosing. Unfortunately, survival for patients with amyloidosis remains dismal at around one to three years. Those with myeloma-associated amyloidosis (AL) have a prognosis largely governed by the underlying haematological disorder and specialist input is warranted to manage the overall condition. Identification of those with ATTR amyloidosis is important as certain cohorts may be eligible for Tafamidis (transthyretin stabiliser) or RNA-interfering agents such as Patisiran based on local funding provisions.

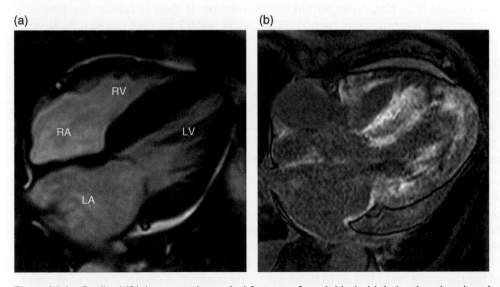

(a) (b)

Figure 14.4 Cardiac MRI demonstrating typical features of amyloidosis. (a) 4-chamber cine view showing concentric LVH, LA dilatation, thickened and aneurysmal interatrial septum (IAS) and small rim of global pericardial effusion. (b) Accompanying late gadolinium enhancement (LGE) suggestive of extensive, diffuse fibrosis in a non-coronary distribution.

14.5.3 Sarcoidosis

14.5.3.1 Pathophysiology

Sarcoidosis is a multi-system disease of unclear aetiology. However, familial aggregation suggests that genetic factors are of influence. It has predilection for adults younger than 40 years and is of higher prevalence in northern Europeans and African-Americans in addition to non-smokers. It may arise from disordered immune regulation in genetically predisposed individuals, with proposed antigens that include viruses, mycobacteria and *Borrelia*. Its pathological hallmark is interstitial deposition of clusters of white blood cells resulting in non-caseating granulomas. Two other microscopic features are presence of Schaumann and asteroid bodies.

14.5.3.2 Diagnosis

The lungs and lymph nodes are primarily involved. Granuloma deposition can eventually result in diffuse fibrosis and a 'honeycomb' lung. Painless enlargement of hilar and paratracheal lymph nodes can coexist. Erythema nodosum of the shins is a feature of acute sarcoidosis with red, raised, tender nodules. Similarly, discoloured plaques may arise in the region of the nose, cheeks and lips (lupus pernio). Lofgren's syndrome is an acute form characterised by bilateral hilar lymphadenopathy, erythema nodosum, pyrexia and polyarthralgia. Other sites of involvement include eyes, lacrimal glands, liver, spleen and bone marrow. Cardiac involvement is uncommon but can arise in around 25% and mainly involves septum and LV free wall.

Sarcoidosis ought to be considered in any young patient presenting with atrioventricular block or ventricular dysrhythmia as there is a strong association. Any presentation with restrictive filling of unclear aetiology should be formally assessed. 12-lead ECG may show atrioventricular conduction disease, ventricular dysrhythmias and/or supraventricular tachycardias. Chest X-ray can show evidence of hilar lymphadenopathy and/or fibrosis. Laboratory profiling is usually suggestive of lymphopenia, elevated ACE and hypercalcaemia due to production of vitamin D by phagocytes within the granulomas. If there is cardiac involvement, elevated myocardial injury markers such as CK, troponin and NT-proBNP can be indicative of active inflammation.

Echocardiography is essential to assess LV systolic and diastolic function. LV hypertrophy and basal thinning of the ventricular septum may be apparent (see Figure 14.5). Cardiac MRI may corroborate structural and functional changes and indicate fibrotic burden. Fluorodeoxyglucose computed tomography-positron emission tomography (FDG CT-PET) scanning is helpful in detecting active sarcoidosis and, crucially, may highlight involvement of extracardiac sites such as hilar lymph nodes for tissue diagnosis. Endomyocardial biopsy has high specificity but is technically challenging and of low sensitivity due to patchy disease involvement.

14.5.3.3 Management

Strategy is dependent upon extent of disease involvement and is established using radiographic findings. For examples of high-grade involvement with active inflammation on CT-PET, corticosteroids are first-line therapy with exploration of biologics in cases of resistance. These should ideally be implemented prior to development of CHF. Otherwise, conventional treatment is required but the use of beta-blockers in those with early conduction disease merits close monitoring. Device therapy in the form of CRT and/or ICD may be considered with adoption of an individualised strategy. Nonetheless, decompensated heart failure remains the primary mode of death in patients with cardiac sarcoidosis.

(a)

(b)

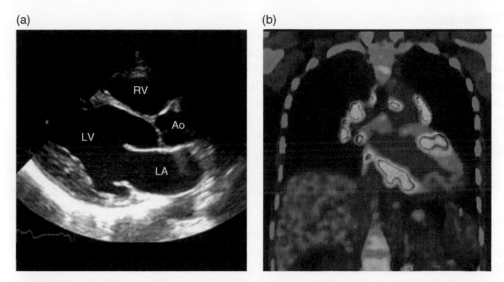

Figure 14.5 Imaging features typical of cardiac sarcoidosis. (a) Parasternal short axis (PSAX) view with LV hypertrophy and basal thinning of septum. (b) FDG CT-PET with grossly abnormal patchy myocardial uptake accompanied by avid hilar and mediastinal lymph nodes. These appearances are consistent with active sarcoidosis. Ao, aorta.

14.5.4 Haemochromatosis

14.5.4.1 Pathophysiology

Primary (hereditary) haemochromatosis is an inherited disorder of iron metabolism resulting in excessive intestinal absorption. 90% of sufferers are male as menstrual blood loss in women is protective. Inheritance is autosomal recessive and in adult-onset cases, gene mutations are predominantly in *HFE* gene on chromosome 6 with variable disease expression. Secondary haemochromatosis can also arise due to multiple blood transfusions, ineffective erythropoiesis or increased iron intake (Bantu siderosis).

14.5.4.2 Diagnosis

It is often asymptomatic in early disease with symptoms classically presenting in fifth or sixth decade of life Multi-organ involvement can occur with predilection for high mitochondrial states. Involvement can extend to myocardium, liver, pancreas, pituitary and adrenal glands, thyroid and parathyroid glands, joints, and skin. Symptoms may include arthralgia, secondary diabetes, amenorrhoea or loss of libido, with signs of chronic liver disease and bronzed skin pigmentation due to epidermal melanin deposition.

Initial joint X-ray may show chondrocalcinosis due to asymmetrical deposition of calcium pyrophosphate (pseudogout). Blood profiling typically exhibits increased transferrin saturation (>50%) in the initial phase. There may be abnormalities in liver function, raised ferritin (albeit non-specific as it is an acute phase reactant), raised serum iron and decreased total iron-binding capacity (TIBC). Blood glucose may be raised. Liver biopsy with Perl's stain is diagnostic and also provides estimation of total iron burden. There is minimal fibrotic deposition within the myocardium and dysrhythmias are not commonly seen. When cardiac involvement does occur, this is initially evident as diastolic dysfunction with restrictive filling. In advanced cases, a typical dilated or restrictive phenotype may occur. Cardiac MRI is of particular use in characterising iron deposition and results in decreased myocardial T1 and T2* mapping times.

14.5.4.3 Management

This involves venesection which is initially performed every one to two weeks until patients become mildly iron-deficient. Maintenance therapy is indicated for life with intended transferrin saturation < 40–50%. It can return life expectancy to normal assuming that patients have not developed secondary diabetes or liver cirrhosis. Indeed, ventricular dysfunction can often reverse entirely. In rare instances where patients are unable to tolerate venesection, chelation therapy with desferrioxamine can be considered. All patients and their first-degree relatives should be offered genetic testing. Additionally, cardiac MRI is a useful imaging modality for surveillance purposes.

14.5.5 Comparison with Constrictive Pericarditis

14.5.5.1 Clinical Features

Constrictive pericarditis tends to affect both parietal and visceral pericardium and is driven by the primary aetiology, being commonest with bacterial causes [particularly tuberculosis (TB)], cardiac injury during surgery and post-radiation. Its clinical presentation is highly variable and has distinct overlap with that of restrictive cardiomyopathy. Patients may describe breathlessness, abdominal distension due to ascites and peripheral oedema.

On examination, features of predominant right-sided heart failure are manifest with raised JVP, ascites, hepatomegaly and pitting oedema. Auscultatory heart sounds may be muffled. Ordinarily, JVP falls during inspiration as reduced intrathoracic pressure allows increased RV expansion for filling in diastole. In cases of constrictive pericarditis, RV is non-compliant and filling is impaired and this results in retrograde propagation of blood into the venous system and JVP that does not fall or paradoxically rises (**Kussmaul's sign**) – see Figure 14.6. However, any condition that impairs RV filling can cause this sign, and therefore, restrictive cardiomyopathy is included in the differential. A separate diagnosis to consider is cardiac tamponade due to acute accumulation of blood in the pericardial cavity, secondary to transmural infarction, for instance (see Section 11.9.4). In these circumstances, features of Beck's triad (i.e. raised JVP, muffled heart sounds and low BP) may be evident.

During inspiration, systolic BP normally decreases by ≤ 10 mmHg and HR rises. Reduced intrathoracic pressure increases venous return and RV filling, and also expands the compliant pulmonary vasculature resulting in pooling of blood in the lungs and reduced LV filling. In addition, RV

NORMAL

RESTRICTED FILLING

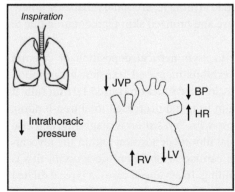
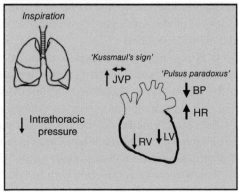

Figure 14.6 Features of restricted ventricular filling.

distension secondary to increased filling directly compromises LV filling. This reduced filling is detectable as a drop in BP with compensatory increase in HR via baroreceptor reflex, which stimulates sympathetic outflow. In cases of constrictive pericarditis, there is evidence of **pulsus paradoxus** where there is more significant drop in BP (>10 mmHg) and rise in HR during inspiration. This occurs because reduced LV filling is compounded by restriction due to exaggerated ventricular interdependence. This phenomenon is also observed in cardiac tamponade but not with restrictive cardiomyopathy.

14.5.5.2 Diagnosis

12-lead ECG is often normal in constrictive pericarditis although low-voltage QRS complexes may be seen. There can be evidence of sinus tachycardia or AF. Chest X-ray may demonstrate pleural effusions without significant alveolar involvement. Pericardial calcification is rarely seen and more prominent when there is a prior history of TB. Even though constrictive pericarditis and restrictive cardiomyopathy have similar clinical presentations, underlying pathophysiology varies. In constrictive pericarditis, impaired ventricular compliance is imposed by external constraints whilst in restrictive cardiomyopathy, it occurs intrinsically as a consequence of abnormal elastic properties of the myocardium itself.

Echocardiography is particularly helpful to differentiate between the two entities assuming adequate hydration status (see Table 14.2). In advanced states, both pathologies demonstrate evidence of severe (grade III) diastolic dysfunction corresponding with shortened DT and increased E : A ratio (see Section 12.8.3). Both may also show preserved LVEF, dilated, unreactive IVC and bi-atrial enlargement, although the latter is usually more pronounced in restrictive cardiomyopathy. With constrictive pericarditis, there may be evidence of pericardial fluid or thickening (>4 mm) although echocardiography is less sensitive than advanced imaging such as cardiac CT and MRI in this regard. In constrictive pericarditis (and tamponade), exaggerated interventricular dependence results in a double component to ventricular septal motion during diastole (**septal bounce**) in around 90% of cases. This manifests as reduced or paradoxical septal movement during diastole, i.e. initial movement towards and then away from LV. Doppler assessment of transvalvular flow across atrioventricular valves to look for exaggerated respiratory variability is also beneficial for discrimination.

Cardiac MRI is an adjunct tool as it enables clear myocardial tissue characterisation to exclude infiltration. With the aid of free-breathing cine sequences, it can also demonstrate

Table 14.2 Discrimination between constrictive pericarditis and restrictive cardiomyopathy on echocardiography.

Constrictive pericarditis	Restrictive cardiomyopathy
Pericardial effusion/thickening/calcification	Normal pericardium
Mildly dilated atria	Severely dilated atria
Septal bounce	No septal bounce
Normal PAP	Raised PAP (>50 mmHg)
Tissue Doppler E$' \geq 8$ cm s^{-1}	Tissue Doppler E$' \leq 8$ cm s^{-1}
Septal E$' >$ lateral E$'$	Septal E$' <$ lateral E$'$
Exaggerated fall ($\geq 25\%$) in transmitral E velocity during inspiration	Physiological fall ($\leq 10\%$) in transmitral E velocity during inspiration

ventricular interdependence to confirm constrictive physiology. In those with suspected constrictive disease where echocardiography and/or cardiac MRI are non-conclusive, invasive evaluation with right heart catheterisation is recommended to aid diagnostic certainty. This will show elevated and equalisation of diastolic pressure in all four chambers with presence of 'dip and plateau' or 'square root' sign as a manifestation of early rapid diastolic filling succeeded by abrupt cessation of flow.

14.5.5.3 Management

The primary objective in constrictive pericarditis is to improve cardiac function and relies on accurate identification and management of the underlying cause. In the context of tuberculous pericarditis, for instance, a six-month anti-tuberculous regimen is adopted with consideration for intrapericardial urokinase and steroids once HIV-associated TB has been excluded. Empirical anti-inflammatories only play a role in cases of transient constriction where inflammatory markers are raised or there is pericardial enhancement on imaging. Cautious use of diuretics may be beneficial in relieving congestion, although rate-limiting agents are generally avoided as coexistent sinus tachycardia is a compensatory mechanism to preserve CO in the setting of fixed SV. The definitive treatment for chronic, permanent constriction is surgical pericardectomy. This leads to rapid haemodynamic and symptomatic improvement in most cases although abnormal diastolic filling can persist for several months post-intervention. It also carries a high risk of major adverse events both peri- and postoperatively.

14.6   Arrhythmogenic Cardiomyopathy (ACM)

14.6.1   Pathophysiology

Arrhythmogenic cardiomyopathy (ACM) is estimated to occur at a population frequency of 1 in 1000 to 1 in 5000, with higher prevalence in victims of SCD. It is genetically heterogeneous but mutations in genes encoding desmosomal proteins such as *JUP, DSP*, and *PKP2* are strongly implicated in a predominantly AD pattern. It is characterised by loss of adhesion between cardiac myocytes which manifests pathologically as fatty or fibrofatty infiltration with preferential involvement of the inflow/outflow tracts and apex. This progresses from epicardium to endocardium and results in gradual wall thinning. It appeared to have preference for the right heart in early cohorts and this informed diagnostic task force criteria for an entity traditionally labelled arrhythmogenic right ventricular cardiomyopathy (ARVC). Our understanding has progressed to now acknowledge presence of biventricular or even left-dominant disease, and in view of this, the generic term of ACM is now preferred.

14.6.2   Diagnosis

This can be challenging as disease expression is variable and right-sided heart failure rarely manifests. The first presentation can be sudden ventricular arrhythmias or SCD, and many patients present within a 'concealed' phase that demonstrates a more predominant electrical phenotype with normal cardiac structure and function. Moreover, transient episodes of dysrhythmia may be well tolerated due to usual preservation of LV function. When symptomatic, this is often with palpitations, syncope and/or SCD due to VT or ventricular fibrillation. It may occur unexpectedly in previously asymptomatic individuals, typically in young patients and competitive athletes, as

Epsilon wave

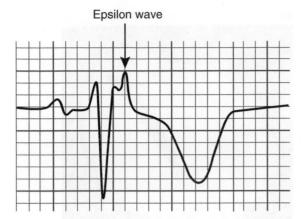

Figure 14.7 Appearance of epsilon wave suggestive of ARVC.

exercise accentuates adhesion defects with greater wall stress on RV compared with LV. Moreover, arrhythmias are potentiated by underlying adrenergic surge. Exploration of a detailed family history in first-degree relatives is therefore vital.

Revised Task Force Criteria are utilised to aid with diagnosis and incorporate multiple features [6]. Unlike other cardiomyopathies, confirmation of a gene mutation is part of the diagnostic criterion in addition to global or regional RV dysfunction, tissue characterisation, repolarisation and depolarisation abnormalities, arrhythmias and family history. 12-lead ECG may show T wave inversion or epsilon waves in precordial leads (see Figure 14.7), visualised as a terminal notch at the end of the QRS complex secondary to late RV activation.

There may be evidence of incomplete or complete RBBB. If VT occurs, tachycardia typically arises from RV where the source of substrate is located. Subsequently, ECGs show a LBBB pattern with right axis deviation. Signal-averaged ECG monitoring may be helpful in clarifying late cardiac potentials (i.e. DAD/EAD), and Holter monitoring can present another diagnostic criterion based on ventricular ectopy burden > 500 extrasystoles in 24 hours. The first indication of underlying disease may relate to incidental echocardiographic findings of isolated RV enlargement without concurrent rise in systolic PAP. In addition, regional RV dyskinesia, akinesia, or aneurysm formation with segmental dilatation and dysfunction may be seen. This can be corroborated with cardiac MRI and provides information on presence, morphology and distribution of scar with greater sensitivity (see Figure 14.8). Endomyocardial biopsy is not routinely practice in view of low sensitivity but can be reserved for instances where diagnostic uncertainty exists or formal assessment of probands is required. Histological diagnosis is more classically used in post-mortem samples where the proband has had a SCD.

14.6.3 Management

Beta-blockers are recommended in all patients with a confirmed diagnosis irrespective of symptoms. If there is survived cardiac arrest due to ventricular arrhythmias, secondary prevention ICD is necessary. No risk stratification criteria exists to guide eligibility for primary prevention implant, but unexplained syncope, NSVT and ventricular dysfunction are generally deemed predictors of poor outcome. The role of EP testing in these contexts is unclear with conflicting data. Anti-arrhythmics such as sotalol and mexiletine can be considered as adjunct therapy to ICD in persistent cases. Catheter ablation can similarly be offered if dysrhythmias remain

(a) (b)

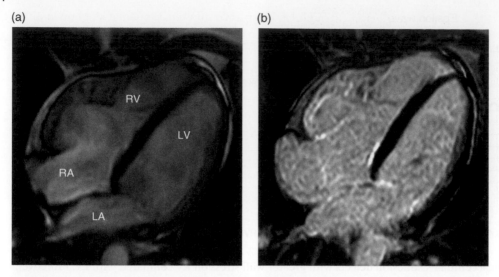

Figure 14.8 Cardiac MRI demonstrating typical features of ACM. (a) 4-chamber cine view showing significant RV dilatation with basal diameter of 5 cm. (b) Accompanying late gadolinium enhancement (LGE) confirming mid-wall fibrosis in RV apex extending to apical lateral segment of the LV.

refractory although effectiveness is limited by multi-locality of substrate, epicardial predisposition and its progressive nature. All those with a confirmed diagnosis, including asymptomatic gene carriers, should be counselled to avoid participation in competitive or endurance exercise. An individualised exercise prescription is often recommended which is best delivered within a specialist ICC centre. If a clear mutation is identified in the proband (see Section 14.7), cascade screening within the family is indicated. In its absence, all first-degree relatives still require phenotypic screening.

14.7 Family Screening

Genetic testing and family evaluation play a key role in the assessment of inherited cardiomyopathies. This is often carried out within a specialist team with expertise in cardiology (adult and paediatric) and clinical genetics. An overarching principle is to identify a three-generation family history and recommend screening of first-degree relatives, with the presenting individual referred to as the **proband**. This includes resting 12-lead ECG and echocardiogram although more detailed phenotyping may be warranted based on underlying condition. In most, this requires serial testing, with periodicity dependent on pathology and tailored to the proband's phenotype as disease expression can occur later in life.

In 30–50% of cardiomyopathies, a pathogenic gene mutation can be identified through a blood test in the proband. In many cases, this will not influence the proband's management. Exceptions include enzyme replacement therapy in HCM patients with *GLA* mutation (i.e. those with Anderson–Fabry disease), or earlier consideration of device therapy in DCM cohorts with lamin mutation. In most families, presence of such a mutation can formulate a role for predicting gene testing in first-degree relatives at risk, with the primary benefit that those without inheritance can be safely discharged from follow-up. Variants of unclear significance can be discovered through testing, however, so careful and expert counselling is mandated. Many individuals with a genetic cardiomyopathy will not have an identifiable mutation so it is paramount for families and clinicians to recognise that a negative result does not automatically exclude genetic aetiology.

Hot Points

- Cardiomyopathy is intrinsic disease of the myocardium and may be considered as primary, secondary or inflammatory.
- HCM is rarely associated with systolic dysfunction. However, there may be coexistent LVOTO (HOCM), propensity for dysrhythmia and abnormal BP response to exercise.
- In comparison with athlete's heart, HCM results in non-dilated LV cavity with diastolic dysfunction and enlarged LA. ECG may show pathological Q waves.
- Classic DCM results in dilatation of all four chambers with associated biventricular dysfunction.
- Constrictive pericarditis may be distinguished from restrictive cardiomyopathy on echocardiography by the presence of septal bounce, normal PAP and exaggerated fall in transmitral E velocity during inspiration.

14.8 Self-assessment Questions

1 Which of the following is not considered a major risk factor in risk stratification of hypertrophic cardiomyopathy?
   A Family history of sudden cardiac death.
   B Unexplained syncope.
   C Reduced left ventricular ejection fraction.
   D Severe left ventricular hypertrophy.
   E Non-sustained ventricular tachycardia.

2 Which of the following statements is true regarding amyloidosis?
   A Primary amyloidosis is most commonly caused by chronic inflammatory conditions.
   B Senile systemic amyloidosis is associated with better prognosis than other forms.
   C The presence of speckled appearance of the myocardium is diagnostic.
   D Digoxin is indicated for patients with amyloidosis and coexistent atrial fibrillation.
   E Amyloidosis is a purely hereditary condition.

3 Which of the following options is not an echocardiographic feature of restrictive cardiomyopathy?
   A Normal appearance of pericardium.
   B Severely dilated atria.
   C Tissue Doppler $E' \leq 8\,\mathrm{cm\,s}^{-1}$.
   D Exaggerated fall ($\geq 25\%$) in transmitral E velocity during inspiration.
   E All of the above.

4   Which of the following statements is true regarding sarcoidosis?
    A Erythema nodosum is commonly seen.
    B Sarcoidosis may result in high-grade AV block.
    C Serum ACE levels can be considered for disease monitoring.
    D A negative endomyocardial biopsy does not exclude diagnosis.
    E All of the above.

5   Which of these options is the commonest cause of dilated cardiomyopathy?
    A Alcohol excess.
    B Genetic mutation.
    C Acute myocarditis.
    D Chemotherapeutic agents.
    E Pregnancy.

References

1 O'Mahony, C., Jichi, F., Pavlou, M. et al. (2014). A novel clinical risk prediction model for sudden cardiac death in hypertrophic cardiomyopathy (HCM risk-SCD). *Eur. Heart J.* 35 (30): 2010–2020.

2 Faber, L., Meissner, A., Ziemssen, P., and Seggewiss, H. (2000). Percutaneous transluminal septal myocardial ablation for hypertrophic obstructive cardiomyopathy: long term follow up of the first series of 25 patients. *Heart* 83 (3): 326–331.

3 Mason, J.W. (2003). Myocarditis and dilated cardiomyopathy: an inflammatory link. *Cardiovasc. Res.* 60 (1): 5–10.

4 Stelken, A.M., Younis, L.T., Jennison, S.H. et al. (1996). Prognostic value of cardiopulmonary exercise testing using percent achieved of predicted peak oxygen uptake for patients with ischemic and dilated cardiomyopathy. *J. Am. Coll. Cardiol.* 27 (2): 345–352.

5 Gillmore, J.D., Maurer, M.S., Falk, R.H. et al. (2016). Nonbiopsy diagnosis of cardiac transthyretin amyloidosis. *Circulation* 133 (24): 2404–2412.

6 Marcus, F.I., McKenna, W.J., Sherrill, D. et al. (2010). Diagnosis of arrhythmogenic right ventricular cardiomyopathy/dysplasia: proposed modification of the task force criteria. *Eur. Heart J.* 31 (7): 806–814.

Further Reading

Adler, Y., Charron, P., Imazio, M. et al. (2015). 2015 ESC guidelines for the diagnosis and management of pericardial diseases: the Task Force for the Diagnosis and Management of Pericardial Diseases of the European Society of Cardiology (ESC) endorsed by: the European Association for Cardio-Thoracic Surgery (EACTS). *Eur. Heart J.* 36 (42): 2921–2964.

Authors/Task Force members, Elliott, P.M., Anastasakis, A. et al. (2014). 2014 ESC guidelines on diagnosis and management of hypertrophic cardiomyopathy: the Task Force for the Diagnosis and Management of Hypertrophic Cardiomyopathy of the European Society of Cardiology (ESC). *Eur. Heart J.* 35 (39): 2733–2779.

Froehlich, W., Bogun, F.M., and Crawford, T.C. (2015). Cardiac sarcoidosis. *Circulation* 132 (10): e137–e138.

Pieroni, M., Moon, J.C., Arbustini, E. et al. (2021). Cardiac involvement in Fabry disease: JACC review topic of the week. *J. Am. Coll. Cardiol.* 77 (7): 922–936.

Priori, S.G., Blomström-Lundqvist, C., Mazzanti, A. et al. (2015). 2015 ESC guidelines for the management of patients with ventricular arrhythmias and the prevention of sudden cardiac death: The Task Force for the Management of Patients with Ventricular Arrhythmias and the Prevention of Sudden Cardiac Death of the European Society of Cardiology (ESC). Endorsed by: Association for European Paediatric and Congenital Cardiology (AEPC). *Eur. Heart J.* 36 (41): 2793–2867.

Rapezzi, C., Arbustini, E., Caforio, A.L. et al. (2013). Diagnostic work-up in cardiomyopathies: bridging the gap between clinical phenotypes and final diagnosis. A position statement from the ESC working group on myocardial and pericardial diseases. *Eur. Heart J.* 34 (19): 1448–1458.

Seward, J.B. and Casaclang-Verzosa, G. (2010). Infiltrative cardiovascular diseases: cardiomyopathies that look alike. *J. Am. Coll. Cardiol.* 55 (17): 1769–1779.

Watkins, H., Ashrafian, H., and Redwood, C. (2011). Inherited cardiomyopathies. *N. Engl. J. Med.* 364 (17): 1643–1656.

Appendix: Answers to Self-assessment Questions

Chapter 1: Electrophysiological Principles

1. B A high concentration of extracellular sodium and intracellular potassium ions result in overall negative electrical potential of around −70 mV. The SAN, rather than AVN, is the dominant pacemaker. Pacemaker cells are not required to reach resting potential prior to depolarisation; they can depolarise once membrane threshold is reached. Finally, pacemaker cells spontaneously depolarise during diastole and have no true resting potential, whereas non-pacemaker myocytes maintain resting potential without spontaneous depolarisation.

2. B The SAN is located at the sulcus terminalis. Koch's triangle is anteriorly bordered by the septal leaflet of the tricuspid valve. Arterial supply for the AVN originates from RCA in 85% of patients, whilst the His–Purkinje system receives dual arterial supply from LAD and PDA.

3. B A normal axis in the coronal plane is between −30° and +90°. The QTc is calculated by dividing the QT interval by the √RR interval. Upright P waves in the inferior leads is normal and indicative of an impulse originating from the SAN. Finally, ventricular activation spreads from endocardium to epicardium.

4. B P-pulmonale generally results from RA enlargement. Right ventricular pacing, in contrast to left ventricular pacing, is a cause of LAD. Partial RBBB is not deemed to be of pathological significance, whereas Wellens syndrome is suggestive of a critical proximal LAD stenosis.

5. C Phase 4 of the action potential in non-pacemaker cells involves activation of sodium–potassium adenosine triphosphate (ATP)ase enzyme. Left-sided carotid sinus massage is generally more effective in dysrhythmia termination due to higher abundance of left-sided efferent fibres to AVN. In the transverse plane, leads V1–V2 correspond roughly to the anterior segment of LV. Finally, PR interval is mediated by the AVN.

Cardiology at its Core, First Edition. Peysh A. Patel.
© 2023 John Wiley & Sons Ltd. Published 2023 by John Wiley & Sons Ltd.

Chapter 2: Atrial Fibrillation

1. B   Left atrial enlargement shortens atrial refractoriness and increases risk of developing AF. Myocardial fibrosis creates intra-atrial conduction block and promotes occurrence of small reentrant circuits, whilst abnormalities in both parasympathetic and sympathetic tone are now recognised as being involved in both genesis and maintenance. Digoxin toxicity is not known to be implicated.

2. D   DC cardioversion must be performed within 48 hours of AF onset to minimise risk of thromboembolism. A pace and ablate strategy is an irreversible procedure which renders patients pacemaker-dependent and may allow rate-limiting therapy to be discontinued; however, the need for long-term anticoagulation remains. Flecainide is contraindicated in patients with coronary artery disease. Pulmonary vein isolation is generally reserved for those with paroxysmal or persistent AF that is associated with symptoms. Digoxin is highly effective at controlling ventricular rate in patients who are ambulatory.

3. E   Hyperlipidaemia is not known to be directly linked to development of AF. Obstructive sleep apnoea increases risk through a combination of hypoxia, hypercapnia and autonomic dysfunction. AF occurs in more than 20% of those who undergo successful atrial flutter ablation. Chronic lung disease can lead to AF through development of hypoxia, cor pulmonale and pulmonary hypertension. Diabetes mellitus is an independent predictor for development of AF.

4. D   High HAS-BLED score does not warrant avoidance of anticoagulation but necessitates more stringent monitoring. Left atrial appendage occlusion is reserved for patients in AF with high thromboembolic risk who are unable to tolerate anticoagulation or refuse it. Following successful AF ablation, all patients should continue oral anticoagulation for a minimum of eight weeks and, if at risk of thromboembolic events (CHA_2DS_2-VASc score ≥ 1), anticoagulation should continue indefinitely. AF ablation is not a cure and episodes of AF can continue to occur. They may not be symptomatic but inherent risk of thromboembolism remains. Coagulation screen is typically abnormal in a patient administered DOAC therapy.

5. E   AF occurs in up to 20% of patients with ventricular pre-excitation caused by an accessory pathway. This is often termed pre-excited AF. Administration of AV nodal blocking agents such as beta-blockers, calcium-channel antagonists and adenosine can increase conduction down the accessory pathway, increasing ventricular rate and predisposing to ventricular fibrillation. These agents should therefore be avoided. If there are signs of haemodynamic compromise, the most appropriate treatment is electrical cardioversion.

Chapter 3: Narrow Complex Tachycardias

1. D   Inadvertent AV block requiring permanent pacing can occur as a consequence of AVNRT ablation, but risk is <1% and risk falls further if cryoablation rather than radiofrequency ablation is used. AVNRT is more common in females and has a prevalence of around 1 in

500, although up to 20% of the general population have dual AV nodal physiology necessary for reentrant arrhythmia to occur. Symptomatic neck pulsation occurs as a consequence of near-simultaneous contraction of atria and ventricles, leading to atria contracting against closed atrioventricular valves.

2. B Flecainide can be used to control atrial flutter but should be given in conjunction with an AV nodal blocking agent such as a beta-blocker. This is because class Ic agents such as flecainide can slow cycle length of the macro reentrant circuit in the atrium without significantly affecting AV nodal conduction. This increases risk of 1:1 atrioventricular conduction and haemodynamic instability.

3. A Adenosine can terminate atrial tachycardias in up to 50%. This can lead to atrial tachycardia being misdiagnosed as an AV reentrant tachycardia. They most commonly cause long RP tachycardia with greater than 1 : 1 A : V conduction. Atrial tachycardias can be challenging to induce, sustain and ablate in the electrophysiology lab. Consequently, anti-arrhythmic drugs are considered first-line with ablation reserved for cases where drug therapy has failed.

4. C Right-sided pathways cause greater degree of pre-excitation on surface ECG. This is due to the accessory pathway being anatomically closer to the sinoatrial node, resulting in the ventricle being pre-excited earlier in comparison to pathways located on the left side of the heart.

5. D Adenosine is of most use in diagnosing and/or treating supraventricular (i.e. narrow complex) tachycardias. It can effectively treat most reentrant tachycardias by transiently blocking AV node. If SVT is not terminated, adenosine momentarily slows ventricular rate to reveal underlying atrial rhythm. It is relatively contraindicated in those with asthma due to risk of inducing bronchospasm and respiratory arrest. Adenosine is occasionally used in patients with a regular broad complex tachycardia and is safe to do so in this setting. However, cardioversion to sinus rhythm in response to adenosine does not necessarily exclude VT, and adenosine should not be used as a diagnostic tool to distinguish VT from SVT with aberrancy. An irregular broad complex tachycardia may reflect pre-excited AF, a condition where adenosine should be avoided due to risk of precipitating ventricular fibrillation. An irregular narrow complex tachycardia is most commonly caused by AF. In this setting, adenosine will not terminate the arrhythmia and is unlikely to provide additional diagnostic information.

Chapter 4: Broad Complex Tachycardias

1. E A rSR′ pattern in lead V1 occurs with typical RBBB whereas RSR′ pattern favours VT. A positive QRS in lead aVR is suggestive of extreme axis deviation, whereas P waves marching through the tachycardia are suggestive of AV dissociation, both of which indicate VT. Negative concordance in the precordial leads occurs when an impulse is initiated in the left ventricular apex and must therefore be VT. A QRS complex that narrows during tachycardia is suggestive of VT as it indicates that the His–Purkinje system is not conducting the impulse. QRS complexes in SVT should remain of the same duration or longer.

2. A Although QTc interval > 470 ms is considered prolonged in females (> 460 ms in males), a value > 500 ms is generally considered to confer increased risk of polymorphic ventricular tachycardia and sudden cardiac death.

3. B Amiodarone prolongs QT interval and can worsen polymorphic VT. It is safe to give a dose of intravenous magnesium prior to blood results being available, even if subsequent value is within normal range. Magnesium reduces risk of early after-depolarisations, and in doing so, reduces risk of VT. If administration of magnesium does not prevent recurrence of polymorphic VT, the next option to consider is overdrive pacing. Beta-blockers can also be added if there are no concerns regarding bradycardia and it is likely non pause-dependent. Finally, if there is a suspicion of acute ischaemia, coronary angiography with intervention can be considered.

4. B RVOT is the commonest site of VT in patients without organic cardiac disease. It is typically a benign condition and ICDs are rarely indicated. Beta-blockers or calcium-channel blockers are commonly used and ablation is reserved for cases where medication has proved ineffective. Imaging modalities such as echocardiography and cardiac MRI typically confirm structurally normal hearts, although RVOT VT can be seen in patients with ARVC.

5. E Papillary muscle and fascicular VT both typically have RBBB morphology. They can be of superior or inferior axis depending on origin and both can exist in the context of a structurally normal heart. Papillary muscle VT tends to result in a distinctly broad QRS morphology. It is typically focal in origin, as opposed to fascicular VT which is both focal and reentrant in mechanism. Ablation of papillary muscle VT can be challenging due to catheter instability and may require concurrent use of intracardiac echocardiography. Verapamil treatment is often effective in management of fascicular VT.

Chapter 5: Bradycardias and Conduction Disease

1. D Carotid sinus massage is a manoeuvre to unveil the cardioinhibitory mechanism behind syncope secondary to neck movements or shaving. It is a class I indication for pacing if systolic BP drop is ≥ 50 mmHg or there is ventricular pause ≥ 3 s. Sinus pause is where there is a failure of sinus impulse generation for < 3 s. Mobitz type II second-degree AV block with a wide QRS rhythm, even without symptoms, is a strong indication for pacing because the wide QRS points to an infranodal origin of ventricular rhythm with higher risk of progression. In complete heart block, impulses originate from the SAN but are unable to propagate beyond AVN. Chronotropic incompetence can cause exercise intolerance because of the heart's inability to increase heart rate in response to physiological stress, thus not producing sufficient cardiac output to meet increased demand.

2. A ECG criteria for incomplete trifascicular block include RBBB plus LAD or RAD, and first- or second-degree AV block or LBBB plus first- or second-degree AV block. Complete trifascicular block based on ECG criteria is reserved for appearance of complete heart block with features of bifascicular block, as escape rhythm is usually originating from one of the two left bundle branches. In those with bifascicular block and syncope, electrophysiological studies showing prolonged HV interval or induction of second- or third-degree AV block by pacing or pharmacological stress identifies cohorts at highest risk. Finally, left axis deviation is a sign of left anterior fascicular block, whereas right axis deviation is a sign of left posterior fascicular block.

3. E Citalopram, a serotonin-selective reuptake inhibitor that is used to treat depression, is associated with prolongation of QTc interval in overdose and can result in TdP. Digoxin slows conduction at the AVN. Chagas disease is secondary to *Trypanasoma cruzi* infection and can affect the myocardium through both direct persistence in cardiac tissue and immune-mediated processes. In amyloidosis, deposition of β-pleated fibrils in the AV node can cause high-grade block. Kearns–Sayre syndrome is a mitochondrial myopathy which causes myocardial fibrosis in addition to retinitis pigmentosa and external ophthalmoplegia.

4. B A vasodepressor response is suppression of sympathetic tone; hence, in tilt testing, as the patient is elevated from a horizontal position, there is a lack of compensatory peripheral vasoconstriction to increase TPR and maintain BP. Patients who show a vasodepressor response include those afflicted by postural hypotension and vasovagal syncope. Unsurprisingly, patients with neutrally mediated syncope usually have normal ECG monitoring and echocardiography. PoTS can cause dizziness, syncope, palpitations and shaking within a few minutes of sitting or standing up. It is more common in females with particular preponderance in those aged 15–50 years. Inferior myocardial infarction is usually the result of RCA occlusion. It supplies the AV node in over 80% and ischaemia in this territory can result in transient arrhythmias.

5. C First-degree AV block is defined by consistently prolonged PR interval > 200 ms but there are no missed beats so there is low immediate risk of asystole. Heart failure (raised jugular venous pressure, pulmonary crackles, pedal oedema) and shock (low blood pressure, prolonged capillary refill, poor urine output and confusion) and syncope (cerebral hypoperfusion causing acute neurological dysfunction) are sequelae of inadequate cardiac output and require immediate action to try to improve heart rate. Atropine, on a short-term basis, will increase SAN automaticity and conduction velocity through the AVN.

Chapter 6: The Cardiac Pump

1. D Muscle fibres within the myocardium consist of tubular myofibrils, which are themselves composed of repeated regions known as sarcomeres. Myocardial contraction is an active process and requires hydrolysis of ATP, thus forming ADP. The two predominant means by which force of contraction can be regulated are via alteration of the amplitude or duration of calcium influx and myofilament sensitivity to calcium. At the termination of systole, phosphorylation of troponin I inhibits binding of calcium to troponin C, allowing tropomyosin to block interaction sites and causing muscle relaxation.

2. C Although it is true that RV and LV pump blood to the pulmonary and systemic circulations respectively, the RV generates a lower pressure of around 25 mmHg. AV opening does not result in total adherence to the wall of the aorta, thus permitting unrestricted perfusion to the right and left coronary arteries. In healthy individuals, only the MV is bicuspid whereas AV, PV and TV are tricuspid. Systolic pressure of 20 mmHg within the LA would be classified as significantly elevated.

3. A Systole represents around three-eighths (37.5%) of total cycle duration. Onset of systole occurs when pressure in LV exceeds aortic pressure, whereas isovolumic relaxation is an active ATP-consuming process. Rapid ventricular filling results in increased chamber volumes, around two-thirds of the total within first one-third of diastole. Whilst patients with significant bradycardia have prolongation of filling duration and relative increase in SV, this is not sufficient to compensate for lower HR and overall CO is impaired.

4. B SV is calculated by subtracting ESV from EDV. Inotropic agents such as digoxin and adrenaline increase myocardial contractility whilst not affecting diastolic compliance. If HR is increased through iatrogenic means using a pacemaker, CO will first rise but then plateau and decline at rates of 120–130 bpm. The Frank–Starling principle states that energy of contraction is a function of the length of the muscle fibre.

5. C The RV receives continuous coronary perfusion in contrast to LV. All other statements are correct.

Chapter 7: Arterial and Venous System

1. A MAP = diastolic BP + 1/3 (systolic BP − diastolic BP).

2. B The reversal of flow from the aorta occurs at end of systole due to blood influx into coronary vasculature and slight regurgitation across aortic valve. The Windkessel effect refers to storage of potential energy, whilst determinants of systemic BP are related in a way that is analogous to Ohm's law. Finally, CVP is a good approximate of right atrial pressure.

3. B Stroke volume is a determinant of systolic blood pressure but does not directly influence diastolic blood pressure.

4. C Mean circulatory pressure can be considered as the difference between MAP and CVP. Upon standing, sequestration of blood in the lower limbs can potentially reduce venous return by up to 20–25%. At low pressure, venous contraction has little effect on flow, whereas at higher pressures, venomotor activity is a more significant contributor. During inspiration, lung expansion increases capacity of the pulmonary vasculature, resulting in pooling, reduced LA filling and impaired SV.

5. D The effect of inspiration on stroke volume is exaggerated in cases of constrictive pericarditis or cardiac tamponade. All other statements are correct.

Chapter 8: Regulation of the Circulatory System

1. C ADH, as its name suggests, inhibits water loss. It acts by enhancing free water resorption in the collecting ducts. In SIADH excess water resorption can lead to hyponatraemia. The adrenal medulla releases adrenaline. Angiotensin II directly mediates arteriolar vasoconstriction and results in secretion of aldosterone. Nitric oxide is synthesised from L-arginine, with L-citrulline a by-product of its formation. ANP only causes natriuresis; it has no chronotropic or inotropic effects.

2. D The sympathetic and parasympathetic nervous systems are two constituents of the autonomic nervous system. Preganglionic nerves of both release acetylcholine. The sympathetic nervous system has an effect on chronotropy and inotropy in the heart. Heart rate responds more gradually to the sympathetic nervous system because it is reliant on production of cAMP; additionally, release of noradrenaline at postganglionic nerve endings is slower than that of acetylcholine. The sympathetic nervous system is dominant in peripheral circulation and causes vasoconstriction through stimulation of α_1-adrenergic receptors.

3. E The Cushing reflex was first described in 1901 by an American neurosurgeon, Henry Cushing. It is usually seen in the final stages of acute head injury where it may be an indicator of imminent brain herniation and death. It is caused by raised intracranial pressure, leading to compression of cerebral vasculature and initiation of a CNS ischaemic response. Thus, there is sympathetic drive and arteriolar vasoconstriction that leads to systemic hypertension.

4. C The cardiovascular control centres are located in the brainstem and include cardiac control centre and vasomotor centre. The cardiostimulatory centre affects the heart through the sympathetic nervous system and can increase HR and BP. The vasomotor centre affects peripheral vasculature. Vasomotor tone is mediated by vascular smooth muscle cells in the media layer which contract slowly but with high force. Basal vasomotor tone is mediated by the sympathetic nervous system.

5. B Autoregulation describes a negative feedback mechanism that provides perfusion to an organ in spite of changes in arterial blood flow; this is mediated by vasoconstriction and vasodilation. This is most prominently seen in the heart, brain and kidneys and, to a lesser extent, in skin. It has not been shown in the liver. In the context of ischaemic stroke, there are alterations in autoregulatory capacity of infarcted tissue. As a consequence, precise control of cerebral blood flow is vital to prevent further injury.

Chapter 9: Coronary Vasculature

1. C The incorrect statement is C as septal branches are supplied by LAD artery.

2. B Coronary vessels originate from the sinuses of Valsalva immediately distal to aortic valve at the aortic root. The Cx artery traverses along the left atrioventricular groove, and collateral vessels arise in the setting of chronic rather than acute ischaemia. Finally, collateral vessels can form between branches of the same coronary artery.

3. E The incorrect statement is E, as the coronary sinus is situated on the posterior and inferior surface of the heart.

4. B Coronary arterial flow is phasic rather than linear, and extrinsic compression has important effects on intramyocardial flow distribution. Coronary perfusion is closely autoregulated and is not generally dependent upon loading conditions. Finally, IABP counterpulsation augments coronary perfusion by raising diastolic BP.

5. D The incorrect statement is D, as hypoxia is deemed to be the primary determinant of coronary arterial vasodilation in the setting of increased metabolic need.

Chapter 10: Stable Angina and Non-invasive Testing

1. **A** Diastolic dysfunction precedes systolic dysfunction, whilst ECG changes are the final perturbation. This cascade explains why stress echocardiography or perfusion scans are more sensitive than exercise ECG testing for identifying ischaemia.

2. **C** The incorrect statement is C, as stunned myocardium often spontaneously recovers contractile function.

3. **C** CT coronary angiography has good spatial resolution and excellent negative predictive value. Beta-blockers are used to maintain HR < 70 bpm. Finally, with the exception of patients with renal failure, coronary calcification correlates well with overall plaque burden.

4. **E** The incorrect statement is E, as a 16- or 17-segment model is used.

5. **E** LGE refers to image acquisition 10–20 minutes after contrast injection, and diffusion of gadolinium occurs from extracellular to intracellular space. Functional improvement from revascularisation is deemed more likely if ≤ 50% mural involvement is seen. Hyperenhancement with LGE is not specific to infarction and can be seen in the context of cardiomyopathies or myocarditis.

Chapter 11: Ischaemic Heart Disease

1. **C** Fatty streaks are manifest in the early 20s, whilst disease states such as diabetes mellitus and hypercholesterolaemia result in a pro-inflammatory milieu. Positive vascular remodelling can result in significant plaques being undetectable via coronary angiography. Finally, vessel occlusion in ACS results from sudden rupture of the fibrous plaque and formation of acute thrombus.

2. **D** Complete resolution of ECG changes is possible if prompt recanalisation or revascularisation occurs.

3. **B** Over-oxygenation may be associated with vasoconstriction and increased infarct burden. As such, therapy is only recommended if saturations are not preserved at ≥ 94%. Glycoprotein inhibitors are no longer recommended for patients with refractory ischaemia, but instead only as a bail-out option during the revascularisation procedure.

4. **C** Significant lesions on angiography are defined as those that cause ≥ 50% in the LMS or ≥ 70% in major epicardial vessels. Access via the radial artery is preferred in view of lower rates of infection, access site complications and major bleeding. CABG is generally preferred in multivessel disease, particularly in diabetic patients. Finally, drug-eluting stents (DES) provide lower rates of in-stent restenosis compared with preceding bare metal stents (BMS).

5. **E** Statins reduce CRP levels via modulation of the inflammatory response and are therefore likely to play a role in abrogating plaque formation and progression.

Chapter 12: Congestive Heart Failure

1. E   Diuretics reduce fluid retention. Furosemide is a loop diuretic which has lower bioavailability than bumetanide. Metolazone is a thiazide-like diuretic and acts on the distal convoluted tubule. Eplerenone is a potassium-sparing diuretic and acts on the collecting ducts. Diuretics are for short-term symptomatic benefit to help patients reach euvolaemia, but chronic use can result in diuretic resistance.

2. D   CRT is an option for patients with refractory symptoms in spite of optimised medical treatment. By achieving biventricular pacing, it will reduce ventricular dyssynchrony which can otherwise impair pump function. The COMPANION and MADIT trials have shown benefit of device therapy over pharmacotherapy alone in terms of both morbidity and mortality. However, most trial evidence for use is in stable patients rather than those with acute decompensation. ICD devices can prevent SCD from life-threating arrhythmias but have impact on driving and can give inappropriate, painful shocks.

3. A   High-output heart failure is where pump function is preserved but cannot meet increased metabolic demand. Diabetes is strongly associated with hypertension and coronary artery disease and also likely has directly deleterious effects on myocardium. The other listed conditions will require augmented cardiac output which the heart may not be able to meet. Paget's disease commonly presents with bone pain and possible bone deformity, with hypervascularity leading to high-output heart failure.

4. C   Diastole is the period between AV closure (end-systole) and MV closure (end-diastole). During this period, there is isovolumic relaxation and, when LV pressure falls below LA pressure, the MV opens and there is rapid filling of LV ('E wave'). As pressure equalises between atria and ventricles with blood flow, there is a period of diastasis before atrial contraction produces late diastolic filling ('A wave'). The 'E wave' can be of larger magnitude than 'A wave' in grade II diastolic dysfunction because there is abnormal relaxation; in these situations, tissue Doppler imaging becomes particularly useful. Patients with HFpEF tend to be older, female and more comorbid and, at present, no specific agents are of proven mortality benefit.

5. C   The NYHA classification of severity is based on functional capacity: I = ordinary physical activity causing no symptoms, II = ordinary physical activity causing symptoms, III = less than ordinary activity causing symptoms, and IV = symptoms present at rest. Breathlessness, orthopnoea, PND, pedal oedema and fatigue are classic symptom constellations. Routine investigation may include ECG, chest radiograph, bloods and echocardiography. BNP, given its low specificity but high sensitivity, is best used as a 'rule out' test.

Chapter 13: Valvular Disease

1. B   Valsalva manoeuvres increase intrathoracic pressure and reduce preload, therefore diminishing intensity of most murmurs. Inspiration causes a fall in intrathoracic pressure and increases preload. This in turn causes right heart murmurs to become louder. Standing from a sitting position results in venous pooling, causing reduction in venous return and decrease in intensity of most murmurs (except for HOCM and MVP). Squatting on the other hand causes the reverse and increases venous return, therefore increasing intensity of most murmurs.

2. B During dobutamine stress echocardiography, as systolic function is accentuated, a significant increase in V_{max} across the AV is noted with only minimal change in AVA. In patients with severe aortic stenosis and severe left ventricular systolic dysfunction, the LV may not be able to generate a significant gradient across the valve, resulting in underestimation of stenosis. AVA measurement may also prove inaccurate as the LV fails to generate enough force to fully open the valve. The LVOT V_{max} would not be helpful in differentiating true severe and pseudo-severe AS.

3. B Surgical AVR is indicated in all patients with at least moderate aortic stenosis undergoing CABG, surgery on the ascending aorta or replacement of another valve. It is also indicated in symptomatic patients with severe AS ($V_{max} > 4.0 \, m \, s^{-1}$ or mean pressure gradient $> 40 \, mmHg$). In an asymptomatic individual with severe aortic stenosis, surgery may be indicated if there is concurrent LV systolic dysfunction due to valvular disease, and if there are symptoms or abnormal BP response on treadmill testing.

4. C Rheumatic disease, endocarditis, systemic lupus erythematosus and Marfan syndrome are well-recognised causes of primary MR in which one or more components of the mitral valve apparatus are directly affected. Dilated cardiomyopathy tends to result in secondary or functional regurgitation in which components of valve apparatus are not directly affected. Regurgitation typically arises due to disparity in closing and tethering forces of the valve as a consequence of alterations in LV geometry.

5. D Rivero-Carvallo's sign is typically seen in TR and is characterised by increased intensity of the pansystolic murmur during inspiration. This is due to increased venous return. Quincke's sign (capillary pulsations seen on light compression of the nail bed), Rosenbach's sign (hepatic pulsations in the absence of tricuspid regurgitation), Duroziez's sign (diastolic murmur heard over the femoral artery) and De Musset's sign (visible nodding of the head in time with aortic pulsation) are all clinical signs associated with aortic regurgitation.

Chapter 14: Cardiomyopathies

1. C Reduced left ventricular ejection fraction does not amount to a major risk factor for SCD in HCM. However, it is a marker of poor prognosis as it is suggestive of end-stage disease. A history of SCD in one or more first-degree relatives < 40 years of age or SCD in a first-degree relative with confirmed HCM at any age, unexplained syncope, severe left ventricular hypertrophy detected on transthoracic echocardiography and non-sustained ventricular tachycardia are all major risk factors.

2. B Senile systemic amyloidosis is slowly progressive and has the best prognosis. Patients with this form typically do not require any specific treatment. Primary amyloidosis is strongly associated with multiple myeloma or monoclonal gammopathies. Secondary amyloidosis is known to be associated with inflammatory conditions such as rheumatoid arthritis. A formal diagnosis of amyloidosis is made by demonstration of apple green birefringence on Congo red staining of histological tissue specimens. Digoxin is relatively contraindicated in amyloidosis as it binds to amyloid fibrils and can cause toxicity even at low dose. Amyloidosis can be either hereditary or acquired.

3. D   A $\geq 25\%$ fall in transmitral E velocity during inspiration is a feature of constrictive pericarditis or cardiac tamponade and is due to exaggerated respiratory variation in filling because of ventricular interdependence. The other features are typically seen in restrictive cardiomyopathy.

4. E   The commonest cutaneous manifestation of sarcoidosis is erythema nodosum. Sarcoidosis should be suspected in any young individual with high-grade AV block. Serum ACE levels can be elevated in up to 70% of cases and may be helpful for monitoring. Endomyocardial biopsy is a useful diagnostic tool and has high specificity but low sensitivity due to patchy nature of the condition. Therefore, an area of granuloma can be missed on biopsy.

5. B   Around 30–50% of cases of dilated cardiomyopathy are secondary to genetic mutations, although the disorder is often polygenic. Alcohol excess, acute myocarditis, chemotherapy and the peri-/postpartum period of pregnancy are among the other recognised causes.

2. D   A 25% fall in transmitral Doppler velocity during inspiration is a feature of constrictive pericarditis or cardiac tamponade and is due to exaggerated respiratory variation in filling. Rise of jugular venous pressure. The effects of these are typically seen in restrictive cardiomyopathy.

4. A   The commonest manifestation of sarcoidosis is erythema nodosum. Sarcoidosis should be suspected in any young patient with heart block with bilateral... AV block. Serum ACE levels can be elevated in up to 75% of cases and may be helpful for monitoring. Endomyocardial biopsy is a useful diagnostic tool and has high specificity but low sensitivity due to patchy nature of the condition. Therefore, an area of granuloma can be missed on biopsy.

5. B   Around 30–50% of cases of dilated cardiomyopathy are secondary to genetic mutations, although the disease is... polygenic. Alcohol excess, acute myocarditis, chemotherapy and the peripartum period of pregnancy are among the other recognised causes.

Index

Cardiology at its Core, First Edition. Peysh A. Patel.
© 2023 John Wiley & Sons Ltd. Published 2023 by John Wiley & Sons Ltd.

Printed and bound by CPI Group (UK) Ltd, Croydon, CR0 4YY

08/05/2024